2005
YEAR BOOK OF
RHEUMATOLOGY, ARTHRITIS, AND MUSCULOSKELETAL DISEASE™

The 2005 Year Book Series

Year Book of Allergy, Asthma, and Clinical Immunology™: Drs Rosenwasser, Boguniewicz, Milgrom, Routes, and Spahn

Year Book of Anesthesiology and Pain Management™: Drs Chestnut, Abram, Black, Gravlee, Mathru, Lee, and Roizen

Year Book of Cardiology®: Drs Gersh, Cheitlin, Graham, Kaplan, Sundt, and Waldo

Year Book of Critical Care Medicine®: Drs Dellinger, Parrillo, Balk, Bekes, Dries, and Dorman

Year Book of Dentistry®: Drs Zakariasen, Hatcher, Horswell, McIntyre, Scott, Victoroff, and Zakariasen

Year Book of Dermatology and Dermatologic Surgery™: Drs Thiers and Lang

Year Book of Diagnostic Radiology®: Drs Osborn, Birdwell, Dalinka, Gardiner, Levy, Maynard, and Oestreich

Year Book of Emergency Medicine®: Drs Burdick, Cydulka, Hamilton, Handly, Werner, and Quintana

Year Book of Endocrinology®: Drs Mazzaferri, Rubin, Molitch, Leahy, Kennedy, Kannan, Bessesen, Rogol, and Meikle

Year Book of Family Practice®: Drs Bowman, Apgar, Dexter, Miser, Neill, and Scherger

Year Book of Gastroenterology™: Drs Lichtenstein, Dempsey, Drebin, Faust, Ginsberg, Katzka, Kochman, Morris, Reddy, and Stein

Year Book of Hand and Upper Limb Surgery®: Drs Berger and Ladd

Year Book of Medicine®: Drs Barkin, Frishman, Klahr, Loehrer, Mazzaferri, Phillips, Pillinger, and Snydman

Year Book of Neonatal and Perinatal Medicine®: Drs Fanaroff, Maisels, and Stevenson

Year Book of Neurology and Neurosurgery®: Drs Gibbs and Verma

Year Book of Nuclear Medicine®: Drs Coleman, Blaufox, Royal, Strauss, and Zubal

Year Book of Obstetrics, Gynecology, and Women's Health®: Dr Shulman

Year Book of Oncology®: Drs Loehrer, Arceci, Glatstein, Gordon, Hanna, Morrow, and Thigpen

Year Book of Ophthalmology®: Drs Rapuano, Cohen, Eagle, Grossman, Hammersmith, Myers, Nelson, Penne, Sergott, Shields, Tipperman, and Vander

Year Book of Orthopedics®: Drs Morrey, Beauchamp, Peterson, Swiontkowski, Trigg, and Yaszemski

Year Book of Otolaryngology-Head and Neck Surgery®: Drs Paparella, Otto, and Keefe

Year Book of Pathology and Laboratory Medicine®: Drs Grzybicki, Raab, Bejarano, Bissell, and Stanley

Year Book of Pediatrics®: Dr Stockman

Year Book of Plastic and Aesthetic Surgery™: Drs Miller, Bartlett, Garner, McKinney, Ruberg, Salisbury, and Smith

Year Book of Psychiatry and Applied Mental Health®: Drs Talbott, Ballenger, Buckley, Frances, Jensen, and Markowitz

Year Book of Pulmonary Disease®: Drs Phillips, Barker, Dunlap, Lewis, Maurer, and Willsie

Year Book of Rheumatology, Arthritis, and Musculoskeletal Disease™: Drs Panush, Hadler, Hellmann, Hochberg, Lahita, and Seibold

Year Book of Sports Medicine®: Drs Shephard, Alexander, Cantu, Feldman, McCrory, Nieman, Rowland, Sanborn, and Shrier

Year Book of Surgery®: Drs Copeland, Bland, Cerfolio, Daly, Eberlein, Fahey, Mozingo, Pruett, and Seeger

Year Book of Urology®: Drs Andriole and Coplen

Year Book of Vascular Surgery®: Dr Moneta

2005

The Year Book of RHEUMATOLOGY, ARTHRITIS, AND MUSCULOSKELETAL DISEASE™

Editor-in-Chief
Richard S. Panush, MD

Associate Editors
Nortin M. Hadler, MD
David B. Hellmann, MD
Marc C. Hochberg, MD
Robert G. Lahita, MD, PhD
James R. Seibold, MD

ELSEVIER

Vice President, Continuity Publishing: Timothy M. Griswold
Managing Editor: David Orzechowski
Developmental Editor: Ali Gavenda
Senior Manager, Continuity Production: Idelle L. Winer
Issue Manager: Donna M. Skelton
Illustrations and Permissions Coordinator: Kimberly E. Hulett

2005 EDITION

Printed in the United States of America
Composition by Thomas Technology Solutions, Inc.
Printing/binding by Sheridan Books, Inc.

Editorial Office:
Elsevier
300 East
170 South Independence Mall West
Philadelphia, PA 19106-3399

International Standard Serial Number: 1070-5406
International Standard Book Number: 0-323-02121-2

Editorial Board

Table of Contents

Journals Represented

Journals represented in this YEAR BOOK are listed below.

American Journal of Cardiology
American Journal of Clinical Pathology
American Journal of Medicine
American Journal of Pathology
American Journal of Respiratory and Critical Care Medicine
American Journal of Roentgenology
American Journal of Sports Medicine
Annals of Internal Medicine
Annals of Rheumatic Diseases
Archives of Dermatology
Archives of Internal Medicine
Arthritis and Rheumatism
Arthroscopy
Brain Research
British Journal of Dermatology
British Medical Journal
Chest
Circulation
Clinical Endocrinology (Oxford)
Endocrinology
Gastroenterology
Human Reproduction
Journal of Bone and Joint Surgery (American Volume)
Journal of Bone and Joint Surgery (British Volume)
Journal of Bone and Mineral Research
Journal of Clinical Endocrinology and Metabolism
Journal of Clinical Investigation
Journal of Clinical Rheumatology
Journal of General Internal Medicine
Journal of Immunology
Journal of Internal Medicine
Journal of Investigative Dermatology
Journal of Neurology, Neurosurgery and Psychiatry
Journal of Pain
Journal of Pediatrics
Journal of Rheumatology
Journal of the American Geriatrics Society
Journal of the American Medical Association
Kidney International
Lancet
Mayo Clinic Proceedings
Medical Care
Medicine
Medicine and Science in Sports and Exercise
Neurology
New England Journal of Medicine
Ophthalmology
Pediatrics
Proceedings of the National Academy of Sciences

Respiratory Medicine
Rheumatology
Scandinavian Journal of Rheumatology
Spine
Spine Journal
The Pharos

STANDARD ABBREVIATIONS

The following terms are abbreviated in this edition: acquired immunodeficiency syndrome (AIDS), cardiopulmonary resuscitation (CPR), central nervous system (CNS), cerebrospinal fluid (CSF), computed tomography (CT), deoxyribonucleic acid (DNA), electrocardiography (ECG), health maintenance organization (HMO), human immunodeficiency virus (HIV), intensive care unit (ICU), intramuscular (IM), intravenous (IV), magnetic resonance (MR) imaging (MRI), rheumatoid arthritis (RA), ribonucleic acid (RNA), and ultrasound (US).

NOTE

The YEAR BOOK OF RHEUMATOLOGY, ARTHRITIS, AND MUSCULOSKELETAL DISEASE™ is a literature survey service providing abstracts of articles published in the professional literature. Every effort is made to assure the accuracy of the information presented in these pages. Neither the editors nor the publisher of the YEAR BOOK OF RHEUMATOLOGY, ARTHRITIS, AND MUSCULOSKELETAL DISEASE™ can be responsible for errors in the original materials. The editors' comments are their own opinions. Mention of specific products within this publication does not constitute endorsement.

To facilitate the use of the YEAR BOOK OF RHEUMATOLOGY, ARTHRITIS, AND MUSCULOSKELETAL DISEASE™ as a reference tool, all illustrations and tables included in this publication are now identified as they appear in the original article. This change is meant to help the reader recognize that any illustration or table appearing in the YEAR BOOK OF RHEUMATOLOGY, ARTHRITIS, AND MUSCULOSKELETAL DISEASE™ may be only one of many in the original article. For this reason, figure and table numbers will often appear to be out of sequence within the YEAR BOOK OF RHEUMATOLOGY, ARTHRITIS, AND MUSCULOSKELETAL DISEASE™.

1 Rheumatoid Arthritis

Introduction

A few years ago I compared the assembling of new weapons in the fight against RA to the massing of battleships for the D day invasion of France. This year, I would summarize the RA literature by saying that many of the troops have now not only landed on the beaches, but have now begun marching across France. The largest troop movements are being transported by TNF-inhibitor vehicles, which now exist in 3 forms. Several generals in RA research report on their power, both alone and in combination with other anti-RA weapons. Other generals are reporting their experience in attacking IL-2 or IL-6 or in increasing the dose of methotrexate. War is never pretty, but the rheumatology literature this year makes it clear that we can now see a winning battle plan emerging that will lead RA patients to victory.

David B. Hellmann, MD

Lead Article

Combination With Etanercept and Anakinra in the Treatment of Patients With Rheumatoid Arthritis Who Have Been Treated Unsuccessfully With Methotrexate

Genovese MC, for the 20000223 Study Group (Stanford Univ, Palo Alto, Calif; et al)

Arthritis Rheum 50:1412-1419, 2004 1–1

Background.—Selective anticytokine treatment has improved outcomes in patients with RA. However, it does not necessarily lead to remission. The effects of combining anticytokine agents have been explored in animal models. The effects of combination therapy with the selective anti-tumor necrosis factor α agent etanercept and the anti-interleukin-1 agent anakinra were determined.

Methods.—In this double-blind study, 41 US centers enrolled a total of 244 patients with active RA despite methotrexate treatment receiving subcutaneous etanercept, 25 mg, twice weekly; this dosage of etanercept plus anakinra, 100 mg/d; or half-dosage etanercept (25 mg once weekly) plus anakinra, 100 mg/d, for 6 months. None of the patients had previously received anticytokine treatment. Responses were assessed by the American

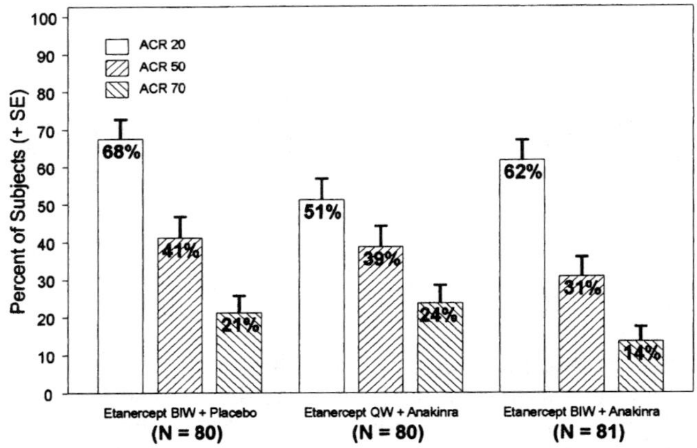

FIGURE 2.—Percent of patients achieving an American College of Rheumatology 20% (ACR20), ACR50, or ACR70 response at week 24. *Abbreviations: BIW*, Twice weekly; *QW*, once weekly. (Courtesy of Genovese MC, for the 20000223 Study Group: Combination with etanercept and anakinra in the treatment of patients with rheumatoid arthritis who have been treated unsuccessfully with methotrexate. *Arthritis Rheum* 50:1412-1419, 2004. Reprinted by permission of John Wiley & Sons, Inc.)

College of Rheumatology (ACR) core set criteria, a health-related quality-of-life questionnaire, and the Disease Activity Score.

Findings.—Combination treatment was not superior to etanercept alone, regardless of regimen. However, combination therapy was associated with increased safety risks. Thirty-one percent of patients given the full dosage of etanercept plus anakinra obtained an ACR 50% response, compared with 41% of patients given etanercept only (Fig 2), a nonsignificant difference. Combination therapy was associated with an increased incidence of serious infections, injection-site reactions, and neutropenia. Combination therapy did not affect the pharmacokinetics or immunogenecity of either agent.

Conclusions.—Combination therapy with etanercept and anakinra does not confer additional benefits over etanercept alone. In addition, it increases the risk of adverse events. Thus, this combination therapy is not recommended for treating RA.

► In the treatment of RA, more is sometimes less. This study, for example, shows that in the treatment of patients with imperfect responses to methotrexate, adding the combination treatment of the anti-tumor necrosis factor agent etanercept and the anti-interleukin-1 agent anakinra was no more effective and was more toxic than adding etanercept alone (Fig 2).

D. B. Hellmann, MD

Experimental Models/Pathophysiology

Autoantibodies to Cyclic Citrullinated Peptides Predict Progression to Rheumatoid Arthritis in Patients With Undifferentiated Arthritis: A Prospective Cohort Study

van Gaalen FA, Linn-Rasker SP, van Venrooij WJ, et al (Leiden Univ, The Netherlands; Univ of Nijmegen, The Netherlands; VU Med Ctr, Amsterdam)
Arthritis Rheum 50:709-715, 2004 1–2

Background.—Approximately 1% of the population is affected by RA. It would appear that recognition of RA as early as possible is important because a significant proportion of the patients have irreversible joint damage after disease onset. However, early diagnosis can be difficult because the disease may initially be indistinguishable from other forms of arthritis. The presence of autoantibodies is a hallmark of RA. Previous retrospective studies have shown that autoantibodies associated with RA can be detected years before clinical symptoms develop. The predictive value of RA-specific autoantibodies to cyclic citrullinated peptides (CCPs) in patients with undifferentiated arthritis (UA) was assessed.

Methods.—Anti-CCP2 antibody tests were performed at baseline in 936 consecutive, newly referred patients with recent-onset arthritis. Patients were classified as having UA when they could not be properly classified 2 weeks after inclusion. Patients with UA were followed up for progression of disease to RA as defined by the American College of Rheumatology (ACR) 1987 revised criteria.

Results.—Of the 936 patients with recent-onset arthritis, 318 (34%) were classified as having UA and were available for analysis. After 3 years of follow-up, 127 (40%) of 318 of these UA patients had been classified as having RA (Table 3). Development of RA had occurred in 63 (25%) of 249 pa-

TABLE 3.—Anti-CCP Antibodies and Prediction of RA in Patients With UA*

	Patients Fulfilling ACR RA Criteria, No. (%)		
	After 1 Year	After 2 Years	After 3 Years
Anti-CCP positive (n = 69)	57 (83)	62 (90)	64 (93)†
Anti-CCP negative (n = 249)	46 (18)	60 (24)	63 (25)
Total (n = 318)	103 (32)	122 (38)	127 (40)

*Of 346 patients with undifferentiated arthritis (UA) at baseline, 28 were lost to follow-up for unknown reasons (24 had tested negative and 4 had tested positive for antibodies to cyclic citrullinated peptide (anti-CCP2 [anti-CCP]). The remaining 318 patients, grouped by their anti-CCP status, were followed up to determine how many of them would fulfill the American College of Rheumatology (ACR) criteria for RA after 1, 2, and 3 years.

†The presence of anti-CCP antibodies was a significant risk factor for RA (odds ratio 37.8 [95% confidence interval, 13.8-111.9]).

(Courtesy of van Gaalen FA, Linn-Rasker SP, van Venrooij WJ, et al: Autoantibodies to cyclic citrullinated peptides predict progression to rheumatoid arthritis in patients with undifferentiated arthritis: A prospective cohort study. *Arthritis Rheum* 50:709-715, 2004. Reprinted by permission of John Wiley & Sons, Inc.)

TABLE 4.—Diagnostic Properties of the Anti-CCP2 Antibody Test*

	Percent (95% Confidence Interval)
Sensitivity	50 (41-59)
Specificity	97 (95-99)
Positive predictive value	93 (87-99)
Negative predictive value	75 (69-80)

*It was determined that anti-CCP antibodies are 16.7 times more likely to be detected in patients with UA that progresses to RA than in those with RA that does not (likelihood ratio for a positive result) (see Results). See Table 3 for definitions.

(Courtesy of van Gaalen FA, Linn-Rasker SP, van Venrooij WJ, et al: Autoantibodies to cyclic citrullinated peptides predict progression to rheumatoid arthritis in patients with undifferentiated arthritis: a prospective cohort study. *Arthritis Rheum* 50:709-715, 2004. Reprinted by permission of John Wiley & Sons, Inc.)

tients with a negative anti-CCP test and in 64 (93%) of 69 with a positive anti-CCP test (Table 4). Significant predictors of RA on multivariate analysis of the presence of anti-CCP antibodies and parameters from the ACR criteria were polyarthritis, symmetric arthritis, erosions on radiographs, and anti-CCP antibodies.

Conclusions.—The presence of anti-CCP antibodies in patients with undifferentiated arthritis is a significant predictor of rheumatoid arthritis.

► Many rheumatologists have been looking for "that easy test" to help diagnose RA. The anti-CCPs can predict the diagnosis of RA in patients who are suspect. But like many of the auto antibodies, it can never be used as a "screening test." Just like the ANA is a terrible screening test for SLE, anti-CCP is never to be used (because of its low predictability in diagnosing RA in the 1% of people who have it) in general screening. After reading this article, I am sold on this test and will use it as a screen for early diagnosis and management in only suspected RA cases. Maybe only in those cases where I am convinced it will likely be positive.

R. G. Lahita, MD, PhD

Specific Autoantibodies Precede the Symptoms of Rheumatoid Arthritis: A Study of Serial Measurements in Blood Donors

Nielen MMJ, van Schaardenburg D, Reesink HW, et al (Jan van Breeman Inst, Amsterdam; Vrije Universiteit Med Centre, Amsterdam; Sanquin Blood Bank Northwest Region, Amsterdam; et al)

Arthritis Rheum 50:380-386, 2004 1–3

Background.—The current goal of management for RA is to recognize early signs and symptoms and provide treatment that halts disease progression. However, 36% to 54% of the patients seen in arthritis clinics after symptoms have begun already have radiographically detected joint damage. Healthy individuals have been found to have autoantibodies in single serum samples taken as long as 10 years before development of RA. Neither the

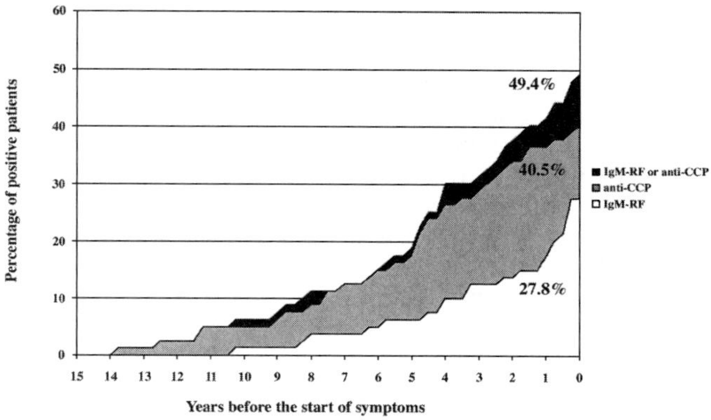

FIGURE 1.—Cumulative percentages of patients with 1 or more positive test results for IgM rheumatoid factor (*IgM-RF*), anticyclic citrullinated peptide (*anti-CCP*), and IgM-RF and/or anti-CCP before the onset of symptoms of RA. (Courtesy of Nielen MMJ, van Schaardenburg D, Reesink HW, et al: Specific autoantibodies precede the symptoms of rheumatoid arthritis: A study of serial measurements in blood donors. *Arthritis Rheum* 50:380-386, 2004. Reprinted by permission of John Wiley & Sons, Inc.)

time course for development of antibodies nor a determination of which antibody or antibody combination is most sensitive or specific for predicting RA has been identified.

The pattern of autoantibodies in the preclinical phase of RA was assessed by using serial measurements and highly specific tests of immunoglobulin M rheumatoid factor (IgM-RF) and anticyclic citrullinated peptide (anti-CCP). Hospital-based groups of patients with early RA have a reported prevalence of RF of 50% to 66%, and that of anti-CCP is between 41% and 48%. Patients who do not have RA have RF prevalences of 7% to 13% and anti-CCP prevalences of 3% to 9%.

Methods.—Frozen serum samples were obtained from 79 patients with RA who had been blood donors before disease symptoms appeared. In addition, 2 serum samples from control subjects matched for age, gender, and date of donation were used, for a total of 2138 samples. All samples underwent testing for IgM-RF and anti-CCP antibodies.

Results.—The earliest serum samples had been collected a median of 7.5 years before the development of RA symptoms. On at least 1 occasion before symptom development, 49.4% of the patients had a sample positive for IgM-RF and/or anti-CCP (Fig 1). This was a median of 4.5 years before the development of symptoms; the range was 0.1 to 13.8 years. Of the control samples, 1.1% tested positive for IgM-RF and 0.6% tested positive for anti-CCP.

Positive tests for IgM-RF persisted in 98% of those with 1 positive test and in 69.2% of those testing positive for anti-CCP. The sensitivity of the IgM-RF test increased with time, but the test for anti-CCP was more sensitive than the IgM-RF test at all time periods evaluated except the 9-year period preceding symptom onset. Anti-CCP tests became positive a maximum of 14 years before symptom onset.

Conclusion.—About half of the patients in whom RA developed were positive for the autoantibodies IgM-RF and anti-CCP considerably earlier than the onset of clinical symptoms. The trigger that activates B lymphocytes to produce RA-specific autoantibodies years before the inflammation causes symptoms remains unknown. Patients who had these early autoantibodies had more severe results on radiographic evaluation, with an increased prevalence of autoantibodies over time. The highest levels were found in the year before symptoms appeared. Tests to detect RA-specific autoantibodies in high-risk populations may predict the development of RA if appropriately high upper limits of normal are established.

► I recently read about a California man who sustained a bat bite to his finger. Unfortunately, the man did not seek treatment, the bat was rabid, and the man died of rabies encephalitis 2 weeks later.

This study reveals that many patients with RA have their B-cells bitten long before clinical disease emerges. Indeed, nearly half of all RA patients develop autoantibodies (IgM-RF or anti-CCP) years before the clinical onset of disease (Fig 1). Sure would be nice to find the "bat" that causes the immunological "bite." Would even be nicer to find a treatment that could prevent rabid joint destruction.

D. B. Hellmann, MD

Antibodies Against Cyclic Citrullinated Peptide and IgA Rheumatoid Factor Predict the Development of Rheumatoid Arthritis

Rantapää-Dahlqvist S, de Jong BAW, Berglin E, et al (Umeå Univ, Sweden; Univ of Nijmegen, The Netherlands; Huddinge Univ, Stockholm)

Arthritis Rheum 48:2741-2749, 2003 1–4

Background.—Some data suggest that posttranslational changes in proteins could be involved in the pathogenesis of autoimmune diseases. For example, the conversion of peptidyl-arginine to peptidyl-citrulline triggers the appearance of antibodies against cyclic citrullinated peptide (CCP), and anti-CCP antibodies are highly specific markers for RA. Rheumatoid factor (RF) is another specific marker that predicts the development of RA. The predictive values of anti-CCP antibodies and RFs (any isotype) for identifying subjects in whom RA subsequently develops were compared.

Methods.—The subjects in this nested case-control study were chosen from 2 national Swedish cohorts. The cases were 86 patients 20 to 67 years old who had provided 98 blood samples a median of 2.5 years before their RA was diagnosed. Each case was matched by age, sex, and geographic region to 3 to 4 control subjects in whom RA had not developed. Serum levels of anti-CCP antibodies and immunoglobulin (Ig) G-RF, IgM-RF, and IgA-RF were analyzed by enzyme immunoassays.

Results.—The stored blood samples of cases had significantly higher levels of anti-CCP antibody (33.7% vs 1.8% in control subjects), IgA-RF (33.7% vs 5.5%), IgM-RF (19.3% vs 6.0%), and IgG-RF (16.9% vs 5.5%)

TABLE 3.—Positive and Negative Predictive Values for Anti-Cyclic Citrullinated Peptide Antibodies and IgM, IgG, and IgA Rheumatoid Factors in 98 Blood Samples From 83 Patients in Whom RA Subsequently Developed at 3 Different Probability Estimates

Antibody	Pretest Probability of 20% for This Study		Calculated Hypothetical Frequency of 8%		Population-based Calculated Frequency of 1%	
	PPV	NPV	PPV	NPV	PPV	NPV
Anti-CCP	82	86	62	94	16	99
IgM-RF	52	83	27	93	4	99
IgG-RF	47	82	23	93	3	99
IgA-RF	65	85	38	94	7	99
Anti-CCP + IgM-RF	83	82	63	93	16	99
Anti-CCP + IgG-RF	83	82	63	93	17	99
Anti-CCP + IgA-RF	87	83	70	94	22	99

Note: Cases were patients with RA whose blood samples were obtained before the onset of any RA symptoms. The positive predictive value (*PPV*) and the negative predictive value (*NPV*) were calculated according to a 20% pretest probability of RA for this study. Values are percentages.

Abbreviations: Anti-CCP, Anti-cyclic citrullinated peptide antibody; *RF*, rheumatoid factor.

(Courtesy of Rantapää-Dahlqvist S, de Jong BAW, Berglin E, et al: Antibodies against cyclic citrullinated peptide and IgA rheumatoid factor predict the development of rheumatoid arthritis. *Arthritis Rheum* 48:2741-2749, 2003. Reprinted by permission of John Wiley & Sons, Inc.)

compared with blood samples from control subjects. By the time the cases presented with RA, more than 70% were positive for anti-CCP antibody, IgM-RF, and IgA-RF, and almost 50% were positive for IgM-RF.

With a calculated pretest probability of RA developing in 20% of patients, the negative predictive value (NPV) of anti-CCP antibodies was similar to that of the 3 RF isotypes (86% vs 82%-85%) (Table 3). However, the positive predictive value (PPV) was much better with anti-CCP antibodies (82% vs 52%-65%).

With a pretest probability of 8% (which is the rate of RA among patients with pain and stiffness referred to the authors' rheumatology clinic), the NPVs were still similar among the 4 markers (93%-94%), but the PPVs were markedly better for anti-CCP antibody (62% vs 23%-38% for RF). Conditional logistic regression analyses showed anti-CCP antibodies (odds ratio, 16.1) and IgA-RF (odds ratio, 5.1) were significant predictors of development of RA more than 1.5 years subsequently (ie, before symptom onset).

Conclusion.—Anti-CCP antibodies and RFs are detectable in the blood of patients with RA long before joint symptoms develop. These findings suggest an important role for anti-CCP antibodies and IgA-RF in the pathogenesis of RA.

► This article taught me several things. First, many patients with RA develop autoantibodies years before they have joint symptoms. And second, in a rheumatology practice where the prevalence of RA may be 8%, anti-CCP antibody has a higher PPV for RA than RF (Table 3).

D. B. Hellmann, MD

Clinical Aspects

Coffee Consumption and Risk of Rheumatoid Arthritis

Karlson EW, Mandl LA, Aweh GN, et al (Harvard Med School, Boston)
Arthritis Rheum 48:3055-3060, 2003 1–5

Background.—The consumption of coffee or decaffeinated coffee and the risk of RA has been linked in recent reports, causing substantial concern in public health sectors. However, these relationships were reported inconsistently, and the studies themselves presented confounding situations. A large, prospective cohort of women was evaluated for any relationship between coffee and tea intake and the risk of RA. In addition to information on beverage consumption, data on potential confounders were collected for 18 years.

Methods.—The 83,124 women completed a food frequency questionnaire at baseline and every 4 years from 1980 through 1998. A connective tissue disease–screening questionnaire and medical record review were used to confirm the diagnosis of incident RA in 480 women. Age-adjusted models and multivariate Cox proportional hazards models were employed to assess any relationships between the intake of various beverages and the risk of RA, with adjustments made for potential confounders such as cigarette smoking.

Results.—The mean age at which the women were given a diagnosis of RA was 53.7 years, with 77% proving rheumatoid factor (RF)–positive. Baseline data indicated that, compared to those who drank no coffee, those consuming 4 cups/d or more were linked to a modest increase in the risk of RA. Adjustments for smoking and other covariates attenuated the relative risk, eliminating the relationship between coffee intake and risk of RA. Similar results were obtained when only RF-positive patients were assessed.

No significant association was found between the intake of 4 or more cups of decaffeinated coffee daily and the risk of RA. The total coffee and total caffeine consumption showed no association with the risk of RA. Tea did not carry any protective effect against development of RA. However, cigarette smoking significantly increased the risk of RA, an effect seen consistently across all analyses.

Conclusion.—No relationship was found between the intake of coffee, decaffeinated coffee, or tea and the risk of RA for women. A significant association was identified between smoking and the risk of RA, as shown in many other studies.

► I previously presented some of the studies first suggesting that coffee, then decaffeinated coffee, was associated with increased risk of RA. These wrought havoc with my beverage consumption habits. Now I can resume my coffee, decaf, or tea without concern. I only hope that soft drinks remain hazard free.

R. S. Panush, MD

Prevalence of Rheumatoid Arthritis in Persons 60 Years of Age and Older in the United States: Effect of Different Methods of Case Classification

Rasch EK, Hirsch R, Paulose-Ram R, et al (Ctrs for Disease Control and Prevention, Hyattsville, Md; Univ of Maryland, Baltimore)

Arthritis Rheum 48:917-926, 2003 1–6

Background.—RA is a multisystem disorder that is characterized by chronic destructive synovitis. The clinical course and outcomes can vary widely among individuals, but it has been well established that persons with persistent RA experience progressive disability and early mortality. The last national prevalence estimates in the United States were derived from the First National Health and Nutrition Examination Survey (NHANES-I). The classification criteria for RA have been revised since that time, and there is a need to update the prevalence estimates for the disease. The prevalence estimates for RA in noninstitutionalized older adults in the United States were investigated. Prevalence estimates were compared by using 3 different classification methods based on the current classification criteria for RA.

Methods.—Data from the NHANES-III were used to create prevalence estimates by the 3 classification methods in 5302 persons 60 years of age and older. Method 1 applied the "n of k" rule, so subjects who met 3 of 6 American College of Rheumatology 1987 criteria were classified as having RA. In method 2, the American College of Rheumatology classification tree algorithm was applied. In method 3, medication data were used to augment case identification by means of method 2. Population prevalence estimates and

TABLE 4.—Stratified Population Prevalence Estimates for RA Using the 3 Classification Methods

	Sample Size	Prevalence of RA, % (95% CI) Method 1 (n of k)	Method 2 (Classification Tree)	Method 3 (Tree/DMARDs)
All subjects	5,302	2.03 (1.30-2.76)	2.15 (1.43-2.87)	2.34 (1.66-3.02)
Sex				
Male	2,587	1.60 (0.84-2.36)	1.59 (0.82-2.36)	1.85 (1.04-2.66)
Female	2,715	2.35 (1.35-3.35)	2.57 (1.58-3.56)	2.71 (1.73-3.69)
Race/ethnicity				
Non-Hispanic white	3,043	2.10 (1.30-2.90)	2.21 (1.42-3.00)	2.41 (1.65-3.17)
Non-Hispanic black	1,073	1.94 (0.48-3.40)	2.26 (0.84-3.68)	2.55 (1.22-3.88)
Mexican American	1,027	2.43 (0.67-4.19)	2.47 (0.71-4.23)	2.80 (1.02-4.58)
Age				
60-69 years	2,309	1.59 (0.98-2.20)	1.66 (1.04-2.28)	1.89 (1.31-2.47)
≥70 years	2,993	2.46 (1.26-3.66)	2.63 (1.42-3.84)	2.80 (1.59-4.01)
Education				
Less than high school	2,990	2.25 (1.44-3.06)	2.49 (1.66-3.32)	2.64 (1.81-3.47)
High school or more	2,274	1.82 (0.90-2.74)	1.86 (0.94-2.78)	2.09 (1.24-2.94)

Note: Separate prevalence estimates for "other" race/ethnicity groups are not reported because of limited sample size. All other prevalence estimates include all race/ethnicity categories.

Abbreviations: *CI*, Confidence interval; *DMARDs*, disease-modifying antirheumatic drugs.

95% confidence intervals were determined by use of the 3 methods on data stratified by sex, race/ethnicity, age, and education.

Results.—The overall prevalence estimates using the 3 classification methods were 2.03%, 2.15%, and 2.34%, respectively (Table 4). The prevalence of RA was generally greater in women, Mexican Americans, respondents with less education, and respondents who were 70 years of age and older.

Conclusion.—This update of prevalence estimates for RA found a prevalence of approximately 2% in persons 60 years of age and older in the United States. This is representative of the proportion of the elderly population in this country who will require medical intervention because of disease activity. Similar prevalence estimates were obtained by 3 different classification methods.

► There are new classification criteria for the diagnosis of RA, but the estimated prevalence of RA in older adults remains the same: about 2% (Table 4).

D. B. Hellmann, MD

Decreases in Rates of Hospitalizations for Manifestations of Severe Rheumatoid Arthritis, 1983-2001

Ward MM (NIH, Bethesda, Md)

Arthritis Rheum 50:1122-1131, 2004 1–7

Background.—In the late 1980s, RA treatment evolved from an approach emphasizing selective use of disease-modifying medications for patients with entrenched synovitis and evidence of joint damage to an approach emphasizing the consistent use of disease-modifying medications in almost all patients from onset of joint inflammation. Whether this change in approach has been associated with improvements in long-term health outcomes is unclear. Whether hospitalization rates for 4 manifestations of severe RA, used as indicators of long-term health outcomes, have changed between 1983 and 2001 was determined.

Methods.—Data were obtained on all patients with RA hospitalized with rheumatoid vasculitis or for splenectomy for Felty's syndrome, cervical spine fusion for myelopathy, or total knee arthroplasty at California hospitals. Changes in hospitalization rates between 1983 and 2001 were sought.

Findings.—Hospitalization rates for rheumatoid vasculitis and splenectomy in Felty's syndrome declined progressively over time (Fig 1). In the period from 1998 to 2001, hospitalization risk for rheumatoid vasculitis was one third lower than in the period from 1983 to 1987. Risk of hospitalization for splenectomy in Felty's syndrome was 71% lower in 1998 to 2001 than in 1983 to 1987. No significant reductions were seen in the rates of hospitalization for cervical spine surgery or total knee arthroplasty. From 1998 to 2001, however, the trend of increasing rates of total knee arthroplasty was reversed. The risk of being hospitalized for primary total knee arthroplasty was significantly lower from 1998 to 2001 than from 1990 to 1993.

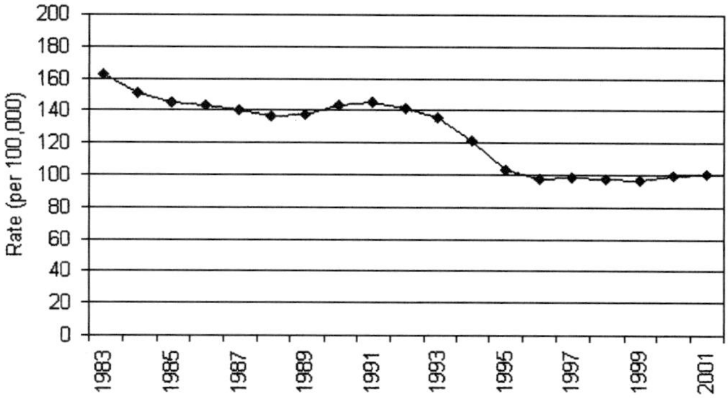

FIGURE 1.—Annual rates of hospitalization for rheumatoid vasculitis per 100,000 persons with RA from 1983 to 2001. Rates are presented as 3-year weighted moving averages. (Courtesy of Ward MM: Decreases in rates of hospitalizations for manifestations of severe rheumatoid arthritis, 1983-2001. *Arthritis Rheum* 50:1122-1131, 2004. Reprinted by permission of John Wiley & Sons, Inc.)

Conclusions.—The rates of hospitalization for rheumatoid vasculitis and splenectomy in Felty's syndrome have declined in the past 19 years. Recently, there has been a reduction in the rates of primary total knee arthroplasty in patients with RA. These findings suggest that long-term health outcomes of patients with RA have improved since the early 1980s.

► I believe this is an important article because it strongly suggests that the new medical therapies introduced in the 1980s really work and have improved the health of patients with RA. Although the reduction in hospitalization rates (Fig 1) could be attributed to a new emphasis on outpatient care, the reduction in rates of knee replacement surgery supports the perceptions of nearly all rheumatologists over the age of 50 years—that the new treatments for RA work better than the old therapies.

D. B. Hellmann, MD

Embolic Complications of a Mitral Valve Rheumatoid Nodule

Kang H, Baron M (McGill Univ, Montreal)
J Rheumatol 31:1001-1003, 2004 1–8

Introduction.—Approximately 25% of cases of definite or classic RA will have rheumatoid nodules, which can occur in all parts of the heart. The thromboembolic complications of a mitral valve rheumatoid nodule in a patient with seropositive RA are illustrated.

Case Report.—A man, 70, came to the hospital with transient dysarthria, left hand weakness, and a pulseless, cool, and painful right leg. The patient's medical history included seropositive nodular RA of 20 years' duration, hypertension, diabetes mellitus type 2, and peptic ulcer disease. Drug therapy had consisted of prednisone, celecoxib, omeprazole, nifedipine, metoprolol, and acetaminophen. The patient was being considered for antitumor necrosis factor therapy because of inadequate response to antirheumatic drugs. On admission, the neurologic examination and sinus rhythm were normal. An ECG, however, showed an incomplete right bundle branch block, and an angiogram of the right leg revealed occlusion of the right profunda femoris and superficial femoral artery. A large mobile lesion attached to the posterior leaflet of the mitral valve was apparent at transesophageal echocardiogram. Treatment consisted of excision of the pedunculated tumor mass and repair of the mitral valve with native pericardium. The patient also underwent a coronary artery bypass for coronary artery disease. Pathologic examination findings were consistent with a rheumatoid nodule. The patient was started on long-term anticoagulation because the potential for a recurrent rheumatoid nodule and thrombus was thought to be present.

Discussion.—This case illustrates the potential for intracardiac rheumatoid nodules to develop in patients with seropositive RA, and these nodules may stimulate the formation of an overlying thrombus and possible embolic sequelae. It is thus important for all patients with RA, especially those who are seropositive, to have regular cardiac evaluations and an ECG if physical examination findings suggest valvular heart disease or conduction abnormalities.

► I have included this case report as a powerful reminder that rheumatoid nodules can develop anywhere.

D. B. Hellmann, MD

Slowing of Bone Loss in Patients With Rheumatoid Arthritis by Long-term High-Intensity Exercise: Results of a Randomized, Controlled Trial

de Jong Z, Munneke M, Lems WF, et al (Leiden Univ, The Netherlands; Vrije Universiteit Med Ctr, Amsterdam; Jan van Breemen Institute, Amsterdam; et al)

Arthritis Rheum 50:1066-1076, 2004 1–9

Background.—The risk of osteoporosis and osteoporotic fractures is higher in patients with RA than in their healthy peers. The effects of a 2-year high-intensity weight-bearing exercise, called the RA-Patients-in-Training (RAPIT) program, on bone mineral density (BMD) compared with usual care physical therapy was investigated.

Methods.—Three hundred nine patients with RA were assigned to RAPIT or usual care physical therapy. Aerobic fitness, muscle strength, and attendance rates were analyzed. One hundred thirty-six patients in the RAPIT group and 145 in the usual care group completed the study and were included in the analysis.

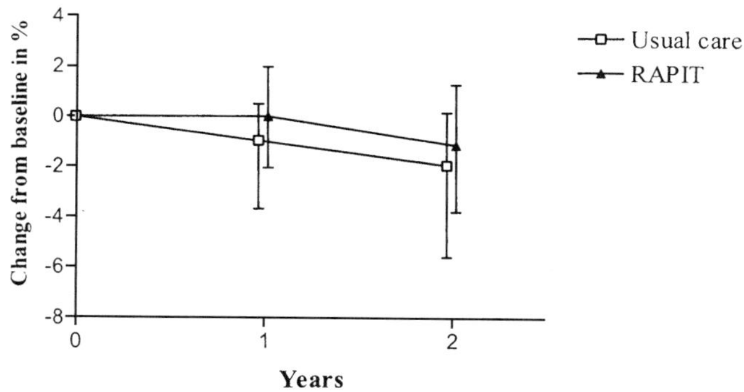

FIGURE 2.—Percentage of change in BMD of the total hip in the 2 years of the trial in patients randomly assigned to receive either usual care physical therapy or to undergo the RAPIT exercise program. *Bars* show the median and interquartile range. (Courtesy of de Jong Z, Munneke M, Lems WF, et al: Slowing of bone loss in patients with rheumatoid arthritis by long-term high-intensity exercise: Results of a randomized, controlled trial. *Arthritis Rheum* 50:1066-1076, 2004. Reprinted by permission of John Wiley & Sons, Inc.)

Findings.—The mean rate of reduction in hip BMD but not in lumbar spine BMD was smaller in the RAPIT group than in the usual care group, with a mean decline of 1.6% in the first year and 0.5% in the second year (Figs 2 and 3). Change in hip BMD was significantly and independently related to changes in muscle strength and aerobic fitness. However, it was not associated with attendance rate.

Conclusions.—A long-term, high-intensity weight-bearing exercise program for patients with RA can slow down BMD loss at the hip. Muscle strength and aerobic fitness are the exercise modalities associated with this effect.

► I am skeptical of the author's conclusions that high-intensity, long-term exercise effectively slows bone loss in RA. Exercise produces a very small benefit in BMD of the hips (Fig 2) and no benefit for the spine (Fig 3). The possibility

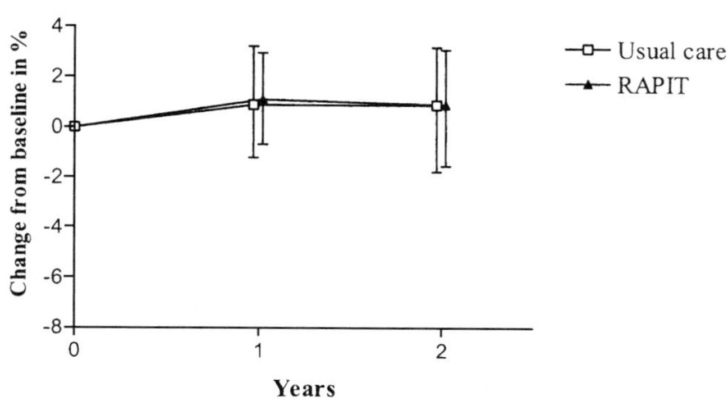

FIGURE 3.—Percentage of change in BMD of the lumbar spine in the 2 years of the trial in patients randomly assigned to receive either usual care physical therapy or to undergo the RAPIT exercise program. *Bars* show the median and interquartile range. (Courtesy of de Jong Z, Munneke M, Lems WF, et al: Slowing of bone loss in patients with rheumatoid arthritis by long-term high-intensity exercise: Results of a randomized, controlled trial. *Arthritis Rheum* 50:1066-1076, 2004. Reprinted by permission of John Wiley & Sons, Inc.)

that intensive exercise may have a deleterious effect on inflamed weight-bearing joints further limits my enthusiasm for these results.

D. B. Hellmann, MD

Prognostic Markers of Radiographic Progression in Early Rheumatoid Arthritis

Goronzy JJ, Matteson EL, Fulbright JW, et al (Mayo Clinic, Rochester, Minn; Roche Molecular Systems, Alameda, Calif)

Arthritis Rheum 50:43-54, 2004 1–10

Background.—About 20% of patients with RA have chronic progressive disease despite treatment and might benefit from early aggressive therapy. Yet, not all patients need aggressive treatment, and many gain disease control with rather minimal treatment. To help identify which patients might benefit more from aggressive therapy, possible prognostic markers of progressive erosive disease in patients with early RA were investigated.

Methods.—The subjects were 111 adults (70% women; mean age, 51.5 years) with RA of less than 1 year's duration. All were treated according to a standardized algorithm designed to avoid overtreatment of mild disease and to accelerate treatment of more aggressive disease. In brief, all patients started receiving hydroxychloroquine (200 mg twice daily), a nonsteroidal anti-inflammatory drug, and (if necessary) low-dose prednisone.

Patients were evaluated at 6, 12, and 24 months, and treatment was adjusted according to response (ie, nonresponders to the initial regimen began taking methotrexate at 6 months). Patients provided blood samples for measuring the frequency of CD4+,CD28^{null} T cells, HLA-DRB1 typing, and genotyping of 26 polymorphisms in 19 candidate genes involved in inflammatory and immune system pathways. These markers were analyzed to examine their association with erosive progression on serial hand/wrist radiographs taken over 2 years.

Results.—Ninety-four patients (84.7%) completed the 2-year study. At the 2-year visit, disease in 49 of these 94 patients (52.1%) was adequately controlled by the initial regimen of hydroxychloroquine, nonsteroidal anti-inflammatory drugs, and (in 7 patients) corticosteroid. Erosions developed

TABLE 4.—Predictive Value of HLA-DRB1* Alleles for Determining Disease Outcome

Parameter	β	Odds Ratio	95% CI	*P*
Shared epitope	0.78	2.18	0.91-5.20	0.079
RA-associated HLA-DRB1*04 allele	0.96	2.60	1.14-5.93	0.023
HLA-DRB1*04/04 versus non-HLA-DRB1*04	1.58	4.87	1.40-16.98	0.013
HLA-DRB1*04/04 versus non-HLA-DRB1*04/04	1.10	3.01	1.01-9.03	0.049
Frequency of CD4+,CD28^{null} T cells†	0.04	1.52	1.00-2.31	0.051

*Per 10% increase.

Abbreviation: CI, Confidence interval

(Courtesy of Goronzy JJ, Matteson EL, Fulbright JW, et al: Prognostic markers of radiographic progression in early rheumatoid arthritis. *Arthritis Rheum* 50:43-54, 2004. Reprinted by permission of John Wiley & Sons, Inc.)

in 25 of these 49 patients (51.0%), and in 49 patients overall (52.1% of total).

Conversely, despite treatment escalation over 2 years, 9 patients (9.6%) were nonresponders. Univariate analyses identified the following predictors of radiographic progression: older age (odds ratio [OR], 1.45 per 10-year increment), rheumatoid factor titer (OR, 1.28 per 100-IU increase), number of erosions at baseline (OR, 4.31), presence of rheumatoid factor (OR, 3.14), and the HLA-DRB1*04 allele (OR, 2.60), particularly homozygosity for this allele (OR, 4.87 vs heterozygotes; OR, 3.01 vs no variante alleles) (Table 4).

The frequency of CD4+,CD28^{null} T cells may also be a significant prognistic indicator of more aggressive disease (OR, 1.52; $P = .51$). In contrast, a polymorphism in the uteroglobulin gene (A587G) was identified as protective of radiographic progression (OR, 10.48 for at least 1 variant allele vs no variant alleles; $P = .026$).

Conclusion.—About half of patients with early RA can be managed with nonaggressive treatment. Only about half of these patients experienced new erosions during follow-up, thus emphasizing the need to avoid unnecessarily aggressive treatment in a large proportion of patients with RA. The HLA-DRB1*04 allele (but not the presence of a shared epitope or HLA-DRB1*01 alone) was strongly associated with more severe erosive disease. On the other hand, homozytosity for the nonvariant allele of the utereoglobulin gene at position 587 was strongly protective against joint erosion, and 9 of the 10 patients homozygous for the nonvariant allele did not have erosions, even though other risk factors (eg, HLA-DRB1*04 allele, high rheumatoid factor titer) were present. Thus, uteroglobulin nucleotide mapping may help identify which patients with RA are less likely to require aggressive therapy.

► The need for early, aggressive treatment for RA has become almost a mantra for rheumatologists. This article reminds us that not every RA patient needs aggressive therapy. Indeed, nearly half of the patients were well controlled on nonaggressive therapy with nonsteroidal anti-inflammatory drugs and hydroxychloroquine. So what we really need to do is identify early those RA patients with a poor prognosis. This article shows that biological markers can help (Table 4) identify the patients who may benefit from aggressive therapy.

D. B. Hellmann, MD

Progression of Radiologic Damage in Patients With Rheumatoid Arthritis in Clinical Remission

Molenaar ETH, Voskuyl AE, Dinant HJ, et al (VU Univ Med Ctr, Amsterdam; Jan van Breemen Instituut Amsterdam)

Arthritis Rheum 50:36-42, 2004 1–11

Background.—Only 10% to 20% of patients with RA achieve clinical remission. But does the cessation of symptoms mean that bone damage has ceased also? Radiologic evidence of disease progression was investigated during follow-up of patients with RA who achieved clinical remission.

Methods.—The subjects were 187 patients (65% women; mean age, 58 years) whose RA was in clinical remission. Clinical remission was defined according to the American College of Rheumatology (ACR) criteria, except that the criterion for fatigue was omitted because fatigue was not routinely assessed. Thus, according to the modification, all patients met at least 4 of the following 5 criteria: duration of morning stiffness less than 15 minutes, no joint pain, no joint tenderness or pain on motion, no soft tissue swelling in joints or tendon sheaths, and an erythrocyte sedimentation rate of less than 30 mm/h for women or less than 20 mm/h for men. Patients were followed up with clinical and laboratory investigations and radiographs at baseline and at 1 and 2 years. Disease progression on radiographs was evaluated according to the Sharp/van der Heijde method.

Results.—Complete radiologic follow-up was available for 179 patients (95.7%). Of these 179 patients, 93 (52.0%) met the revised ACR criteria for persistent clinical remission at 2 years. Median radiologic joint damage scores (comparing 2-year images with baseline) were significantly lower in the patients with persistent clinical remission than in the 86 patients (48.0%) with disease exacerbation (scores 0 and 1.0, respectively). The situation was similar when the radiographs from 104 patients who met the stan-

TABLE 2.—Radiologic Joint Damage Scores in Patients With RA in Clinical Remission as Defined by the American College of Rheumatology Criteria

	Sharp/van der Heijde Score				
Patient Group	Baseline	1-Year Followup	2-Year Followup	Difference Between Baseline and 1-Year Followup	Difference Between Baseline and 2-Year Followup
Complete cohort (n = 110)*					
Mean ± SD	44 ± 62	46 ± 64	43 ± 58	0.7 ± 2.3	1.4 ± 3.3
Median (range)	17 (0, 273)	20 (0, 270)†	21 (0, 272)‡	0 (−6, 11)	0.5 (−5, 18)
Interquartile range	4-48	6-53	6-52	0-1	0-2
Persistent remission (n = 65)					
Mean ± SD	44 ± 60	46 ± 60	46 ± 60	0.7 ± 2.5	1.2 ± 3.6
Median (range)	21 (0, 273)	22 (0, 271)†	23 (0, 272)§	0 (−5, 11)	0 (−5, 18)‖
Interquartile range	7-46	7-53	7-55	0-0.5	0-2
Exacerbation of RA (n = 39)					
Mean ± SD	43 ± 66	47 ± 71	39 ± 52	0.8 ± 1.9	1.7 ± 2.3
Median (range)	14 (0, 267)	15 (0, 267)†	16 (0, 224)‡	0.5 (−6, 6)	1.0 (−3, 9)
Interquartile range	4-48	5-53	5-51	0-1.5	0-4

Note: Except where indicated otherwise, *P* values were determined by Wilcoxon's signed rank test.
*Radiologic data were available for only 104 patients.
†$P < .05$ versus baseline.
‡$P < .05$ versus baseline and 1-year follow-up.
§$P < .05$ versus 1-year follow-up.
‖$P < .05$ by Mann-Whitney U test versus patients with exacerbation.
Abbreviation: SD, Standard deviation.
(Courtesy of Molenaar ETH, Voskuyl AE, Dinant HJ, et al: Progression of radiologic damage in patients with rheumatoid arthritis in clinical remission. *Arthritis Rheum* 50:36-42, 2004. Reprinted by permission of John Wiley & Sons, Inc.)

dard ACR criteria at baseline (ie, they met all 5 of the modified criteria) were evaluated:

Median radiologic joint damage scores were significantly lower in the 65 patients (62.5%) still in remission than in the 39 patients (37.5%) with disease exacerbation (scores 0 and 1.0, respectively) (Table 2). Still, in 14 patients who had remained in clinical remission for 2 years (15.1% of those meeting revised ACR criteria, 21.5% of those meeting standard ACR criteria), an erosion had developed in a previously unaffected joint.

Conclusion.—About half of patients with RA in clinical remission had a relapse during 2 years of follow-up. Patients whose RA stayed in clinical remission for 2 years had less radiologic bone damage than patients whose RA reactivated during follow-up. Still, in 15% to 20% of the patients with persistent clinical remission, an erosion developed in a previously unaffected joint. Thus, even long-term clinical remission does not protect fully against radiologic progression.

► In the early 1980s, before the time of biological therapies, the chief of my rheumatology fellowship program used to contend that "disease-modifying antirheumatic drug" was a misnomer. He doubted that any drug truly produced remission in RA. The current study suggests that even in the time of biologics, his skepticism might be well placed.

D. B. Hellmann, MD

Relative Sensitivity to Change of the Erythrocyte Sedimentation Rate and Serum C-Reactive Protein Concentration in Rheumatoid Arthritis

Ward MM (NIH, Bethesda, Md)

J Rheumatol 31:884-895, 2003 1–12

Introduction.—Both the erythrocyte sedimentation rate (ESR) and the serum C-reactive protein (CRP) concentration tests are used to evaluate treatment response in patients with RA. Little is known, however, about the relative sensitivity to change of these tests. Studies that used both tests were analyzed to compare how well ESR and CRP show changes in clinical status after treatment with disease-modifying agents.

Methods.—The Cochrane Database and MEDLINE were searched for clinical trials and observational studies that measured both ESR and CRP in the same patients at the start of treatment and after 4 to 24 weeks of treatment. Reference lists of retrieved articles were also searched for additional studies. Excluded from analysis were studies of IV corticosteroids, which typically measured responses after several days, and those in which patients with RA were combined with patients with other diagnoses. A pooled analysis was carried out on the paired differences in effect sizes for ESR and CRP within each study.

Results.—The literature search identified 123 potentially eligible studies, 63 of which provided sufficient data to permit calculation of effect sizes for both tests. Another 16 studies became eligible after their authors or sponsors provided additional data. The median number of patients in treatment arms was 42. In the 36 treatment arms that reported results at 12 weeks, the ESR was more sensitive to change than the CRP, with a paired difference in effect sizes of 0.09 units. The ESR was also more sensitive to change than the CRP in the 76 treatment arms that reported results at 24 weeks, with a paired difference in effect sizes of 0.11 units. Some treatment arms indicated that the CRP was more sensitive to change early, yet this effect was lost by 24 weeks. There were differences among medications, with the CRP more sensitive to change in studies of cyclosporine and the ESR much more sensitive in studies of sulfasalazine and combination therapy.

Conclusion.—An analysis of studies of disease-modifying medications in RA suggests that the sensitivity to change of the ESR is approximately 15% to 20% greater than that of the CRP. The ESR may thus be the preferred measure of the acute phase response in RA.

► I'm often asked by physicians outside of rheumatology, "Which is the better test, ESR or CRP?" I generally respond by noting that the data are too exiguous to give a definitive answer. Practical issues, however, often loom large in the choice: ESR is accurate only if performed within a short time of collection. If the blood sample has to travel for testing, then CRP is the better test.

D. B. Hellmann, MD

Therapy

Is a Long-term High-Intensity Exercise Program Effective and Safe in Patients With Rheumatoid Arthritis? Results of a Randomized Controlled Trial

de Jong Z, Munneke M, Zwinderman AH, et al (Leiden Univ, The Netherlands; Jan van Breemen Instituut, Amsterdam; Leyenburg Hosp, The Hague, The Netherlands; et al)

Arthritis Rheum 48:2415-2424, 2003 1–13

Introduction.—Data are insufficient concerning the effect of long-term intensive exercise in patients with rheumatoid arthritis (RA). A randomized, controlled, multicenter trial was performed to compare the effectiveness and safety of a 2-year intensive exercise program (Rheumatoid Arthritis Patients in Training [RAPIT]) with those of physical therapy (UC, usual care).

Methods.—A total of 309 patients with RA were randomized to participate in either the RAPIT or UC program. The major end point was functional ability (evaluated by the McMaster Toronto Arthritis [MACTAR] Patient Preference Disability Questionnaire [HAQ]) and the effects on radiographic progression in large joints. Secondary end points addressed emotional status and disease activity.

Results.—At the 2-year follow-up examination, participants in the RAPIT program demonstrated greater improvement in functional ability, aerobic fitness, and muscle strength than did those in UC. The mean difference in change of the MACTAR Questionnaire score was 2.6 (95% confidence interval [CI], 0.1, 5.2) over the first year and 3.1 (95% CI, 0.7, -5.5) over the next year. At the 2-year follow-up examination, the mean difference in change of the HAQ score was −0.09 (95% CI, −0.18, −0.01). The median radiographic damage of the large joints did not increase during follow-up for either group. For both RAPIT and UC, participants with considerable baseline damage had slightly more progression in damage that was more obvious in the RAPIT group. Emotional status was improved in both groups and no detrimental effects on disease activity were seen for either group.

Conclusion.—A long-term high-intensity exercise program is more effective than UC in improving functional ability in patients with RA. Intensive exercise does not increase radiographic damage in the large joints; the exception is patients with considerable baseline damage of the large joints.

▶ The arthritis foundation recently asked me for a statement about exercise for arthritis. I thought the following recommendation fit available information: "Most arthritis patients should be encouraged to participate in judicious exercise programs. They should select activities they enjoy and be as physically active as possible without causing or increasing joint symptoms. This should be done with the benefit of expert advice. Patients usually experience salutary psychological, physical, and functional benefits from proper exercise programs. These include improved sense of well being, better aerobic capacity, greater strength, increased joint mobility, and more functional ability." Jim Fries' continued observations of his cohorts have been great, offering extremely valuable data about the benefits of exercise (running) generally. I haven't seen him at the American College of Rheumatogy annual 5k races lately though (where I must boast that I won a silver medal for 2nd place for my age group the last time I ran, which speaks more about my age than ability, unfortunately).

R. S. Panush, MD

Recommendations on Screening for Chloroquine and Hydroxychloroquine Retinopathy: A Report by the American Academy of Ophthalmology

Marmor MF, for the American Academy of Ophthalmology
Ophthalmology 109:1377-1382, 2002 1–14

Introduction.—Retinal toxicity from chloroquine and its analogue, hydroxychloroquine, is well known. A diversity of screening regimens has been proposed. They vary in practicality, cost, and cost/benefit ratio. It would be useful to have a consensus recommendation. Screening programs for chloroquine and hydroxychloroquine were examined.

Screening Programs.—Screening helps recognize toxicity early, before damage is too great. It cannot prevent toxicity or guarantee that there will be no visual loss. Although toxicities occur and can be serious, their incidence is very low. There seems to be a minimal risk of toxicity for persons using less than 6.5 mg/kg of hydroxychloroquine or 3 mg/kg of chloroquine for less

TABLE 1.—Criteria of Low and Higher Risk for Development of Retinopathy

	Low Risk	Higher Risk
Dosage	<6.5 mg/kg hydroxychloroquine <3 mg/kg chloroquine	>6.5 mg/kg hydroxychloroquine >3 mg/kg chloroquine
Duration of Use	<5 years	>5 years
Habitus	Lean or average fat	High fat level (unless dosage is appropriately low)
Renal/liver disease	None	Present
Concomitant retinal disease	None	Present
Age	<60 years	>60 years

(Reprinted from *Ophthalmology* courtesy of Marmor MF, for the American Academy of Ophthalmology: Recommendations on screening for chloroquine and hydroxychloroquine retinopathy: A report by the American Academy of Ophthalmology. *Ophthalmology* 109:1377-1382, 2002. Copyright 2002, with permission from Elsevier Science.)

than 5 years (Table 1). Screening practices can be modified to consider these facts and to be maximally cost effective.

If baseline examination is normal at initiation of therapy and dosages are at relatively safe levels, screening during the next 5 years can be performed at the frequency of regular ophthalmic examinations recommended by the American Academy of Ophthalmology Preferred Practice Pattern for the patient's age (Table 2). Both drugs are cleared from the body renally and hepatically. Severe failure of these symptoms could cause greater drug retention and toxicity. All patients starting hydroxychloroquine or chloroquine therapy should have a baseline examination within the first year of therapy to document any complicating ocular conditions and to establish a record of the fundus appearance and visual field. It allows a risk status (low/high) to be established.

Annual screening is recommended for patients in the high-risk category. More careful examination is needed for patients with suggestive visual symptoms and for those for whom any screening examination raises a question of early toxicity. There is no proven medical therapy that is effective in treating toxicity other than cessation of the drug. If toxicity is recognized at a very early stage of functional versus pigmentary loss, some recovery may be possible. Reevaluation is recommended every 3 months after a diagnosis of toxicity is made, even after discontinuation of the drug.

TABLE 2.—Comprehensive Eye Evaluation for Patients With No Risk Factors

Age	Frequency of Examination
20-29 years	at least once during period
30-39 years	at least twice during period
40-64 years	every 2-4 years
65 years or older	every 1-2 years

(Reprinted from *Ophthalmology* courtesy of Marmor MF, for the American Academy of Ophthalmology: Recommendations on screening for chloroquine and hydroxychloroquine retinopathy: A report by the American Academy of Ophthalmology. *Ophthalmology* 109:1377-1382, 2002. Copyright 2002, with permission from Elsevier Science.)

Conclusion.—Patients in a high-risk category for toxicity from chloroquine or hydroxychloroquine and patients with toxicity must be followed up carefully.

Rheumatologists' Attitudes Toward Routine Screening for Hydroxychloroquine Retinopathy

Fraenkel L, Felson DT (Yale Univ, New Haven, Conn; VA Connecticut Health Care System, West Haven)

J Rheumatol 28:1218-1221, 2001 1–15

Introduction.—Routine annual or biannual ophthalmologic screening is recommended in the United States for all patients taking hydroxychloroquine (HCQ), based on the belief that screening will identify early signs of toxicity. Several trials have demonstrated that retinal toxicity is exceedingly rare in patients taking HCQ at below 6.5 mg/kg lean body weight/d. Rheumatologists' attitudes toward routine ophthalmologic screening for HCQ retinopathy was examined. The acceptability of hypothetical guidelines discouraging this practice were also assessed.

Methods.—A random sample of 300 US rheumatologists listed in the American College of Rheumatology (ACR) Directory who treated adults were sent a survey by e-mail. Rheumatologists were queried regarding current screening practices, reasons for screening, and the effect of hypothetical guidelines discouraging routine screening or future practice. Associations between adherence to guidelines and clinical variables were examined by multiple logistic regression.

Results.—The response rate was 56%. Nearly all (94%) respondents screened their patients at least once each year. Seventy-five percent stated that they would continue to screen due to unwillingness to accept any risk of visual loss among their patients; 74% screened due to legal liability; and 56% believed their patients would insist on screening regardless of physician opinion (Table 1). Even if ACR published guidelines discouraged routine screening, 45% indicated that they would continue to screen regularly. Rheumatologists unwilling to accept any risk of retinopathy were not as likely to follow guidelines that discouraged screening (46% vs 77%; adjusted odds ratio, 0.2; 95% confidence interval, 0.1-0.6). Patient insistence

TABLE 1.—Distribution of Reasons for Continued Routine Screening

	N	Strongly Agree	Agree	Neutral	Disagree	Strongly Agree	Missing
Unwillingness to accept any risk	155	52 (34)	63 (41)	25 (16)	11 (7)	2 (1)	2 (1)
Fear of legal liability	155	53 (34)	62 (40)	27 (17)	10 (7)	1 (1)	2 (1)
Patient insistence	155	31 (20)	56 (36)	35 (23)	23 (15)	8 (5)	2 (1)

Note: Percentages are shown in parentheses.
(Courtesy of Fraenkel L, Felson DT: Rheumatologists' attitudes toward routine screening for hydroxychloroquine retinopathy. *J Rheumatol* 28:1218-1221, 2001.)

and fear of legal liability were not significantly linked with predicted adherence to guidelines.

Conclusion.—Most rheumatologists currently routinely screen their patients for HCQ retinopathy. Many would not follow ACR guidelines that discourage this practice, at least in part since they are unwilling to accept any risk of visual damage.

▶ The ophthalmology recommendations are pretty minimal, although some rheumatologists have advocated that no screening at all is necessary. I'm like most rheumatologists here; I feel comfortable having my patients checked about once a year and recognize that, for me, this is reflective of what I learned as a fellow, not based on current data or recommendations.

R. S. Panush, MD

Safety of Hydroxychloroquine in Pregnant Patients With Connective Tissue Diseases: A Study of One Hundred Thirty-Three Cases Compared With a Control Group

Costedoat-Chalumeau N, Amoura Z, Duhaut P, et al (Centre Hospitalier Universitaire Pitié-Salpêtrière, Paris; Centre Hospitalier Universitaire Robert Debré, Paris)

Arthritis Rheum 48:3207-3211, 2003 1–16

Background.—The antimalarial drug hydroxychloroquine (HCQ) is given as part of the treatment for systemic lupus erythematosus (SLE). Discontinuing HCQ doubles the risk of experiencing an SLE flare during the next 6 months in nonpregnant women. Pregnancy itself is acknowledged to increase disease activity among patients with SLE. The use of HCQ during pregnancy is controversial in light of evidence that it crosses the placenta and cord blood concentrations are almost the same as those in maternal blood. Few cases of pregnant women with SLE who are receiving HCQ have been reported. The 133 pregnancies of 90 women receiving HCQ were evaluated in comparison to those of control subjects.

Methods.—In 122 pregnancies, the 90 women were given 200 mg of HCQ twice daily, and 11 received this dose once a day. Outcomes were compared with those of 70 pregnancies in 53 women who had similar disorders but did not take HCQ. Forty-seven children of women in the HCQ group and 45 of those in the control group underwent electrocardiography.

Results.—A live birth was achieved in 88% of the women taking HCQ and 84% of the control women. In the HCQ group there were 15 spontaneous abortions, one fetal death, 33 premature births, and 84 full-term births. The mean gestational age of infants born to women taking HCQ was 37.1 weeks, with a range of 26 to 41 weeks. The only difference between these infants and those in the control group was a slightly lower mean gestational age (Table 2).

Three malformations developed in the HCQ group and 4 in the control group. Mean PR intervals were 91.4 ms for the HCG infants and 92.1 ms for

TABLE 2.—Pregnancy Outcomes

Outcome	Group A (133 Pregnancies)	Group B (70 Pregnancies)	*P*
Spontaneous abortion	15 (11.3)	7 (10)	0.78
Fetal death	1 (0.8)	2 (2.9)	0.27
Therapeutic abortion	0 (0)	2 (2.9)	0.12
Live birth*	117 (88)	59 (84.3)	0.46
Premature birth	33 (28)	12 (17)	0.21
Full-term birth	84 (72)	47 (67)	0.21
Gestational age, mean (range) weeks	37.1 (26-41)	38.1 (29-41)	<0.02
Weight, mean (range) grams	2,754 (500-4,300)	2,897 (1,200-4,250)	0.15

Note: Except where indicated otherwise, values are the number (percentage) of pregnancies. Group A includes patients with connective tissue disease who received hydroxychloroquine; group B includes patients with connective tissue disease who did not receive hydroxychloroquine.

*Two twin pregnancies occurred in each group.

(Courtesy of Costedoat-Chalumeau N, Amoura Z, Duhaut P, et al: Safety of hydroxychloroquine in pregnant patients with connective tissue diseases: A study of one hundred thirty-three cases compared with a control group. *Arthritis Rheum* 48:3207-3211, 2003. Reprinted by permission of John Wiley & Sons, Inc.)

the control infants. Mean QTc intervals were 406 ms for the HCG infants and 407 ms for the control subjects. All other ECG findings were normal for age in both groups. At a mean of 26 months after birth, follow-up evaluations detected no visual, hearing, growth, or developmental abnormalities in the infants born to mothers taking HCQ.

Conclusion.—HCQ appears to be safe for use during pregnancy. Unless adverse effects develop during pregnancy and to avoid SLE flares that often occur when HCQ is discontinued, this treatment should probably be continued throughout the gestational period for patients with SLE.

► This study is useful because it suggests that if a patient who really needs to take HCQ becomes pregnant, then that patient should probably continue the medicine since her risk of poor pregnancy outcomes appears no different from control subjects (Table 2).

D. B. Hellmann, MD

Dose Escalation of Parenteral Methotrexate in Active Rheumatoid Arthritis That Has Been Unresponsive to Conventional Doses of Methotrexate: A Randomized, Controlled Trial

Lambert CM, Sandhu S, Lochhead A, et al (Univ of Edinburgh, Scotland)

Arthritis Rheum 50:364-371, 2004 1–17

Background.—Many patients with active RA do not have an optimal response to low-dose (15-20 mg/wk) oral methotrexate (MTX) therapy. Whether switching to parenteral administration or increasing the MTX dose might benefit this subset of patients was examined.

Methods.—The subjects were 64 adults with active RA (defined as a European League Against Rheumatism [EULAR] Disease Activity Score in 28 joints [DAS28] of greater than 3.2). None of the patients had optimal re-

TABLE 3.—Change in Disease Activity Score in 28 Joints and American College of Rheumatology Core Disease Activity Set Measures in the Study Groups by Week 22

Disease Activity Measure	Controls (n = 27)	MTX Escalation (n = 27)
DAS28		
Baseline	5.4 ± 1.1	5.4 ± 0.97
Absolute change	−0.7 ± 1.3	−0.5 ± 1.0
Percentage change	−13	−9
Erythrocyte sedimentation rate, mm/hour		
Baseline	33 ± 19.1	34 ± 23.5
Absolute change	−5.4 ± 14.8	2.2 ± 14.3
Percentage change	−16	6.4
Swollen joint count (range 0-28 joints)		
Baseline	11 ± 6	9 ± 5
Absolute change	−2 ± 5	−1 ± 4
Percentage change	−16	−7
Tender joint count (range 0-28 joints)		
Baseline	9 ± 7	9 ± 7
Absolute change	−3 ± 7	−4 ± 6
Percentage change	−34	−40
Patient's global disease assessment		
Baseline	49 ± 25	54 ± 18
Absolute change	−10 ± 35	−12 ± 27
Percentage change	−20	−22
Physician's global disease assessment		
Baseline	46 ± 20	40 ± 18
Absolute change	−6.6 ± 20	−3.5 ± 24
Percentage change	−14	−9
Pain (VAS scale 0-100)		
Baseline	56 ± 21	55 ± 18
Absolute change	−18 ± 36	−9 ± 14
Percentage change	−32	−16
HAQ (scale 0-3)		
Baseline	1.2 ± 0.65	1.4 ± 0.47
Absolute change	0.14 ± 1.0	−0.05 ± 0.44
Percentage change	12	−4

Note: Values are the mean ± standard deviation, with last observation carried forward for noncompleters. A negative absolute change or percentage change indicates improvement in the response criterion. No significant difference between groups for any variable ($P > .1$). The visual analogue scale for pain ranges from 0 = no pain to 100 = extreme pain. Patient and physician global assessments of disease activity range from 0 = no disease activity to 100 = extreme disease activity. The Health Assessment Questionnaire scale ranges from 0 = no difficulty to 3 = unable to perform activity.

Abbreviations: MTX, Methotrexate; *DAS28*, Disease Activity Score in 28 joints; *VAS*, visual analogue scale; *HAQ*, Health Assessment Questionnaire.

(Courtesy of Lambert CM, Sandhu S, Lochhead A, et al: Dose escalation of parenteral methotrexate in active rheumatoid arthritis that has been unresponsive to conventional doses of methotrexate: A randomized, controlled trial. *Arthritis Rheum* 50:364-371, 2004. Reprinted by permission of John Wiley & Sons, Inc.)

sponses to oral MTX, 15 to 20 mg/wk, for more than 2 weeks, nor to other disease-modifying antirheumatic drugs for more than 4 months. Patients were switched to IM MTX (15 mg/wk) for 6 weeks. Patients whose DAS28 was greater than 3.2 at both weeks 4 and 6 were randomly assigned to either the same 15-mg/wk dose of IM MTX or escalating doses of IM MTX monthly up to 45 mg/wk.

Safety assessments were performed every 2 weeks, and DAS28 scores were assessed every month. Additionally, disease activity parameters (the American College of Rheumatology [ACR] core disease activity set and the Medical Outcome Study Short-Form 12) were evaluated at baseline (week 0) and the end of the study (week 22). The primary outcome was the percentage of patients whose DAS28 was greater than 3.2. Secondary outcomes were the percentage of patients in whom the DAS28 improved by more than 1.2, the percentage of patients who achieved a 20% improvement in the ACR core disease activity (ACR20) score, and the percentage of patients with a good, moderate, or no response (according to the EULAR response criteria).

Results.—The mean DAS28 was 5.6 at week 0 but improved to 0.42 after 6 weeks of IM MTX. Ten patients were excluded (4 for a DAS28 less than 3.2, 6 declined to participate), leaving 54 patients to enter the randomization phase at 6 weeks. The median dose of IM MTX was 45 mg/wk, and 21 of the 27 patients in the dose-escalation group (78%) received the maximum dose. Only 1 patient each in the stable 15-mg/wk and the dose-escalation groups (3.7%) achieved a DAS28 of greater than 3.2. Five patients in each group (18.4%) had an improvement of more than 1.2 in the DAS28.

Furthermore, while 1 patient in each group (3.7%) achieved an ACR20 response, none had a good EULAR response. Physical or mental health components of the Medical Outcome Study Short-Form 12 changes in DAS28 scores, and changes in individual components of the ACR core disease activity set did not differ significantly between the 2 groups (Table 3). One patient in each group discontinued therapy due to serious adverse events.

Conclusion.—Disease control improved in 4 of 64 patients (6.2%) with refractory RA who switched from oral to IM therapy with MTX, 15 mg/wk. However, increasing the dose up to 45 mg/wk did not improve disease control appreciably. Thus, for most patients with RA who do not respond to switching from oral to IM MTX, escalating the dose above 45 mg/wk is not likely to provide additional benefit, and alternative strategies should be sought.

► I frequently have patients with RA who have suboptimal responses to oral MTX. For such patients, should I change to IM MTX or increase beyond the arbitrary maximal dose of 20 to 25 mg/wk? This study addresses those questions and shows that a few patients will benefit from switching from oral to IM MTX. Surprisingly, increasing the MTX dose to 45 mg/wk rarely benefits patients (Table 3). This study suggests that if MTX does not work at the standard doses, it's usually time to move on or add another agent.

D. B. Hellmann, MD

Lymphoma in Rheumatoid Arthritis: The Effect of Methotrexate and Anti–Tumor Necrosis Factor Therapy in 18,572 Patients

Wolfe F, Michaud K (Univ of Kansas, Wichita; Natl Data Bank for Rheumatic Diseases, Wichita, Kan)

Arthritis Rheum 50:1740-1751, 2004 1–18

Introduction.—Most studies indicate that the risk of lymphoma is increased in patients with RA. This increased risk has been attributed to RA severity, yet there is concern that medications may contribute to the devel-

TABLE 4.—SIR and Incidence Rate for Lymphoma in RA Patients According to Exposure Group*

Treatment Group	No. of Lymphomas		SIR	95% CI	No. of Patients at Risk	Time at Risk	Incidence Rate
	Actual	Expected					
All patients/treatments	29	15.5	1.9	1.3-2.7	18,572	29,314	98.9
All biologics	14	4.9	2.9	1.7-4.9	8,614	10,012	139.8
Infliximab or infliximab + etanercept	9	3.4	2.6	1.4-4.5	6,465	6,538	137.7
Etanercept or etanercept + infliximab	8	2.1	3.8	1.9-7.5	3,381	5,099	156.9
Infliximab	6	2.7	2.2	1.0-4.9	5,233	4,913	122.1
Etanercept	5	1.4	3.5	1.5-8.4	2,149	3,474	143.9
Infliximab + etanercept	3	0.7	4.3	1.4-13.2	1,232	1,624	184.7
Anakinra	0	0.2	0.0	—	58	33	0
Leflunomide only	0	0.5	0	—	758	1,024	0.0
Leflunomide only (switched)	0	0.9	0	—	1,184	1,850	0.0
No MTX/no biologics	5	3.9	1.3	0.5-3.1	3,504	7,122	70.2
No MTX/no biologics (switched)	5	4.8	1.0	0.4-2.5	4,399	8,938	55.9
MTX only	10	6.8	1.5	0.8-2.7	6,396	12,147	82.3
MTX only (switched)	10	5.8	1.7	0.9-3.2	5,501	10,331	96.8

*Time at risk is expressed in years. Incidence rates are expressed per 100,000 patient-years of exposure. For leflunomide, *switched* means patients in the leflunomide-only group who did not receive leflunomide during NDB follow-up were counted as being in the no methotrexate (MTX)/no biologics group. For MTX, *switched* means patients in the MTX-only group who did not receive MTX during NDB follow-up were counted as being in the no MTX/no biologics group.

(Courtesy of Wolfe F, Michaud K: Lymphoma in rheumatoid arthritis: The effect of methotrexate and anti-tumor necrosis factor therapy in 18,572 patients. *Arthritis Rheum* 50:1740-1751, 2004. Reprinted by permission of John Wiley & Sons, Inc.)

opment of lymphoproliferative cancer by altering immune function. The rate of and standardized incidence ratio (SIR) for lymphoma in patients with RA and potential predictors of lymphoma in RA was examined.

Methods.—The National Data Bank for Rheumatic Diseases (NDB) is an open cohort with continuous enrollment. Included in the study were 18,572 patients with RA and without previous lymphoma. All had completed biannual questionnaires during consecutive 6-month assessment periods from January 1999 until June 2002. A validation process was initiated when a patient reported a lymphoma or a description suggestive of lymphoma. Patients were classified into 4 treatment groups: infliximab, etanercept, methotrexate (MTX)/no biologic, and no MTX/no biologic. The expected number of lymphoma cases and the SIRs were calculated on the basis of age- and sex-matched data from the National Cancer Institute Surveillance, Epidemiology, and End Results resource.

Results.—Eighty-eight lymphomas were identified, 29 of which occurred after NDB enrollment and during the period of intensive follow-up. Eight of these patients received infliximab (3 also received etanercept), 8 received etanercept (3 also received infliximab), 10 received MTX/no biologic, and 5 received no MTX/no biologic. The overall SIR for lymphoma was 1.9. For specific therapies, SIRs were 2.9 for biologic use, 2.6 for infliximab use (with or without etanercept), 3.8 for etanercept (with or without infliximab), 1.7 for MTX, and 1.0 for no MTX/no biologic (Table 4). Development of lymphoma was associated with increasing age, male sex, and level of education.

Discussion.—Lymphoma is increased in RA compared with the general population. Differences in lymphoma risk are slight when various treatments are compared, but the SIR is greatest for antitumor necrosis factor therapies. No causal relationship between RA treatment and the development of lymphoma could be established, however.

► The increased risk of lymphoma in RA has been well known. What grabbed my attention in this article are the data suggesting an association of lymphoma and biologic therapies (Table 4). Whereas methotrexate alone was not associated with an increased risk of lymphoma, all biologic therapies were associated with a nearly 3-fold increased risk (Table 4). Clearly more studies are needed to determine whether a causal role exists. But data such as these help me believe that biologic agents should not replace methotrexate as the number 1 second-line treatment for RA. The long-term effects of biologic therapies are not yet defined.

D. B. Hellmann, MD

Impact of Initial Aggressive Drug Treatment With a Combination of Disease-Modifying Antirheumatic Drugs on the Development of Work Disability in Early Rheumatoid Arthritis: A Five-Year Randomized Followup Trial

Puolakka K, for the FIN-RACo Trial Group (Lappeenranta Central Hosp, Finland; et al)

Arthritis Rheum 50:55-62, 2004 1–19

Background.—Some studies suggest that early use of a disease-modifying antirheumatic drug (DMARD) protects against work disability in patients with RA. Whether a combination of DMARDs would be more effective than a single DMARD in maintaining the patient's ability to work was investigated.

Methods.—The subjects were 162 patients with RA of less than 2 years' duration who were still working or available for work at baseline. Patients were randomly assigned to receive either DMARD combination therapy (sulfasalazine, methotrexate, and hydroxychloroquine) plus prednisolone (80 patients) or DMARD monotherapy with or without prednisolone (82 patients) for 2 years.

After 2 years, the treatment strategy became unrestricted, and about two thirds of the patients randomly assigned to DMARD monotherapy switched to DMARD combination therapy. Patients were followed up for 5 years to determine sick leave and retirement. The primary end point was the cumulative duration of all sick leaves and RA-related disability pensions for each patient, divided by the period during follow-up when the patient was not retired because of age or other co-morbidity.

Results.—The cumulative duration of work disability per patient-year was significantly lower in the patients randomly allotted to early DMARD combination therapy (median, 12.4 days per patient-year) than in those randomly assigned to early DMARD monotherapy (median, 32.2 days per patient-year). Most of this difference was due to significantly fewer sick leaves (ie, work disability periods of 300 days or less) for patients receiving early DMARD combination therapy (median, 11.7 vs 30.0 days per patient-year). The proportion of patients with an RA-related disability pension was similar in the combination and monotherapy groups (17 of 80 patients, or 21%, vs 28 of 82 patients, or 34%).

Conclusion.—For patients with early RA, early aggressive treatment with DMARD combination therapy improves the patient's ability to work and is associated with fewer days off work due to disability over a 5-year follow-up, compared with early DMARD monotherapy.

▶ This study, together with the results of the etanercept trial (Abstract 1–20) reinforces the idea that aggressive treatment of RA not only saves bones but also saves jobs.

D. B. Hellmann, MD

Association Between Etanercept Use and Employment Outcomes Among Patients With Rheumatoid Arthritis

Yelin E, Trupin L, Katz P, et al (Univ of California, San Francisco; Amgen Inc, Thousand Oaks, Calif)

Arthritis Rheum 48:3046-3054, 2003 1–20

Background.—Between one fourth and one half of patients with RA stop working within 10 years of being diagnosed, and from 50% to 90% stop working before age 65 years, or retirement age. Thus, the indirect costs associated with lost work or lost functionality in nonwork activities may exceed the direct costs of RA linked to medical care expenditures. Whether medical therapy for RA can have a notable impact on this situation has rarely been addressed. An investigation was carried out to see whether etanercept therapy shows any relationship to employment outcomes in patients with RA.

Methods.—The employment status of 497 RA patients at diagnosis and in 1999, when they reported their employment status, was determined via structured telephone interviews. In 1999, they were aged 18 to 64 years. Two hundred thirty-eight had been in clinical trials of etanercept and were taking that medication. Two hundred fifty-nine had not taken etanercept. Regression techniques were used to determine whether employment outcomes in 1999 among the 379 patients employed when they were diagnosed with RA changed with etanercept use. Adjustments were also made for demographic data, RA status, overall health status, and the type of job held when the diagnosis was made.

Results.—Characteristics of the etanercept group in comparison to the control subjects included fewer in fair or poor health, significantly more comorbid conditions, slightly shorter disease duration, and fewer major anatomical sites with painful joints. Those using etanercept reported improved RA compared with the previous year more often than did control subjects. Control subjects were less likely to have an hour or more of daily morning stiffness and had a better mean self-reported fatigue score.

At the time of diagnosis, the number of hours worked each week, weeks of work per year, and hours of work per year did not differ between the employed patients in the etanercept group and those in the control group. More of the etanercept patients reported being employed both at diagnosis and at the current time. Fewer of these patients were not currently employed but had been employed at diagnosis compared with controls. Seventy-one percent of the etanercept patients reported being employed as compared with only 55% of control subjects (Table 3).

Older patients, those with less than a high school education, those with longer durations of disease, and those who were poorer had lower employment rates. Higher rates were seen among patients with a greater number of painful joints. Patients who were taking etanercept, whether or not they participated in etanercept trials, had an employment rate 10 percentage points higher than those not taking etanercept. Those who were in etanercept trials had a current employment rate 16 percentage points higher than those not in

TABLE 3.—Probability of Employment at Latest Interview Among Patients With RA, Aged 18 to 64 Years, Who Were Employed at the Time of Diagnosis, by Study Group, With and Without Adjustment for Demographic and Health Characteristics and Occupation and Industry of Respondent at the Time of Diagnosis

Independent Variables	RAPANEL (n = 194)	RAPOLO (n = 185)	Difference (95% CI)
Study group	0.55	0.71	−0.16 (−0.26, −0.07)*
Study group and demographics	0.55	0.72	−0.17 (−0.26, −0.08)*
Study group, demographics, overall health status	0.52	0.74	−0.22 (−0.32, −0.12)*
Study group, demographics, overall health status, duration of RA	0.54	0.72	−0.18 (−0.29, −0.09)*
Study group, demographics, overall health status, duration of RA, occupation and industry	0.53	0.72	−0.19 (−0.29, −0.09)*
Study group, demographics, overall health status, duration of RA, RA status	0.53	0.73	−0.20 (−0.31, −0.08)*
Study group, demographics, overall health status, duration of RA, RA status, occupation and industry	0.53	0.73	−0.20 (−0.32, −0.09)*

*$P < .05$.

Abbreviations: RAPANEL, RA panel study; *RAPOLO*, RA Pharmacoeconomic and Outcomes Longitudinal Observational Study; *CI*, confidence interval.

(Courtesy of Yelin E, Trupin L, Katz P, et al: Association between etanercept use and employment outcomes among patients with rheumatoid arthritis. *Arthritis Rheum* 48:3046-3054, 2003. Reprinted by permission of John Wiley & Sons, Inc.)

the trials. Making full adjustments for various factors yielded a difference of 20%. Those taking etanercept worked 7.4 more hours per week (adjusted) than those not taking it.

Conclusion.—Patients who were in the etanercept clinical trials had higher employment rates in 1999 and worked more hours per year than those who had not been in an etanercept trial. Randomized clinical trials of sufficient duration are advised to evaluate the employment effects of RA medications more definitively.

► This study is important because it is the only publication (beyond an abstract) to suggest that treatment of RA with a biological agent increases the chance that a patient will continue to be able to work. RA has a devastating impact on employment. As the authors note, as many as one half of patients stop working within 10 years of disease onset. In that context, it is striking that employment of participants in an etanercept trial was 20% higher that nonparticipants who appear to have had similar severity of disease (Table 3). Controlled trials will need to confirm these results, but it appears that etanercept "really works"!

D. B. Hellmann, MD

Once-Weekly Administration of 50 mg Etanercerpt in Patients With Active Rheumatoid Arthritis: Results of a Multicenter, Randomized, Double-Blind, Placebo-Controlled Trial

Keystone EC, Schiff MH, Kremer JM, et al (Mt Sinai Hosp, Toronto; Denver Arthritis Clinic, Colo; Ctr for Rhematology, Albany, NY; et al)

Arthritis Rheum 50:353-363, 2004 1–21

Background.—Etanercept is approved in the United States for the treatment of moderate to severe active RA. In most studies, etanercept has been administered as a twice-weekly, 25-mg subcutaneous injection. Whether once-weekly, 50-mg etanercept would be as effective and safe as the standard twice-weekly 25-mg dosing was examined.

Methods.—The subjects were 420 adults with active RA who had not used disease-modifying antirheumatic drugs (other than methotrexate) for 28 days or more. During a 16-week study, 214 patients received once-weekly 50-mg etanercept; 153 patients received twice-weekly 25-mg etanercept; and 53 patients received placebo for 8 weeks, then received twice-weekly 25-mg etanercept for 8 weeks. The primary outcome was the proportion of patients achieving a 20% improvement in American College of Rheumatology criteria (ACR20) by week 8. Safety was evaluated at 8 and 16 weeks. Additionally, 44 patients provided serum samples for pharmacokinetic analyses.

Results.—Disease activity at baseline was similar in the 3 groups (Table 3). In all, 46 patients (87%) in the placebo group, 195 patients (91%) in the once-daily 50-mg etanercept group, and 140 patients (92%) in the twice-daily, 25-mg etanercept group completed therapy. By week 8, significantly more patients in the once-weekly group and the twice-weekly group had achieved an ACR20 than did patients in the placebo group (50%, 49% , and

TABLE 3.—Individual Measures of Disease Activity at Baseline

Parameter	Placebo (n = 53)	Etanercept 50 mg qw (n = 214)	Etanercept 25 mg biw (n = 153)
Tender joint count (range 0-71)	24.6 (19.5)	26.0 (22.0)	29.2 (28.0)
Swollen joint count (range 0-68)	19.2 (18.0)	19.2 (16.0)	19.2 (17.0)
Physician global assessment (scale 0 [best]–10 [worst])	5.9 (6.0)	6.3 (6.0)	6.3 (6.0)
Patient global assessment (scale 0 [best]–10 [worst])	6.2 (7.0)	6.0 (6.0)	6.1 (6.0)
Pain assessment (scale 0 [best]–10 [worst])	5.3 (4.9)	5.3 (5.4)	5.7 (5.9)
HAQ Disability Index (scale 0 [best]–3 [worst])	1.4 (1.4)	1.4 (1.4)	1.4 (1.5)
CRP, mg/dl*	1.4 (0.5)	1.7 (0.5)	1.9 (0.7)
Morning stiffness, minutes/day	245.8 (120)	237.8 (90)	252.9 (120)

Note: Values are the mean (median).

*Normal range of C-reactive protein (*CRP*) is 0-0.79 mg/dL.

Abbreviations: qw, Once weekly; *biw*, twice weekly; *HAQ*, Health Assessment Questionnaire.

19%, respectively). Similarly, significantly more patients in the active drug groups had achieved an ACR50 response by week 8 (18% in both active drug groups vs 6% in the placebo group). The safety profile of the 2 active drug groups was also similar, except that twice-weekly 25-mg etanercept caused more nausea than once-weekly 50-mg dosing (12% vs 6%). Pharmacokinetic characteristics at steady-state were similar in the 2 etanercept groups.

Conclusion.—The efficacy, safety, and pharmacokinetics of once-weekly 50-mg etanercept are similar to those of twice-weekly 25-mg etanercept, and thus clinical outcomes with these 2 regimens would be expected to be similar also.

▶ Etanercept 50 mg once weekly is as effective and safe as 25 mg twice weekly (Table 3).

D. B. Hellmann, MD

Radiographic, Clinical, and Functional Outcomes of Treatment With Adalimumab (a Human Anti-Tumor Necrosis Factor Monoclonal Antibody) in Patients With Active Rheumatoid Arthritis Receiving Concomitant Methotrexate Therapy: A Randomized, Placebo-Controlled, 52-Week Trial

Keystone EC, Kavanaugh AF, Sharp JT, et al (Univ of Toronto; Univ of California, San Diego; Univ of Washington, Seattle; et al)

Arthritis Rheum 50:1400-1411, 2004 1–22

Background.—Tumor necrosis factor, an important proinflammatory cytokine, mediates inflammatory synovitis and articular matrix degradation in RA. Adalimumab is a human anti-tumor necrosis factor monoclonal antibody. The ability of adalimumab to inhibit the progression of structural joint damage, decrease signs and symptoms, and improve physical functioning in patients with active RA receiving concomitant methotrexate (MTX) treatment was determined.

Methods.—Six hundred nineteen patients with active RA were enrolled in the multicenter, 52-week, double-blind, placebo-controlled study. All had previously had an inadequate response to MTX. By random assignment, they received adalimumab, 40 mg, subcutaneously every other week; adalimumab, 20 mg, subcutaneously every week; or placebo plus MTX.

Findings.—Patients in the 2 adalimumab groups had significantly less radiographic progression at 52 weeks than patients in the placebo group. Significant changes in the components of the total Sharp score were also observed. At 24 weeks, American College of Rheumatology core criteria (ACR20) responses were obtained in 63% of those receiving adalimumab 40 mg every other week and in 61% of those receiving adalimumab 20 mg weekly, compared with 30% of those receiving placebo. At 52 weeks, ACR20 responses were achieved in 59%, 55%, and 24%, respectively (Fig 3). Physical function at week 52 was significantly improved in the active

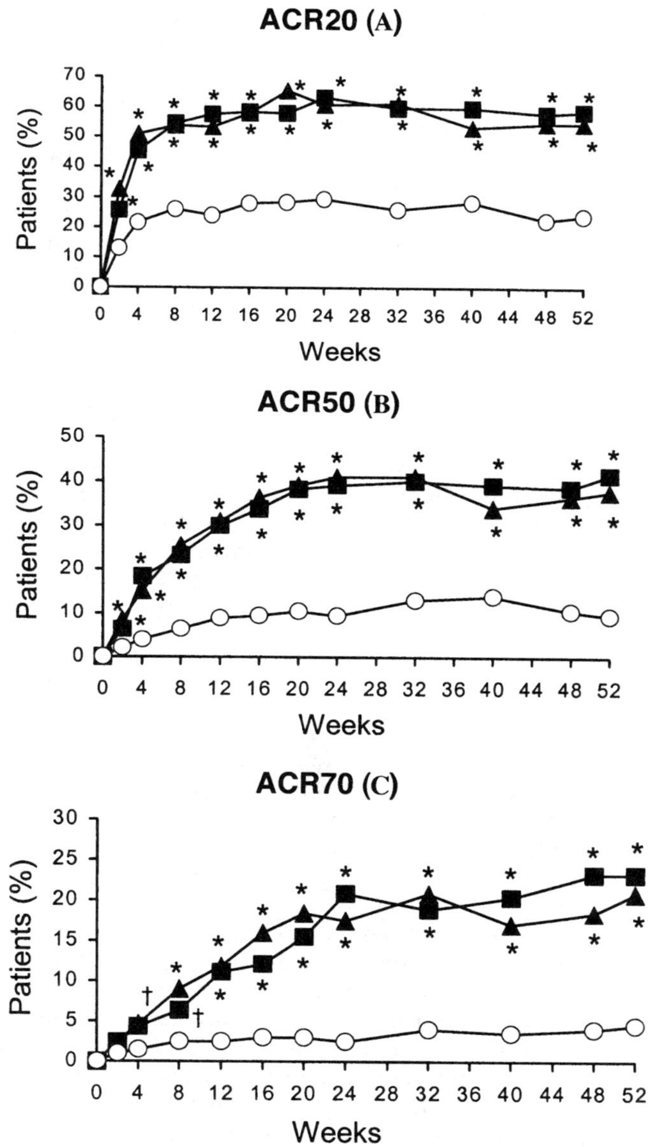

FIGURE 3.—Distribution of patients who showed improvement in the American College of Rheumatology (ACR) criteria of at least 20%, 50%, and 70% (**A**, **B**, and **C**, respectively) (using nonresponders imputation), among the patients receiving adalimumab 40 mg every other week plus methotrexate (MTX) (■), adalimemab 20 mg weekly plus MTX (▲), and placebo plus MTX (○). *$P \leq .001$, and †$P \leq .01$ vs plecabo (by Pearson's chi-square test). (Courtesy of Keystone EC, Kavanaugh AF, Sharp JT, et al: Radiographic, clinical, and functional outcomes of treatment with adalimumab [a human anti-tumor necrosis factor monoclonal antibody] in patients with active rheumatoid arthritis receiving concomitant methotrexate therapy: A randomized, placebo-controlled, 52-week trial. *Arthritis Rheum* 50:1400-1411, 2004. Reprinted by permission of John Wiley & Sons, Inc.)

treatment groups versus the placebo group. Three fourths of the patients completed the 52 weeks of treatment. In general, adalimumab was well tolerated. Twenty-two percent of patients discontinued adalimumab, and 30% discontinued placebo. A greater proportion of patients receiving adalimumab had serious infections than those receiving placebo.

Conclusions.—Adalimumab appears to be more effective than placebo at inhibiting the progression of structural joint damage in patients with active RA and an inadequate response to MTX. Adalimumab also reduces signs and symptoms and improves physical function in this patient population.

▶ On the basis of this study, I will add adalimumab to the list of agents that help patients who have partial responses to methotrexate (Fig 3). That expanding list of "methotrexate-enhancers" now includes infliximab, etanercept, anakinra, cyclosporine, sulfasalazine, hydroxychloroquine, and leflunomide.

D. B. Hellmann, MD

Sustained Improvement Over Two Years in Physical Function, Structural Damage, and Signs and Symptoms Among Patients With Rheumatoid Arthritis Treated With Infliximab and Methotrexate

Maini RN, for the Anti-Tumor Necrosis Factor Trial in Rheumatoid Arthritis With Concomitant Therapy Study Group (Kennedy Inst of Rheumatology, Hammersmith, London; et al)

Arthritis Rheum 50:1051-1065, 2004 1–23

Background.—Disease-modifying antirheumatic drugs (DMARDs), including weekly methotrexate (MTX), is currently the gold standard for treating RA. However, in a large proportion of patients, this approach fails to control disease activity, prevent structural damage, or maintain quality of life. The safety and efficacy of repeated administration of infliximab plus MTX for 2 years in patients with RA previously experiencing an incomplete response to MTX were reported.

Methods.—Four hundred twenty-eight patients were assigned randomly to MTX plus placebo or infliximab, 3 or 10 mg/kg, plus MTX for 54 weeks, with an additional year of follow-up. Subsequently, the protocol was amended to allow for continued treatment during year 2. Of the 259 patients entering year 2 of treatment, 216 continued to receive infliximab plus MTX for 102 weeks. Ninety-four of these patients had a greater than 8-week gap in treatment before continuing. Infusions were given in weeks 0, 2, and 6, followed by treatment every 4 or 8 weeks at the 3 or 10 mg/kg dose for a total of 102 weeks. Efficacy measures were the Health Assessment Questionnaire (HAQ), Short Form 36 health survey (SF-36), total radiographic scores, and American College of Rheumatology 20% improvement criteria (ACR20).

Findings.—Compared with the MTX-only group, the infliximab plus MTX groups had significantly greater improvement in HAQ and SF-36 physical component summary scores. Patients receiving infliximab plus MTX regimens also had stability in SF-36 mental component summary

TABLE 4.—Change from Baseline to Week 102 in Radiographic Parameters Among Patients Treated With MTX Only Compared With Those Treated With the Infliximab Plus MTX Regimens

Radiographic Scores	MTX + Placebo	Infliximab 3 mg/kg + MTX q8 Weeks	Infliximab 3 mg/kg + MTX q4 Weeks	Infliximab 10 mg/kg + MTX q8 Weeks	Infliximab 10 mg/kg + MTX q4 Weeks
Total radiographic score*					
No. of patients evaluated	50	58	66	69	66
Mean ± SD change	12.59 ± 20.05	1.02 ± 7.13	1.03 ± 11.65	1.14 ± 4.92	−0.42 ± 6.10
Median change	4.25	0.43	0.50	1.00	0.00
Interquartile range	0.50, 17.50	−1.50, 3.67	−2.95, 3.05	−0.50, 3.73	−3.08, 1.93
P	Referent	<0.001	<0.001	<0.001	<0.001
Erosion score					
No. of patients evaluated	51	59	70	71	68
Mean ± SD change	6.65 ± 11.20	0.25 ± 4.38	0.50 ± 9.05	0.43 ± 2.61	−0.57 ± 3.85
Median change	2.00	0.00	0.13	0.50	−0.04
Interquartile range	0.50, 10.63	−1.77, 1.97	−1.50, 2.00	−1.00, 1.55	−1.67, 0.65
P	Referent	<0.001	<0.001	<0.001	<0.001
Joint space narrowing score					
No. of patients evaluated	50	58	66	69	66
Mean ± SD change	5.91 ± 10.59	0.77 ± 3.68	0.10 ± 4.81	0.63 ± 3.25	0.17 ± 3.60
Median change	2.00	0.50	0.00	0.00	0.00
Interquartile range	0.00, 8.50	−0.50, 2.50	−2.00, 1.50	−0.50, 2.00	−1.50, 1.00
P	Referent	0.002	<0.001	<0.001	<0.001

*Total radiographic score of the hands and feet is based on the van der Heijde-modified Sharp score. At baseline, the median radiographic scores were 61.8 (MTX plus placebo), 55.5 (infliximab 3 mg/kg plus MTX q8 weeks), 45.5 (infliximab 3 mg/kg plus MTX q4 weeks), 49.5 (infliximab 10 mg/kg plus MTX 8.8 weeks), and 48.8 (infliximab 10 mg/kg plus MTX q4 weeks).

Abbreviations: q4 weeks, Administered every 4 weeks after initial infusion; *q8 weeks*, administered every 8 weeks after initial infusions, with placebo administered in the 4-week intervals.

(Courtesy of Maini RN, for the Anti-Tumor Necrosis Factor Trial in Rheumatoid Arthritis With Concomitant Therapy Study Group: Sustained improvement over two years in physical function, structural damage, and signs and symptoms among patients with rheumatoid arthritis treated with infliximab and methotrexate. *Arthritis Rheum* 50:1051-1065, 2004. Reprinted by permission of John Wiley & Sons, Inc.)

TABLE 5.—Comparison of Clinical Responses Among Patients Treated With MTX Only and Infliximab Plus MTX Regimens at Week 102*

Response	MTX + Placebo	Infliximab 3 mg/kg + MTX q8 Weeks	Infliximab 3 mg/kg + MTX q4 Weeks	Infliximab 10 mg/kg + MTX q8 Weeks	Infliximab 10 mg/kg + MTX q4 Weeks
ACR criteria*					
ACR20					
% of responders	16	42	40	48	40
P	Referent	<0.001	<0.001	<0.001	<0.001
ACR50					
% of responders	6	21	30	36	20
P	Referent	0.003	<0.001	<0.001	0.006
ACR70					
% of responders	1	10	21	20	10
P	Referent	0.008	<0.001	<0.001	0.011
Median % decrease in no. of swollen joints	20.0	52.5	65.1	69.1	72.2
P	Referent	<0.001	<0.001	<0.001	<0.001
Median % decrease in no. of tender joints	29.2	63.8	68.8	75.3	63.2
P	Referent	0.005	<0.001	<0.001	<0.001
Median % decrease in serum C-reactive protein	8.4	45.4	58.7	55.7	73.3
P	Referent	0.002	<0.001	0.002	<0.001

*ACR20 indicates a decrease of at least 20% in the number of tender joints and a decrease of at least 20% in the number of swollen joints, along with a 20% improvement in 3 of the following: the patient's global assessment of disease status, the patient's assessment of pain, and the physician's global assessment of disease status, all of which were assessed with the use of visual analog scales (range 0-10 cm, with higher scores indicating poorer status or more severe pain), the Health Assessment Questionnaire estimate of disability, and the erythrocyte sedimentation rate or C-reactive protein concentration. The percentages of patients with an improvement of 50% (ACR50) and 70% (ACR70) according to the American College of Rheumatology (ACR) criteria were assessed in a similar manner.

Abbreviations: q4 weeks, Administered every 4 weeks after initial infusion; *q8 weeks*, administered every 8 weeks after initial infusions, with placebo administered in the 4-week intervals.

(Courtesy of Maini RN, for the Anti-Tumor Necrosis Factor Trial in Rheumatoid Arthritis With Concomitant Therapy Study Group: Sustained improvement over two years in physical function, structural damage, and signs and symptoms among patients with rheumatoid arthritis treated with infliximab and methotrexate. *Arthritis Rheum* 50:1051-1065, 2004. Reprinted by permission of John Wiley & Sons, Inc.)

scores. The total radiographic score showed median changes of 4.25 from baseline to week 102 in patients receiving the MTX-only regimen and 0.50 for those receiving infliximab plus MTX regimen (Table 4). The percentage of patients obtaining an ACR20 response at week 102 ranged from 40% to 48% in the infliximab plus MTX group, compared with 16% in the MTX-only group (Table 5).

Conclusions.—During 102 weeks of treatment, infliximab plus MTX provided significant, clinically relevant improvement in physical function and quality of life in patients with RA and a previous incomplete response to MTX alone. These outcomes were accompanied by inhibition of progressive joint damage and sustained improvement in the signs and symptoms of RA.

▶ This treatment trial addresses the important issue of whether the benefits of infliximab and MTX for RA extend beyond 1 year. Happily, the answer from this 2-year study is "yes." Both the clinical response and the radiographic benefit were sustained for 2 years (Tables 4 and 5).

D. B. Hellmann, MD

Anti-Tumor Necrosis Factor-α Therapy-Induced Vasculitis: Case Series
Jarrett SJ, Cunnane G, Conaghan PG, et al (Univ of Leeds, England)
J Rheumatol 30:2287-2291, 2003 1–24

Introduction.—Patients with RA who fail to respond well to conventional disease modifying drugs may be treated with tumor necrosis factor α (TNF-α) blockade. A variety of complications have been reported, however, after treatment with TNF-blocking agents. Vasculitis and vasculitic rashes developed in the 8 patients.

> *Case Report.*—Man, 55, had seropositive, erosive RA of 13 years' duration and was being treated with 10 to 15 mg/day of oral prednisone. The patient received 2 infusions of leflunomide and infliximab before lesions developed on his hands and legs (Fig 2). Infliximab was withdrawn and the lesions were biopsied, revealing a leukocytoclastic vasculitis. Treatment with oral prednisone led to resolution of the rash, but vasculitis recurred at the same site when etanercept therapy was started.

Discussion.—Seven of the patients in this series were initially treated with infliximab and 1 with etanercept. The vasculitis and/or vasculitic rash reappeared in 2 patients switched from infliximab to etanercept, suggesting a class effect of TNF blockade. Two patients showed an increase in autoantibodies while receiving TNF-blocking agents. Complications that occur in patients with RA may be attributed to ongoing disease activity evolution into other disease states, drug-induced autoimmunity, or drug reaction. Because of mounting evidence that vasculitis is a Th2 lymphocyte-mediated disease, patients with preexisting autoantibodies may be reflecting the pre-

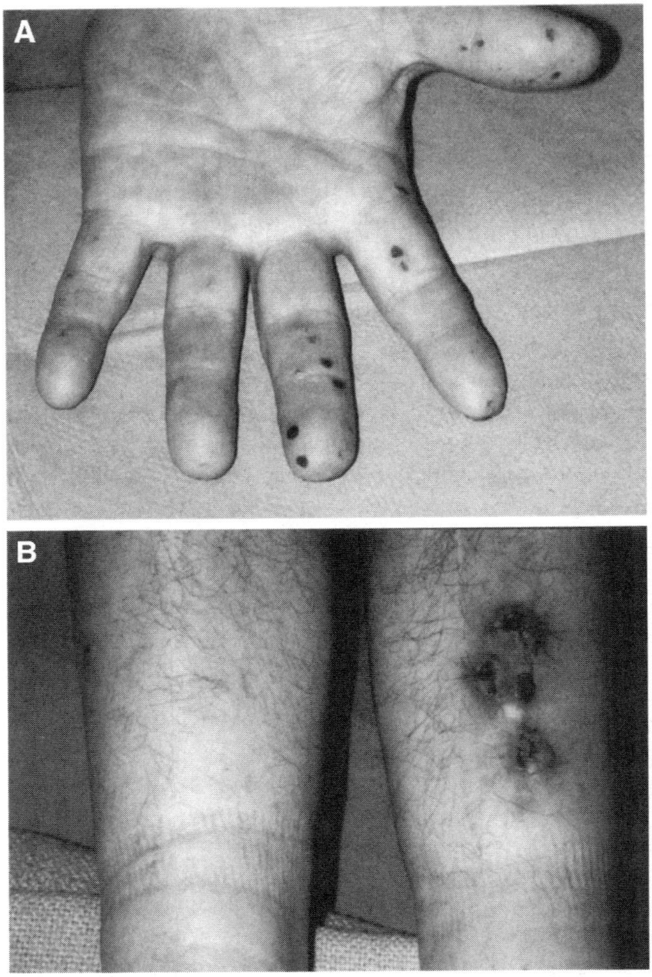

FIGURE 2.—Patient 4. Biopsy proven vasculitic rash (A) on hands and (B) on legs. (Courtesy of Jarrett SJ, Cunnane G, Conaghan PG, et al: Anti-tumor necrosis factor-α therapy-induced vasculitis: Case series. *J Rheumatol* 30:2287-2291, 2003.)

dominance of the Th2 response. Increased expression of this phenotype, with consequent vasculitis, may be promoted in such patients by the addition of anti-TNF therapy.

► I am not sure I buy the title of this article. That is, I cannot be sure anti-TNF therapy really caused vasculitis (Fig 2) or was merely associated with it. After all, it is the sicker patients with RA who are more likely to have vasculitis develop and to receive anti-TNF therapy.

D. B. Hellmann, MD

Tuberculosis Infection in Patients With Rheumatoid Arthritis and the Effect of Infliximab Therapy

Wolfe F, Michaud K, Anderson J, et al (Univ of Kansas, Wichita; Natl Data Bank for Rheumatic Diseases, Wichita, Kan)

Arthritis Rheum 50:372-379, 2004 1–25

Background.—Several case studies suggest an increased incidence of tuberculosis (TB) in patients with RA. In particular, the rate of TB seems high in patients with RA who use infliximab. Two nationwide surveys were undertaken to determine the incidence of TB in patients with RA, both before and after the widespread use of infliximab.

Methods.—Patients were participants in the National Data Bank for Rheumatic Diseases. The first study involved 10,782 patients (77% women; mean age, 59.8 years) evaluated from July 1998 through December 1999, before infliximab became widely available in 2000. The second study involved 6460 patients (73.5% women; mean age, 61.4 years) with RA who were treated with infliximab from January 2000 through June 2002. In both studies, patients completed questionnaires regarding their history of tuberculin skin testing and any diagnosis of TB. Patients with positive responses received further follow-up in the form of another survey, medical record reviews, and physician reports.

Results.—In study 1, 7412 patients (68.7%) had received a tuberculin skin test, and 681 patients (9.2%) had tested positive for TB. Of these, 75 patients had had active TB during their lifetime (lifetime rate, 696 cases per 100,000 persons). In the majority of these cases (76.8%), TB had occurred before the onset of RA. During 16,173 patient-years of follow-up, only 1 patient had been diagnosed with TB, for an incidence rate of 6.2 cases per 100,000 persons. Multivariate analyses revealed that the only significant independent predictor of lifetime TB was being nonwhite (odds ratio, 2.26).

In study 2, 4 cases of TB occurred during the observation period, for an incidence rate of 52.5 cases per 100,000 patient-years, or 61.9 cases per 100,000 patients. All 4 cases occurred in older women (65-78 years of age), and in 3 cases TB developed 1 to 7 months after the patients began infliximab therapy (after 12 months of infliximab in the fourth patient). Three of these 4 patients had previously had a positive skin test for TB, but none had received TB prophylaxis. The status of the fourth patient before developing TB is unknown, but none of these 4 patients had had a TB skin test in 2001 or 2002, before the symptoms of TB developed. Furthermore, 3 of these 4 cases of TB were extrapulmonary.

Conclusion.—The incidence rate of TB among patients with RA not receiving infliximab (6.2 cases per 100,000 patients) is similar to rates in the general United States population (6.4 cases per 100,000 persons in 1999; 5.8 cases per 100,000 persons in 2000). For patients with RA taking infliximab, however, the incidence rate jumps 10-fold, to 61.9 cases per 100,000 patients. TB typically developed within a few months of the initiation of infliximab therapy. This is consistent with results of another study reporting a median interval of 12 weeks from the start of infliximab therapy to the development of TB. None of the 4 patients in whom TB developed in study 2 had been completely screened for TB, and none were receiving TB prophylaxis. Thus, it is crucial to follow the recommendations of infliximab's manufacturer to screen patients for TB before beginning infliximab therapy.

▶ This instructive study shows that infliximab increases the risk of TB about 10-fold, to 52.5 cases per 100,000 patient years. This means that every year about 1 out of every 2000 RA patients on infliximab will develop TB. These results emphasize the need for screening for TB before starting infliximab therapy.

D. B. Hellmann, MD

Onset of Multiple Sclerosis Associated With Anti-TNF Therapy

Sicotte NL, Voskuhl RR (Univ of California, Los Angeles)
Neurology 57:1885-1888, 2001 1–26

Background.—The proinflammatory cytokine tumor necrosis factor (TNF)is involved in lymphocyte signaling and has an important role in cell-mediated immunity. TNF is thought to be an important mediator in several autoimmune diseases, including RA, ulcerative colitis, and multiple sclerosis (MS). Anti-TNF therapy was initially considered for the treatment of MS on the basis of studies of experimental autoimmune encephalomyelitis (EAE) and from data in human studies. High levels of TNF-α have been found in MS plaques and in CSF in humans. However, despite these findings, anti-TNF treatments for MS may worsen disease. Etanercept (Enbrel) is a fusion protein that consists of the extracellular portion of the human TNF receptor linked to the Fc portion of the human IgG. Etanercept has been widely used in the treatment of refractory RA, but there have been observations of worsening of established MS activity in some persons treated with etanercept, and a drug warning was issued by the manufacturer in 2000. A case of a patient with new-onset MS that coincided with the initiation of etanercept treatment for juvenile rheumatoid arthritis is reported.

Case Report.—Woman, 21, with juvenile RA was seen with a 1-week history of pain and decreased vision in her right eye. She had no previous visual symptoms or other neurologic dysfunction and had no recent illness or travel history. The patient had been diagnosed with juvenile RA at 8 years old. Administration of oral and IM gold, methotrexate, and sulfasalazine were only partially effective. Her arthritis was significantly improved after 9 months of treatment with etanercept; the patient was also taking celecoxib and lansoprazole. The family history was significant for RA, but there was no family history of MS. An MRI evaluation of the brain showed several T2 hyperintensities within the white matter. Visual evoked responses showed significant slowing on the right. The eye pain resolved after a 5-day course of high-dose IV methylprednisolone. No warnings were given regarding the use of etanercept at this time, and the patient was reluctant to stop therapy. No new symptoms were observed at an evaluation 2 months later. However, an MRI study of the brain at that time showed 2 large enhancing lesions, and etanercept was discontinued. Another high-dose course of steroids was initiated, and leflunomide was started for her arthritis. The patient was reevaluated at 6 weeks. She had worsening arthritis symptoms, numbness in her right foot, and dysequilibrium. Physical examination showed a new up-going toe on the right. Two new enhancing lesions were seen on another brain MRI. A diagnosis of MS was made, and treatment with interferon β-1a was initiated.

Conclusions.—Therapies aimed at inhibition of TNF are effective in the treatment of RA but may be associated with the development of MS.

► TNF is a proinflammatory cytokine that is involved in a variety of functions, which include lymphocyte signaling and cell-mediated immunity. We all know that TNF has multiple effects on the induction of adhesion molecules and a variety of other things. This article really goes into a discussion of the onset of MS associated with anti-TNF therapy. We now know that TNF is an important mediator in autoimmune diseases like RA, ulcerative colitis and perhaps MS. But this is an unusual article that describes the onset of MS in a patient taking etanercept for RA. The difficult aspect of this article is that there are reported some 20 to 25 cases of CNS demyelination associated with the use of etanercept. The bottom line is that patients who have any new neurologic findings while taking TNF inhibitors should be scrutinized with MRI and a clinical examination to ensure that no new cases of demyelination occur with this new biotherapy for RA and other autoimmune diseases.

R. G. Lahita, MD, PhD

Induction of Autoantibodies During Prolonged Treatment With Infliximab

Louis M, Rauch J, Armstrong M, et al (McGill Univ, Montreal)
J Rheumatol 30:2557-2562, 2003 1–27

Background.—Infliximab is a monoclonal antibody that binds tumor necrosis factor-α (TNF-α) and has been successfully used to treat numerous inflammatory arthritic diseases. This agent, however, has also been linked with the development of autoantibodies in some patients. Thus, the autoantibody profiles of patients with inflammatory rheumatic disease who received infliximab were analyzed.

Methods.—The study included 42 patients (88% women; mean age, 53 years) with severe rheumatic disease (79% had RA) not responsive to disease-modifying antirheumatic drugs. Patients were given 5 infusions or more of infliximab. Blood samples obtained before each infliximab infusion were assayed to measure levels of antinuclear antibody (ANA), anti-DNA, anti-Sm, anti-RNP, rheumatoid factor, anti-SSA, and anti-SSB. Antibody levels were analyzed in relation to the response to infliximab and the development of adverse events.

Results.—Of these 42 patients, a new autoantibody developed in 32 (76%) after starting infliximab therapy, and 2 or more new autoantibodies developed in 20 (48%). These autoantibodies appeared as early as after the first infliximab infusion. In 24 (57%) patients, levels of these autoantibodies persisted for 2 or more infliximab infusions. Among the patients who had new autoantibodies, ANA developed in 45%, anti-DNA developed in 33%, anti-SM developed in 31%, and anti-RNP developed in 29%. New autoantibody formation increased significantly as the number of infliximab infusions increased, and as the total dose of infliximab increased. Patients who had new autoantibodies were similar to those who did not have new autoantibodies as a result of other treatments, disease characteristics, and loss of response to infliximab. Despite the presence of these new autoantibodies, none of the patients showed clinical evidence of a new connective tissue disease. Ultimately, 16 (38%) patients stopped taking infliximab, 9 (21%) because of an inadequate response and 7 (17%) because of adverse events.

Conclusion.—New autoantibodies developed in 3 of 4 patients with rheumatic disease receiving successive infliximab infusions. In particular, concomitant use of immunosuppressants did not prevent the formation of these autoantibodies. The clinical significance of new autoantibody formation remains unclear, but these results suggest patients receiving infliximab should be carefully monitored for the development of autoimmune disease.

► One collective concern is the production of autoantibodies with the use of tumor necrosis factor (TNF) inhibitors like infliximab which is highlighted in this interesting article. Roughly 57% of the patients who received this monoclonal antibody developed autoantibodies, not necessarily to the monoclonal therapeutic. Surprisingly, some of these were quite specific for lupus since, of 42 patients, the incidence of anti-SM was 31% and anti-RNP was 29%. The mechanisms for this specific repertoire are not clear and should be further explored. To say that we are simply changing cytokine profiles from TH1 to TH2 is probably too simplistic, and the real mechanism needs definition. Also worrisome is the description elsewhere of demyelination after use of these agents, which is also possibly due to an autoantibody.

R. G. Lahita, MD, PhD

The Safety of Anakinra in the High-Risk Patients With Active Rheumatoid Arthritis: Six-Month Observations of Patients With Comorbid Conditions

Schiff MH, DiVittorio G, Tesser J, et al (Denver Arthritis Clinic; Coastal Clinical Research Inc, Mobile, Ala; Phoenix Ctr for Clinical Research, Ariz; et al)

Arthritis Rheum 50:1752-1760, 2004 1–28

Introduction.—Both clinical and animals studies have implicated the proinflammatory cytokine interleukin-1 (IL-1) in the pathogenesis of RA, and

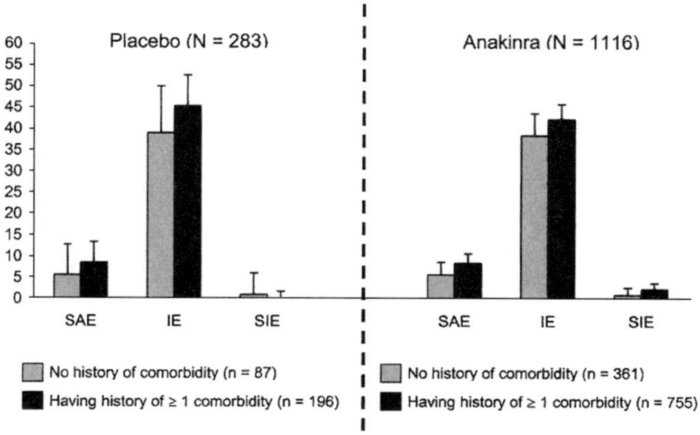

FIGURE 1.—Incidence of serious adverse events (SAEs), infectious events (IEs), and serious IEs (SIEs) by treatment group (placebo or anakinra) and comorbidity status (with or without). *Bars* show the 95% exact confidence intervals. (Courtesy of Schiff MH, DiVittorio G, Tesser J, et al: The safety of anakinra in high-risk patients with active rheumatoid arthritis: Six-month observations of patients with comorbid conditions. *Arthritis Rheum* 50:1752-1760, 2004. Reprinted by permission of John Wiley & Sons, Inc.)

regulation of this cytokine is an important component of RA management. A naturally occurring, specific blocker of the IL-1 receptor, IL-1Ra, is available in a recombinant form (anakinra) that blocks IL-1 cell signaling and has been approved for treatment of RA. The safety profile of daily anakinra use was assessed in patients with active RA and concurrent comorbidities that would put them at high risk for therapy-related adverse events.

Methods.—The multicenter trial randomly assigned patients in a 4:1 ratio into double-blinded treatment with anakinra (100 mg/day) or placebo for 6 months. A post hoc analysis identified a subpopulation of the patients with comorbid conditions. Safety end points were the incidence rates of serious adverse events, infectious events, and serious infectious events.

Results.—A total of 1399 of 1414 enrolled patients received at least 1 dose of the study drug and were included in the safety analysis. Comorbidity was present in 755 patients randomly assigned to anakinra and 196 randomly assigned to placebo. Overall, the incidence rates of adverse events were similar regardless of treatment group or comorbidity status (Fig 1). Most adverse events in both comorbidity and no comorbidity groups were injection-site reactions that were more common with anakinra (72.5%) than with placebo (29.6%). The incidence of serious infectious events with anakinra use was similar in patients with (2.5%) and without (2.1%) comorbidity and not attributed to any single comorbidity.

Conclusion.—The use of anakinra was found to minimally increase the risk of serious infectious events in a diverse population of patients with RA. In this study, a modest increase in the incidence of such events in high-risk patients was similar to that seen in the total study population. Thus, the safety profile of anakinra is confirmed, even in high-risk populations.

► Patients with RA and comorbidities tolerated anakinra (Fig 1).

D. B. Hellmann, MD

Tacrolimus in Rheumatoid Arthritis Patients Receiving Concomitant Methotrexate: A Six-Month, Open-Label Study

Kremer JM, for Tacrolimus-Methotrexate Rheumatoid Arthritis Study Group (Ctr for Rheumatology, Albany, NY; et al)

Arthritis Rheum 48:2763-2768, 2003 1–29

Background.—Combination therapy with methotrexate (MTX) is a popular option for patients with RA who cannot tolerate MTX doses high enough to achieve disease control. Tacrolimus is a macrolide that suppresses the activation and proliferation of antigen-specific T cells but is much more potent than similar dugs (such as cyclosporin A). Whether combination tacrolimus plus MTX therapy would be effective and safe for patients with RA was examined.

Methods.—The subjects were 80 patients (74% female; 93% white; mean age, 55 years) with active RA despite maximally tolerated doses of oral MTX (5-20 mg/wk) for 1 month or longer. Patients continued their MTX dosage and their usual nonsteroidal anti-inflammatory drugs and corticosteroids during the study, but they stopped taking other disease-modifying antirheumatic drugs 2 weeks or longer before study entry. Patients agreed to try oral tacrolimus (1-mg tablet 3 times daily) for 6 months, and safety was monitored throughout the study. The primary end point was the percentage of patients with at least 20% improvement in American College of Rheumatology criteria (ACR20) by the end of treatment.

Results.—All patients took at least 1 dose of tacrolimus while they were receiving MTX, and all but 5 patients had 1or more efficacy assessments. Most patients (69, or 86.3%) had 1 or more tacrolimus-related adverse events. Tacrolimus-related adverse events prompted 10 patients (12.5%) to withdraw from the study (including 1 in whom pancreatitis, possibly related to tacrolimus, developed); another 4 patients (5.0%) withdrew because of lack of efficacy, and 3 patients (3.7%) were withdrawn for administrative reasons. Thus, 63 patients (78.8%) completed 6 months of combination tacrolimus plus MTX therapy.

At study end, 42 of 80 patients (52.5%) had achieved an ACR20 response. Creatinine (Cr) levels were monitored in all patients, and mean levels increased from 0.74 mg/dL at baseline to 0.81 mg/dL at the end of treatment. At some point during treatment, 23 patients (28.3%) had a maximum increase in Cr level of 30% or greater (Table 2). These increases, however, normalized within a mean of 30 days, even when tacrolimus therapy was not interrupted. Also, 3 patients (3.8%) had a Cr level of more than 1.4 mg/dL, but levels returned to normal within 17 days.

TABLE 2.—Incidence of Increase in Serum Creatinine Among Patients Who Received at Least 1 Dose of Study Drug and for Whom a Baseline and at Least 1 On-Treatment Creatinine Measurement Were Available

Serum Cr	Tacrolimus 3 mg + MTX 5-12.5 mg/week (n = 35)	Tacrolimus 3 mg + MTX 15-20 mg/week (n = 45)	Total (n = 80)
% increase from baseline			
≥30% to <40%			
Maximum*	4 (11.4)	5 (11.1)	9 (11.3)
End of treatment	2 (5.7)	4 (8.9)	6 (7.5)
≥40%			
Maximum*	7 (20)	7 (15.6)	14 (17.5)
End of treatment	3 (8.6)	3 (6.7)	6 (7.5)
Maximum on-treatment value			
≥0.5 mg/dl to ≤1.4 mg/dl†	34 (97.1)	43 (95.6)	77 (96.3)
>1.4 mg/dl to ≤1.8 mg/dl	1 (2.9)	2 (4.4)	3 (3.7)
>1.8 mg/dl	0	0	0

Note: Values are the number (percentage) of patients.
*Maximum increase during treatment, from baseline.
†Normal range.
Abbreviations: MTX, Methotrexate; *CR*, creatinine.
(Courtesy of Kremer JM, for the Tacrolimus-Methotrexate Rheumatoid Arthritis Study Group: Tacrolimus in rheumatoid arthritis patients receiving concomitant methotrexate: A six-month, open-label study. *Arthritis Rheum* 48:2763-2768, 2003. Reprinted by permission of John Wiley & Sons, Inc.)

Conclusion.—For patients with active RA whose disease is not adequately controlled by maximally tolerated doses of MTX, adding tacrolimus to therapy is effective and safe. In particular, tacrolimus and MTX combination therapy carries a lower risk of hypertension (3 patients, or 3.8%) compared with other macrolide combinations such as cyclosporin A plus MTX.

▶ Tacrolimus, a macrotide immunosuppressant that inhibits the activation and proliferations of antigen-specific T cells, appears to be effective for RA. Although it appears safer than its cousin cyclosporine, the renal toxicity of tacrolimus limits the drug's appeal to me. Nearly 30% of patients experienced a 30% or greater increase in serum Cr (Table 2). Although the apparent reversibility of the elevation is reassuring, I want to see good results from long-term studies before I warm up to the tacrolimus option.

D. B. Hellmann, MD

Efficacy and Safety of Tacrolimus in Patients With Rheumatoid Arthritis: A Double-Blind Trial

Borton MA, for the Tacrolimus Rheumatoid Arthritis Study Group (Univ of Arizona, Tucson; et al)

Arthritis Rheum 48:3328-3337, 2003 1–30

Background.—Tacrolimus is an oral macrolide that inhibits the synthesis of inflammatory cytokines and has been studied as a treatment for RA. Thus, the efficacy and safety of tacrolimus as monotherapy for patients with RA were investigated in a phase III study.

Methods.—The subjects were 464 adults with active RA (77% women; mean age, about 56 years) who were resistant to or intolerant of at least 1 disease-modifying antirheumatic drug (DMARD). All patients discontinued DMARDs for 1 to 4 months (depending on the drug) and had a stable joint count (10 or more tender or painful joints and 7 or more swollen joints) before enrollment.

Patients were stratified according to whether they were DMARD resistant (193 patients) or DMARD intolerant (171 patients), then were randomly assigned to 6 months of once-daily oral treatment with placebo, tacrolimus 2 mg, or tacrolimus 3 mg. The primary outcome was the American College of Rheumatology (ACR) success rate, defined as the proportion of patients who completed 6 months of treatment and had achieved a 20% improvement according to ACR criteria (ACR20).

Results.—In all, 45 patients (29%) in the placebo group, 64 patients (42%) in the tacrolimus 2-mg group, and 80 patients (52%) in the tacrolimus 3-mg group completed 6 months of therapy. The ACR success rate was significantly higher in the 2-mg tacrolimus group (29 patients, or 18.8%) than in the placebo group (16 patients, or 10.2%) and was significantly higher with the 3-mg tacrolimus dose (41 patients, or 26.8%) than with the lower dose. Also, at the end of treatment, compared with placebo, significantly more of the patients in the 3-mg tacrolimus group had achieved an ACR20 (32.0% vs 13.4%), and there was a trend for a higher ACR20 response rate in the 2-mg group as well (21.4%; P = .0595). And significantly more of the tacrolimus groups had achieved an ACR50 (11.7% in the 2-mg group; 11.8% in the 3-mg group) than did the control subjects (4.5%).

With both active drugs, ACR response rates were better in DMARD-intolerant patients than in DMARD-resistant patients. As for safety, only 3 patients had a serious drug-related adverse event, all of which resolved without residual effects. At some point during the study, 20.1% of patients in the 2-mg tacrolimus group and 29.1% of those in the 3-mg tacrolimus group had an increase in serum creatinine level of 40% or greater compared with baseline. Nonetheless, in 90.9% of patients in the 2-mg group and in 87.6% of those in the 3-mg group, the serum creatinine level remained within or below the normal range throughout the study.

Conclusion.—Oral tacrolimus, at either 2 or 3 mg/d, is effective and safe as monotherapy for patients with active RA who are resistant to or intolerant of DMARDs. The 3-mg tacrolimus dose was associated with better ACR success rates and ACR20 and ACR50 response rates than the lower dose, but both active drug regimens were superior to placebo in controlling disease.

► If you are my age, you will remember the debates that raged in the 1970s over whether cyclophosphamide was better than prednisone in treatment of lupus nephritis. The debate raged because of inconclusive short-term studies and was settled (in cyclophosphamide's favor) by long-term studies.

Toxicity—like efficacy—may take time to become evident. That is why this study makes me nervous. Tacrolimus is a nephrotoxin. Although the short-term nephrotoxicity may seem modest, the long-term renal effects of tacrolimus must be defined before it can be embraced in the treatment of a chronic disease.

D. B. Hellmann, MD

Treatment of Rheumatoid Arthritis With Humanized Anti–Interleukin-6 Receptor Antibody: A Multicenter, Double-Blind, Placebo-Controlled Trial

Nishimoto N, Yoshizaki K, Miyasaka N, et al (Osaka Univ, Japan; Tokyo Med and Dental Univ; Unv of Tokyo; et al)

Arthritis Rheum 50:1761-1769, 2004 1–31

Introduction.—Proinflammatory cytokines are involved in the development of RA and may be potential targets of treatment. Because overproduction of interleukin-6 (IL-6) plays pathologic roles in RA, blockade of this pleiotropic cytokine may prove therapeutically effective. The effectiveness of MRA, a humanized anti-IL-6 receptor antibody, was evaluated.

Methods.—The 164 patients in the double-blind trial were randomly assigned to receive either MRA (4 mg/kg body weight or 8 mg/kg body weight) or placebo. Treatment was administered IV every 4 weeks for a total of 3 months. During a 4-week washout period before the first dose and throughout the study period, patients were not allowed to take disease-modifying antirheumatic drugs, immumosuppressants, or corticosteroids or to undergo plasma exchange therapies or surgical treatment. Clinical response to MRA was measured according to American College of Rheumatology criteria.

Results.—A total of 162 patients (125 women and 37 men) were included in the full analysis set. The median age of the MRA and placebo groups was 54 years and the median disease duration was 7.6 years. All patients had relatively severe disease. Only 53% of patients in the placebo group completed treatment, whereas 95% of those who received MRA did so. Treatment with MRA significantly improved all measures of disease in a dose-response relationship (Fig 2). Efficacy of the drug was noted at week 4 and most pronounced by week 12. The active treatment resulted in increases in total cholesterol, triglycerides (Fig 3), and high-density lipoprotein cholesterol. There were also mild and transient liver function disorders and decreases in white blood cell counts in MRA groups. Treatment tolerance of MRA was good, but 5 serious adverse events were reported, 3 in the MRA group and 2 in the placebo group.

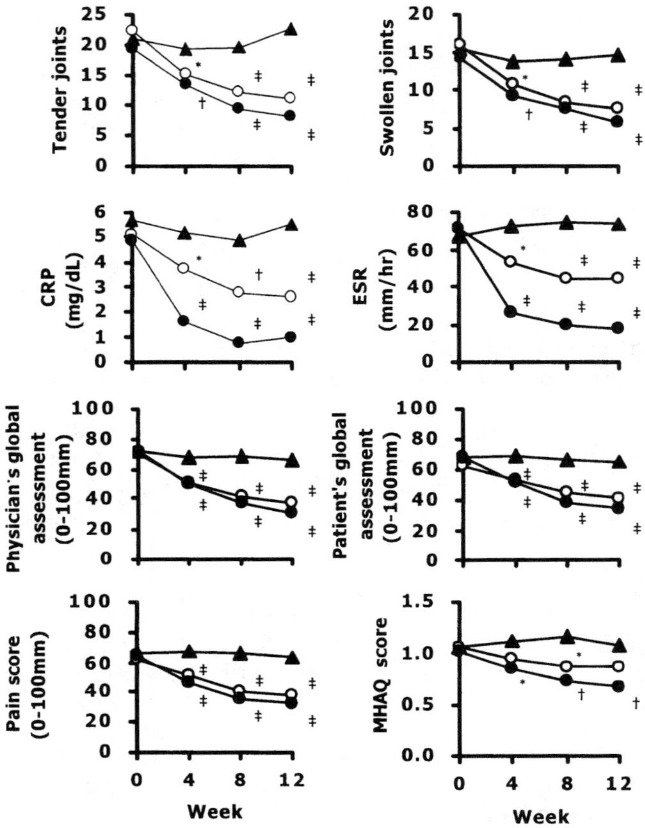

FIGURE 2.—RA disease activity assessments. *Solid triangles* indicate placebo-treated group. *Open circles* indicate group treated with 4 mg/kg humanized anti-IL-6 receptor antibody (MRA). *Solid circles* indicate 8 mg/kg MRA-treated group. Values are the mean for each group at each time point. *$P < .05$; †$P < .01$; ‡$P < .001$ vs placebo, by Student *t* test. *Abbreviations: CRP*, C-reactive protein; *ESR*, erythrocyte sedimentation rate; *M-HAQ*, modified Health Assessment Questionnaire. (Courtesy of Nishimoto N, Yoshizaki K, Miyasaka N, et al: Treatment of rheumatoid arthritis with humanized anti–interleukin-6 receptor antibody: A multicenter, double-blind, placebo-controlled trial. *Arthritis Rheum* 50:1761-1769, 2004. Reprinted by permission of John Wiley & Sons, Inc.)

Conclusion.—Treatment with MRA rapidly reduced disease activity in patients with refractory RA. The efficacy was dose-related, and safety was considered acceptable relative to clinical benefit. But serum cholesterol increases will need to be examined, for patients with RA are reportedly at increased risk for development of cardiac complications.

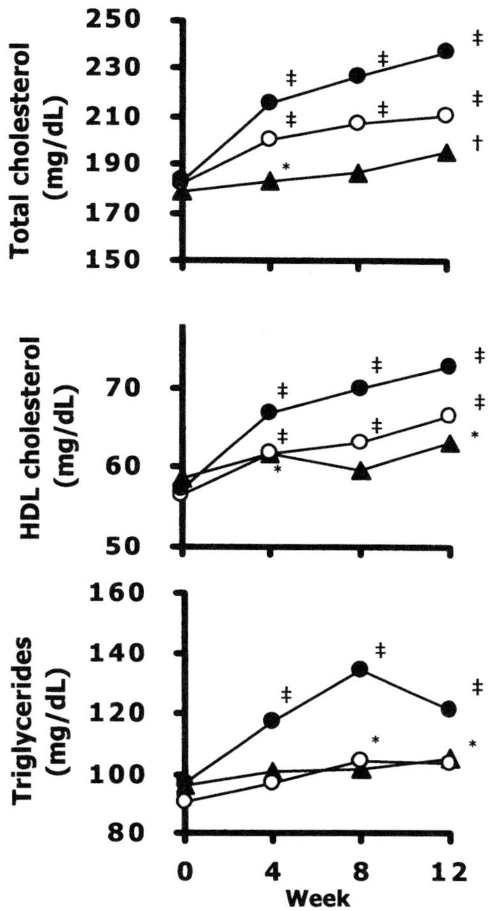

FIGURE 3.—Changes from baseline in serum levels of total cholesterol, high-density lipoprotein (HDL) cholesterol, and triglycerides in patients with RA. *Solid triangles* indicate placebo-treated group. *Open circles* indicate group treated with 4 mg/kg humanized anti-IL-6 receptor antibody (MRA). *Solid circles* indicate 8 mg/kg MRA-treated group. Each parameter was compared with its baseline value. Values are the mean for each group at each time point. **P* < .05; †*P* < .01; ‡*P* < .001 vs baseline, by paired *t* test. (Courtesy of Nishimoto N, Yoshizaki K, Miyasaka N, et al: Treatment of rheumatoid arthritis with humanized anti–interleukin-6 receptor antibody: A multicenter, double-blind, placebo-controlled trial. *Arthritis Rheum* 50:1761-1769, 2004. Reprinted by permission of John Wiley & Sons, Inc.)

► This is the first large, double-blind, placebo-controlled trial of a novel biologic therapy—anti-IL-6 receptor antibody (MRA)—in patients with RA. MRA was impressively effective (Fig 2) but also had impressive negative effects on lipids (Fig 3). Given the accelerated atherosclerosis that bedevils patients with RA, the increases in cholesterol levels caused by MRA may be important.

D. B. Hellmann, MD

Efficacy of Etanercept for the Treatment of Juvenile Idiopathic Arthritis According to the Onset Type

Quartier P, Taupin P, Bourdeaut F, et al (Hôpital Necker-Enfants Malades, Paris; Centre Hospitalo-Universitaire de Nancy, France; Centre Hospitalo-Universitaire de Bordeaux, France; et al)

Arthritis Rheum 48:1093-1101, 2003 1–32

Background.—Juvenile idiopathic arthritis (JIA) is a designation applied to several conditions that are characterized by early-onset arthritis (before age 16 years) that persists in 1 or more joints for at least 6 weeks and in which infectious arthritis and other well-defined illnesses have been actively excluded. JIA may be associated with severe disability and life-threatening complications, particularly in patients in whom polyarthritis develops and who are not sufficiently responsive to treatment. Etanercept is a soluble tumor necrosis factor receptor fusion protein that has been shown to be effective and well tolerated in patients with RA. The efficacy of etanercept for the treatment of patients with JIA and their tolerance of this drug were assessed.

Methods.—Included in the study were all JIA patients with active chronic polyarthritis who were first treated with etanercept between November 1999 and June 2001 in 18 French centers after poor response or intolerance to methotrexate. Treating physicians were asked to complete a standardized questionnaire. The validated international core-set score for JIA activity was assessed every 3 months, and in intent-to-treat analysis was performed. The study also compared the risk of treatment failure in patients defined as having systemic onset, oligoarticular onset, or polyarticular onset JIA.

Results.—A total of 61 patients were enrolled and followed up for a median of 13 months. Treatment was stopped in 1 patient who became pregnant and in 12 patients as a result of severe side effects, including neurologic or psychiatric disorders, retrobulbar optic neuropathy, major weight gain, and severe infection, among others (Table 2). All adverse side effects ceased after discontinuation of etanercept. One child was subsequently given a diagnosis of Crohn's disease. Scores improved by 30% or greater in 73% of patients after 3 months, but this patient percentage decreased to 39% after 12 months (Fig 2). The response rate was significantly lower in patients with systemic onset JIA than in patients with oligoarticular or polyarticular onset JIA.

Conclusion.—A wide spectrum of severe side effects was associated with the use of etanercept in patients with JIA. Most patients in this study were responsive to the drug initially, but this response was not always followed by sustained improvement over time. A higher rate of treatment failures in the patients with systemic onset JIA indicates that these patients may require additional treatments.

TABLE 2.—Main Side Effects and Unexpected Events During Etanercept Therapy for Patients With Juvenile Idiopathic Arthritis

	No. of Patients	JIA Onset Type	No. of Months Receiving Etanercept
Events that justified etanercept withdrawal			
Pancytopenia	2	Both systemic-onset	0.5, 12*
Severe psychiatric disorders	2	Both oligo-onset	3, 3
Uveitis flare	2	Poly-onset, oligo-onset	12, 12.5
Retrobulbar optic neuropathy	1	Oligo-onset	3
Headaches and marked dysesthesia	1	Poly-onset	14
Hemorrhagic diarrhea (revealing Crohn's disease)	1	Oligo-onset	0.5
Vasculitic skin rash + systemic symptoms	1	Systemic-onset	0.5
Major weight gain (20 kg)†	1	Psoriatic	9
Appendicular abscess and weight gain (6 kg)‡	1	Systemic-onset	7
Pregnancy (1 month)§	1	Systemic-onset	2
Events that resolved spontaneously			
Mild reactions at injection site	17	7 systemic-onset, 5 oligo-onset, 5 poly-onset	1-9
Cutaneous rash	10	4 systemic-onset, 2 oligo-onset, 4 poly-onset	<2 months
Mild gastrointestinal disorders	10	5 systemic-onset, 3 oligo-onset, 2 poly-onset	<2 months
Headaches	7	3 oligo-onset, 4 poly-onset	2-6
Mild mood changes	6	4 systemic-onset, 2 oligo-onset	1-9
Asthenia, anorexia	2	1 systemic-onset, 1 oligo-onset	3, 3
Thoracic pain	1	Systemic-onset	2
Chronic cough	1	Poly-onset	5
Hematoma	1	Oligo-onset	3

*One of these patients had macrophage activation syndrome; etanercept was successfully reintroduced 2 months later.

†Patient had gained a large amount of weight 3 years previously, while receiving methotrexate.

‡Occurrence while patient was receiving methotrexate, which had been reintroduced 2 months previously, and a combination oral contraceptive.

§No obstetric complication; patient had a healthy 9-month-old child at last follow-up.

Abbreviations: Oligo-onset, Oligoarticular onset; *poly-onset*, polyarticular onset.

(Courtesy of Quartier P, Taupin P, Bordeaut F, et al: Efficacy of etanercept for the treatment of juvenile idiopathic arthritis according to the onset type. *Arthritis Rheum* 48:1093-1101, 2003. Reprinted by permission of John Wiley & Sons, Inc.)

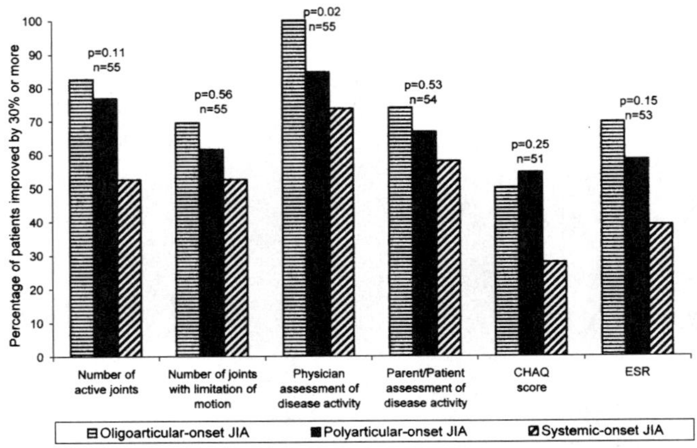

FIGURE 2.—Percentage of patients who achieved at least 30% improvement at 3 months, for each of the constitutive items of the core-set score, according to the type of onset of juvenile idiopathic arthritis (*JIA*). Results were derived from the relationship between the changes in each item of the core-set (adjusted according to the baseline value of the item), as continuous variables, and the type of JIA. The differences between the values at month 3 and at baseline were computed. *P* values were determined by Fisher's exact test. *Abbreviations: CHAQ*, Childhood Health Assessment Questionnaire; *ESR*, erythrocyte sedimentation rate. (Courtesy of Quartier P, Taupin P, Bordeaut F, et al: Efficacy of etanercept for the treatment of juvenile idiopathic arthritis according to the onset type. *Arthritis Rheum* 48:1093-1101, 2003. Reprinted by permission of John Wiley & Sons, Inc.)

► The main results of this study are that etanercept works less well in systemic onset JIA than in oligoarticular or polyarticular JIA (Fig 2), and etanercept is less well tolerated in children (Table 2).

D. B. Hellmann, MD

2 Systemic Lupus Erythematosus and Related Disorders

Introduction

This was a fascinating year for papers in the area of systemic lupus erythematosus (SLE) and related syndromes. I have selected articles focusing on drug therapy of lupus and related syndromes, the various antibodies that are important to various presentations of lupus and related conditions, the strange assortment of risk factors and mechanisms for the development of the disease entity, and the various comments on pathogenesis of the disease. I have also chosen as the lead article one that suggests, yet again, that autoimmunity is involved directly in that most common of conditions, atherosclerosis.

In previous volumes of this YEAR BOOK, we commented on the suggestion that accelerated atherosclerosis and antiphospholipid antibodies were intertwined and that the pathogenesis of atherosclerosis was a condition associated with autoimmunity. I strongly believe that to be the case and have included this paper as the lead article to emphasize that again. There are, of course, no specific drugs for the disease SLE at this writing and no specific ideas regarding the cause of the disease. However, there are a lot of ideas concerning pathogenesis and risk of developing SLE, antiphospholipid antibody syndrome, or related conditions. I am sure that you will enjoy these selections and come to your own conclusions about the rapid pace with which this area is progressing.

Robert G. Lahita, MD, PhD

Lead Article

Association of Serum Antibodies to Heat-Shock Protein 65 With Coronary Calcification Levels: Suggestion of Pathogen-Triggered Autoimmunity in Early Atherosclerosis

Zhu J, Katz RJ, Quyyumi AA, et al (Washington Hosp Ctr, Washington, DC; George Washington Univ, Washington, DC; Emory Univ, Atlanta, Ga; et al)
Circulation 109:36-41, 2004 2–1

Background.—Heat-shock protein (HSP) has been identified as a possible autoantigenic determinant operating in atherogenesis. HSPs help to mediate the correct folding of intracellular proteins, transporting these proteins across membranes and protecting cellular proteins from denaturation as a result of environmental insults. A specific association has been demonstrated between antibodies to mycobacterial HSP 65 (mHSP65) and carotid artery thickening. It was hypothesized that early coronary vascular changes in the host that predispose to the development of coronary artery disease (CAD) are triggered by infection.

The causative agent was believed to be antibodies targeted to pathogen HSP that cross-react with human HSP50 on cells of the vascular wall. An investigation looked at the links between levels of coronary calcification that may reflect preclinical CAD and mHSP65 antibody levels.

Methods.—Two hundred one subjects aged 27 to 79 years (mean, 56.6 years) were studied; 52% were men. Serum specimens were obtained, and all patients had electron-beam CT imaging. Levels of mHSP65 and human HSP60 antibodies plus antibodies to several infectious pathogens were measured and the findings evaluated statistically.

Results.—A correlation was found between HSP65 and HSP60 antibody levels. Compared with the low calcium score group, the high calcium score group had a higher prevalence of anti-mHSP65 antibodies but not anti-HSP60 antibodies. Twenty-two percent of individuals in the anti-mHSP65 seropositive group had high coronary calcium scores. Only 6% of those seronegative for anti-mHSP65 had elevated calcium scores.

Higher mean titers of mHSP65 were present in those with high coronary calcium than in those without these high calcium levels. The association between mHSP65 antibodies and high coronary calcification was independent of established risk factors for CAD, such as age, male gender, smoking, diabetes, hypercholesterolemia, hypertension, family history of CAD, and serum C-reactive protein levels.

A significant association was also found between increasing titers of mHSP65 antibodies and coronary calcification on multivariate analysis. Neither the presence of human HSP60 antibodies nor increasing human HSP60 antibody titers were linked to elevated levels of coronary calcification. Serum titers to mHSP65 showed a correlation with *Helicobacter pylori* infection. After adjusting for CAD risk factors, *H pylori* immunoglobulin G seropositivity and mHSP65 antibody titers remained significantly associated. *H pylori* Immunoglobulin G antibodies were not significantly linked to

TABLE 4.—Association of Coronary Calcification Scores of Less Than 150 or 150 or More With Immunoglobulin G Seropositivity to 6 Infectious Pathogens

	Coronary Calcification Score			
Antibodies, %	<150	≥150	*P*	Adjusted* *P*
Cytomegalovirus	49.1	56.4	0.410	0.968
Chlamydia pneumoniae	76.6	67.6	0.255	0.494
Helicobacter pylori	10.7	20.5	0.110	0.050
Hepatitis A virus	27.2	46.2	0.026	0.333
Herpes simplex virus type 1	56.0	64.1	0.357	0.713
Herpes simplex virus type 2	32.7	43.6	0.201	0.254

*Adjusted covariates: age, male gender, smoking, diabetes, hypercholesterolemia, hypertension, family history of coronary artery disease, elevated C-reactive protein levels, and seropositivities to other infectious pathogens as described in Table 4.

(Courtesy of Zhu J, Katz RJ, Quyyumi AA, et al: Association of serum antibodies to heat-shock protein 65 with coronary calcification levels: Suggestion of pathogen-triggered autoimmunity in early atherosclerosis. *Circulation* 109:36-41, 2004.)

increased levels of coronary calcification on univariate analysis but were associated on multivariate analysis after adjustment for CAD risk factors and seropositivity to other infectious pathogens (Table 4).

Conclusion.—In clinically healthy persons, the levels of mHSP65 antibodies were significantly associated with elevated levels of coronary calcification. There was also a correlation with *H pylori* infection. Thus, pathogen-triggered autoimmunity derived from the generation of anti-mHSP65 antibodies that cross-react to host HSP60 is involved in producing early atherosclerosis. Autoreactivity to self-HSP60 may develop over the course of the disease's progression.

▶ This is a remarkable article that deals with HSP antibodies associated with levels of coronary calcification. This appears to reflect preclinical CAD. The interesting aspect of this is this presumes that atherosclerosis is developed as a result of an autoimmune process. Moreover, *H pylori* was the only organism that maintained significance after adjustment for CAD risk factors and zero positivity to other pathogens. The other pathogens are viruses for various types of herpes simplex, hepatitis A, *Chlamydia* pneumonia, and cytomegalovirus, to name but a few.

If this study is correct and it is one of those that is really out there, this would mean that the presence of *H pylori* infections, as with other infections, can promote the appearance of the HSP antigen. The subsequent autoimmune reaction to the HSP and further deleterious effects of this antigen-antibody response on the endothelium of the vascular wall result in CAD. It is curious that the authors picked coronary calcification and not just fat deposition to examine with regard to this immune response.

Nevertheless, this is really a fascinating study, with ramifications that go far beyond immunology, and cardiology, for that matter. It is of particular interest that prior data suggested the findings of mRNA in the endothelial plaque for herpesvirus, which was not the case in this study since herpesvirus was not associated or correlated with immunoglobulin G zero positivity and coronary calcification.

R. G. Lahita, MD, PhD

Immunogenetics and Pathophysiology

Hydralazine May Induce Autoimmunity by Inhibiting Extracellular Signal–Regulated Kinase Pathway Signaling

Deng C, Lu Q, Zhang Z, et al (Astrozeneca, Boston; Univ of Michigan, Ann Arbor; Guanxi Med Univ, China; et al)
Arthritis Rheum 48:746-756, 2003 2–2

Background.—Multiple T-cell biochemical abnormalities and autoantibody production are characteristic of systemic lupus erythematosus (SLE), but the mechanisms producing this disorder are unclear. Some drugs cause a lupuslike disease in genetically predisposed individuals; understanding how these drugs produce these findings may help in understanding what causes SLE. One mechanism implicated in lupus pathogenesis is T-cell DNA methylation. Whether the drug hydralazine can decrease DNA methyltransferase (DNMT) expression and induce autoimmunity by inhibiting extracellular signal–regulated kinase (ERK) pathway signaling was explored.

Methods.—In vitro, enzyme inhibition studies were performed to determine the effect of hydralazine on DNMT. In vivo, mRNA levels and enzyme activity were measured. Immunoblotting techniques were used to evaluate

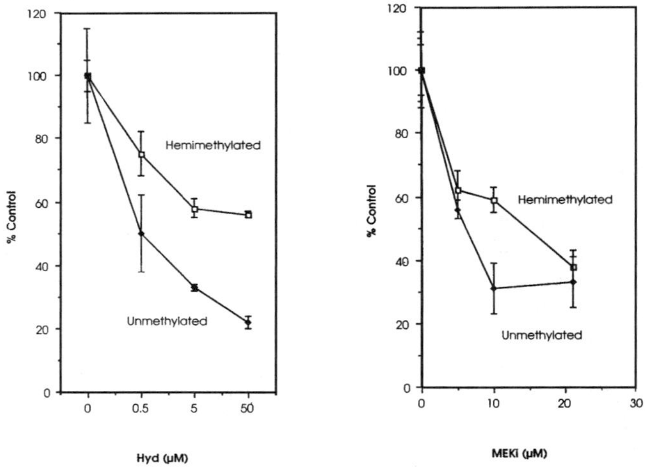

FIGURE 1.—Hydralazine (*Hyd*)-induced decrease in DNMT activity. **A**, Jurkat cells were treated with indicated concentrations of Hyd, and then DNMT activity was measured. **B**, Jurkat cells were treated with indicated concentrations of a mitogen-activated protein kinase inhibitor (MEKi; PD98059), and DNMT activity was measured as in **A**. Results are the mean ± SEM of triplicate determinations. (Courtesy of Deng C, Lu Q, Zhang Z, et al: Hydralazine may induce autoimmunity by inhibiting extracellular signal–regulated kinase pathway signaling. *Arthritis Rheum* 48:746-756, 2003. Reprinted by permission of John Wiley & Sons, Inc.)

HYDRALAZINE

↓

ERK PATHWAY INHIBITION

↓

DECREASED DNA METHYLTRANSFERASE EXPRESSION

↓

DNA HYPOMETHYLATION

↓

LFA-1 OVEREXPRESSION

↓

T CELL AUTOREACTIVITY

↓

LUPUS-LIKE DISEASE

FIGURE 7.—Proposed mechanism for hydralazine-induced lupus. *Abbreviation: LFA-1*, Lymphocyte function–associated antigen 1. (Courtesy of Deng C, Lu Q, Zhang Z, et al: Hydralazine may induce autoimmunity by inhibiting extracellular signal(regulated kinase pathway signaling. *Arthritis Rheum* 48:746-756, 2003. Reprinted by permission of John Wiley & Sons, Inc.)

the effects on ERK, c-Jun N-terminal kinase, and p32 pathway signaling. T cells from the mouse model were treated with hydralazine or an ERK pathway inhibitor was injected into mice; the anti-DNA antibody levels were then measured by enzyme-linked immunosorbent assay.

Results.—Hydralazine did not inhibit DNMT activity in vitro but did decrease in vivo DNMT expression at the protein level. Both hydralazine and PD98059 lowered DNMT enzyme activity (Fig 1). Hydralazine produced significant decreases in DNMT1 mRNA but phthalazine did not. DNMT3a levels were also significantly decreased by hydralazine but not phthalazine. The DNMT3b levels were too low to be accurately quantified. ERK phosphorylation in T cells was inhibited by hydralazine. The inhibition of T-cell ERK pathway signaling in vitro induced autoreactivity. In vivo it induced autoimmunity (Fig 7).

Conclusions.—The effects of the lupus-inducing drug hydralazine included decreasing T-cell ERK pathway signaling, decreasing DNMT activity, inducing DNA hypomethylation, increasing the expression of lymphocyte function–associated antigen 1, and inducing T-cell autoreactivity. Thus, hydralazine produces inhibition of T-cell DNA methylation through influences on DNMT enzyme expression rather than direct inhibition. Signals through the ERK pathway partly regulate DNMT1 and DNMT3a transcripts but do not regulate DNMt3b transcripts.

► This study is quite important regarding the little-known mechanisms that are now proposed for drug-induced SLE. In this particular report, hydralazine, better known to clinicians as Apresoline (an antihypertensive), inhibits T-cell DNA methylation to effect a specific enzyme. Most of the other drugs, like procainamide, affect these enzymes directly, but this expression is affected by hydralazine indirectly, which affects T-cell methylation. In fact, when T cells are hypomethylated (that is, the DNA of the T-cell are hypomethylated), there is expression of lymphocyte factors and increased T-cell activity. These authors propose this mechanism as being the true one for the induction of drug-induced SLE, which as we all know is reversible. We had a significant interest in acetylation after procainamide administration and showed that slow acetylation predisposed one to develop drug-induced lupus. Hydralazine, however, is very specific as a double-ring structure and has a hydrazine side chain, which is important for signaling inhibition. Many of us have studied hydrazine induction of SLE in the past. One such article about a technician that developed SLE, who was a chemist's assistant, recognized the effect of this hydrazine side chain as a later cause of drug-induced SLE. The exciting aspect of this report is that the same observations can be demonstrated in patients who develop idiopathic SLE, so that the mechanisms between both idiopathic and drug induced, specifically hydralazine-induced systemic SLE, are extremely similar. This is a very interesting hypothesis and one that should be explored further in human beings, since the data described in the paper are largely in a mouse model.

R. G. Lahita, MD, PhD

Interferon-Inducible Gene Expression Signature in Peripheral Blood Cells of Patients With Severe Lupus

Baechler EC, Batliwalla FM, Karypis G, et al (Univ of Minnesota, Minneapolis; North Shore Long Island Jewish Research Inst, Manhasset, NY)

Proc Natl Acad Sci U S A 100:2610-2615, 2003 2–3

Introduction.—Systemic lupus erythematosus (SLE) is characterized by the production of antibodies with specificity for a broad range of self-antigens. The SLE autoantibodies mediate organ damage by binding to host tissues and forming immune complexes that deposit in vascular tissues and activate immune system cells. Global gene expression profiling of peripheral blood mononuclear cells was used to identify particular patterns of gene expression that distinguish most patients with SLE from healthy control subjects.

Findings.—About half of the patients evaluated exhibited dysregulated expression of genes in the interferon (IFN) pathway (Fig 4). This IFN gene expression "signature" acted as a marker for more severe disease involving the kidneys, hematopoietic cells, or the CNS.

Conclusion.—These findings offer insights into the genetic pathways underlying SLE. There is a subgroup of patients who may benefit from therapies that target the IFN pathway.

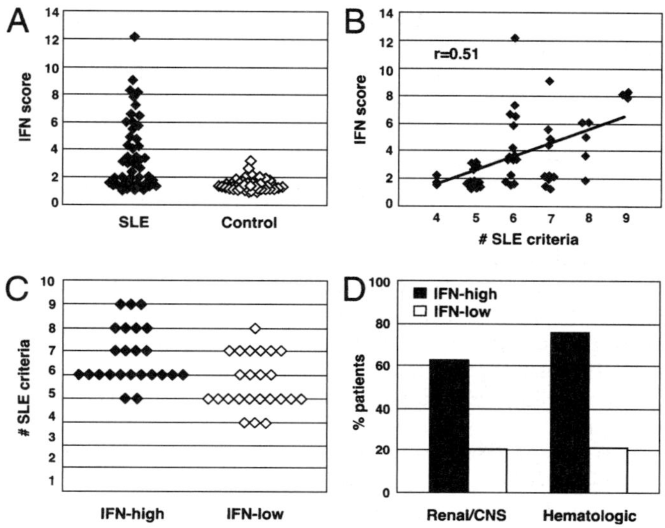

FIGURE 4.—The interferon (*IFN*) expression signature identifies a clinical subset of systemic lupus erythematosus (*SLE*) patients with severe disease. **A**, A numerical score was calculated by using the normalized expression levels of the 14 IFN-regulated genes that compose the IFN signature. The differences between patients and control subjects were significant ($P = 2.8 \times 10^{-7}$). **B**, Linear regression analysis demonstrates a significant correlation between IFN score and the number of SLE disease criteria (r = 0.51; $P = .0002$). **C**, Patients were divided into 2 groups: *IFN-high*, the 24 patients with the highest IFN scores, and the *IFN-low*, the 24 patients with the lowest scores. The data compare the 2 groups for number of American College of Rheumatology criteria for SLE (minimum of 4 to establish the disease, maximum of 11) ($P = .002$). **D**, The data compare the percentage of patients in the IFN-high and IFN-low groups with American College of Rheumatology–defined criteria for renal or CNS disease ($P = 7.7 \times 10^{-6}$) or hematologic involvement ($P = 6.1 \times 10^{-9}$). (Courtesy of Baechler EC, Batliwalla FM, Karypis G, et al: Interferon-induced gene expression signature in peripheral blood cells of patients with severe lupus. *Proc Natl Acad Sci U S A* 100:2610-1615, 2003. Copyright 2003 National Academy of Sciences, USA.)

► In many ways, this article may be the most important of those cited for the year 2004. Using gene arrays, the authors describe an upregulated expression of IFN genes in severe SLE. Very recently, IFN-α has been marked as an indicator of severe infection in patients with influenza or other systemic viral infection. The case with IFN-γ expression and also IFN-γ increases points strongly to an infectious etiology as the cause of this disease. The data are very suggestive and impressive. The use of the gene array technology has revolutionized the study of gene expression for a variety of enzymes and protein products of disease. This is very important and deserves our collective clinical attention.

R. G. Lahita, MD, PhD

N-Acetyl Transferase Genotypes in Relation to Risk of Developing Systemic Lupus Erythematosus

Cooper GS, Treadwell EL, Dooley MA, et al (Natl Inst of Environmental Health Sciences, Durham, NC; Univ of North Carolina, Chapel Hill; East Carolina Univ, Greenville, NC; et al)
J Rheumatol 31:76-80, 2004 2–4

Background.—A complex process is involved in the metabolism of arylamines, which are products of hair dye and smoking. N-acetylation and O-acetylation are accomplished by 2 N-acetyl transferase (NAT) isozymes, designated NAT1 and NAT2. When several relatively common alleles of NAT2 are inherited together, a "slow" acetylation phenotype activity is conferred, in contrast to normal activity, which is dubbed "fast." NAT1 expression occurs in the bladder and in leukocytes but varies and is tissue specific as well as polymorphic. NAT activity has been linked to drug-induced lupus. Slow acetylation is believed to carry a higher risk for development of specific autoantibodies or other aspects of lupus.

In the Carolina Lupus Study, the role of hormonal, environmental, and genetic risk factors for systemic lupus erythematosus (SLE) are evaluated. Smoking was not linked to increased risk for SLE but the use of permanent hair dyes was weakly correlated with an increased SLE risk. Data from this study were assessed to illuminate the link between NAT1 and NAT2 genotypes and SLE and to study the interaction between these genotypes and the use of permanent hair dyes. It was hypothesized that the risk of SLE would be related to the presence of a *10 NAT1 allele and slow-acetylation NAT2 genotype, with the highest risk found in those who use permanent hair dyes.

Methods.—The population-based case-control Carolina Lupus Study was conducted in 60 counties in North and South Carolina. Samples of DNA obtained from 243 patients recently diagnosed with SLE and 298 control subjects were analyzed.

Results.—Compared with African American sample subjects, white sample subjects more often contained the wild-type NAT1 genotype and the slow-acetylation NAT2 genotypes. Neither gender nor age showed any link with the NAT1 or NAT2 genotype. No association was noted between SLE and the NAT1 or NAT2 genotype. The NAT1*10 genotype and the use of hair dyes showed an interaction, with a higher risk among hair dye users than nonusers who were carriers of the *10 allele, but this was not statistically significant.

The strongest association was among NAT2 slow-acetylation genotypes. With the combined presence of the NAT*10 allele plus the slow NAT2 acetylation genotype and hair dye use, the risk of SLE was increased. In patients, the NAT2 genotype and the prevalence of clinical and immunologic features showed no relationship. Anti–double-stranded DNA antibodies and renal involvement were somewhat more common among patients with the NAT2 slow-acetylation genotype.

Conclusion.—Some indication of an interaction with hair dyes was noted in conjunction with slow NAT2 activity and the *10 NAT1 allele. This relationship was a chance finding and should be evaluated in other studies.

► This study really negates the association of NAT genotype and the development of SLE. The NAT enzymes catalyze N-acetylation and O-acetylation of arylamines. We know from previous work with drug-induced SLE that slow acetylators tend to develop more procainamide-induced SLE than fast acetylators. I suppose that these authors want to explore the acetylation pathway in idiopathic SLE, since there was a suggestion made in previous literature many years ago that patients who were slow acetylators or had the slow acetylation genotype were those patients who had a tendency to develop not just SLE, but other autoimmune diseases as well.

This study, even though negative, eliminates the possibility that slow acetylation is associated with the risk of SLE. Moreover, these authors tackle the hair dye issue, which I thought was put to bed many years ago. Unfortunately, the hair dye issue keeps surfacing, that is, the association of the use of hair dye in young women with the slow acetylation genotype that predisposes young women to the development of SLE. Apparently, this has also been eliminated in this article as any possible cause of idiopathic SLE.

R. G. Lahita, MD, PhD

Increased Serum Matrix Metalloproteinase 9 Levels in Systemic Lupus Erythematosus Patients With Neuropsychiatric Manifestations and Brain Magnetic Resonance Imaging Abnormalities

Ainiala H, Hietaharju A, Dastidar P, et al (Tampere Univ, Finland)

Arthritis Rheum 50:858-865, 2004 2–5

Introduction.—Neuropsychiatric manifestations of systemic lupus erythematosus (SLE) are common and may impact up to two thirds of patients so affected. The diagnosis of neuropsychiatric SLE (NSLE) is challenging to establish since no single laboratory marker or imaging modality has been reported that can serve as a gold standard. Increased activity of matrix metalloproteinases (MMPs) has been implicated in several disease processes. Serum MMP-9 levels were obtained to determine whether they are associated with neuropsychiatric manifestations, especially cognitive dysfunction, or cerebral MRI abnormalities in patients with SLE.

Methods.—The study included 44 patients with SLE and 43 healthy control subjects who underwent clinical neurologic and neuropsychological evaluations to identify neuropsychiatric manifestations. Participants underwent determination of MMP-9 levels, in addition to cerebral MRI scans with volumetric estimation of intracranial cerebral fluid spaces, T1-weighted lesions, and T2-weighted lesions. The European Consensus Lupus Activity Measure (ECLAM) index was used to evaluate SLE activity. The Systemic Lupus International Collaborating Clinics (SLICC)/American Col-

TABLE 4.—Comparison Of Serum MMP-9 Levels (μg/L) in 44 SLE Patients, by Presence or Absence of Specific Neuropsychiatric Manifestations*

	Neuropsychiatric Manifestations		No Neuropsychiatric Manifestations		
Manifestation	No. of Patients	MMP-9 Level	No. of Patients	MMP-9 Level	P
Cognitive dysfunction	11	80.8 ± 45.8	33	48.6 ± 34.2	0.027
Cerebrovascular disease	7	76.3 ± 43.9	37	53.0 ± 38.1	0.092
Seizure disorder	4	82.9 ± 50.1	40	54.0 ± 38.0	0.111
Severe depression	4	27.9 ± 12.2	40	59.5 ± 40.1	0.072
Polyneuropathy	3	106.2 ± 56.3	41	53.0 ± 36.3	0.081
Acute confusional state	3	62.4 ± 26.0	41	56.2 ± 40.4	0.442
Neuropathy, cranial	2	43.9 ± 45.6	42	57.3 ± 39.6	0.652
Aseptic meningitis	1	11.6	43	57.7 ± 39.3	0.106
Demyelinating syndrome	1	137.8	43	54.8 ± 37.8	0.125
Movement disorder	1	79.2	43	56.1 ± 39.7	0.288
Myasthenia gravis	1	64.1	43	56.5 ± 39.9	0.503

*Values are the mean SD. *P* values were determined by nonparametric analysis of variance.

Abbreviations: MMP, Matrix metalloproteinase; *SLE*, systemic lupus erythematosus.

(Courtesy of Ainiala H, Hietaharju A, Dastidar P, et al: Increased serum matrix metalloproteinase 9 levels in systemic lupus erythematosus patients with neuropsychiatric manifestations and brain magnetic resonance imaging abnormalities. *Arthritis Rheum* 50:858-865, 2004. Reprinted by permission of John Wiley & Sons, Inc.)

lege of Rheumatology damaging index was used to assess accumulated neuropsychiatric abnormality.

Results.—No significant differences were observed in serum MMP-9 levels between patients with SLE and control subjects. Patients with SLE who had at least 1 neuropsychiatric manifestation (NSLE patients) had significantly higher serum MMP-9 concentrations, compared with those of SLE patients without neuropsychiatric syndromes ($P = .009$). Serum concentrations of MMP-9 were significantly increased among patients with NPSLE who had cognitive deficits, compared with those with normal cognitive function ($P = .027$) (Table 4). Serum MMP-9 levels were significantly positively correlated with the volumes of T1-weighted and T2-weighted lesions in the brain MRI ($P = .031$ and $P = .015$, respectively). The concentration of serum MMP-9 was significantly correlated with the SLICC index and not the ECLAM index.

Conclusion.—Increased levels of serum MMP-9 in patients with SLE may indicate neuropsychiatric involvement, especially cognitive dysfunction. Serum MMP-9 concentration may be linked with small-vessel cerebral vasculopathy and increased risk of cerebral ischemic events in patients with SLE.

► There is no end to the fascinating molecular associations of clinical conditions related to lupus and various enzymes and molecules within the body. The current article documents an increase in MMP9 in patients with neuropsychiatric lupus. I learned something about MMP9 and its relationship to T cells and findings, such as demyelination. It looks and sounds like a cerebral C-reactive protein. Since neuropsychiatric lupus is so hard to diagnose, the levels of MMP9 might prove useful as an adjunctive laboratory test in this disease manifestation. I have some problems with the author's interpretation of the data since this molecule is so commonly elevated in so many other conditions. The most amazing aspect of this article is the author's correlation of the MMP9 levels with the MRI findings. I can see a rapid CNS diagnostic test on the horizon!

R. G. Lahita, MD, PhD

Experimental Models

An ACE Inhibitor Reduces Th2 Cytokines and TGF-β1 and TGF-β2 Isoforms in Murine Lupus Nephritis

De Albuquerque DA, Saxena V, Adams DE, et al (Univ of Cincinnati, Ohio)
Kidney Int 65:846-859, 2004 2–6

Background.—One of the most serious consequences of systemic lupus erythematosus is the development of kidney disease. Lupus nephritis is thought to result mainly from renal deposition of autoantibodies and immune complexes, which then triggers an acute inflammatory response characterized by the activation of leukocytes and renal parenchymal cells and the production of cytokines and growth factors. The chronic phase of nephritis can develop and is characterized by excessive deposition of collagen and other extracellular matrix macromolecules. Angiotensin-converting enzyme (ACE) inhibitors, such as captopril, are used to control hypertension. These agents by their beneficial effect on hypertension have been shown to improve renal function to a greater degree than would be expected. The effects of treatment with captopril on lupus nephritis were assessed, and the potential mechanisms of this agent's renoprotective effects were determined.

Methods.—Lupus-prone NZB/NZW F1 and MRL-*lpr*/*lpr* mice were treated with captopril or with verapamil, a control antihypertensive agent. The mice were monitored for nephritis, and their sera and tissues were analyzed for cytokine and transforming growth factor-β (TGF-β) expression.

Results.—The onset of proteinuria in prenephritic mice was delayed by captopril treatment but not by treatment with verapamil (Fig 1). Captopril treatment was also observed to retard disease progression when administered to lupus mice that had early disease and even to reverse severe proteinuria in some older animals with advanced disease. Captopril treatment also reduced chronic renal lesions but had no effect on the production of autoantibodies. A correlation was observed between improvement in renal disease and reduced expression of TGF-β in the kidneys. The in-vivo or in-vitro exposure to captopril was found to reduce splenic levels of type 2 cytokines (IL-4 and IL-10), which is suggestive of a possible role of the immune system in captopril-mediated disease modulation.

Conclusions.—Type 2 cytokines are known to promote lupus glomerulosclerosis; therefore, the finding of decreased IL-4 and IL-10 production in mice treated with captopril may be related to the renoprotective effects of captopril. It is suggested that ACE inhibitors act not only as selective TGF-β inhibitors but also as selective immunomodulators, for the improvement of lupus nephritis.

FIGURE 1

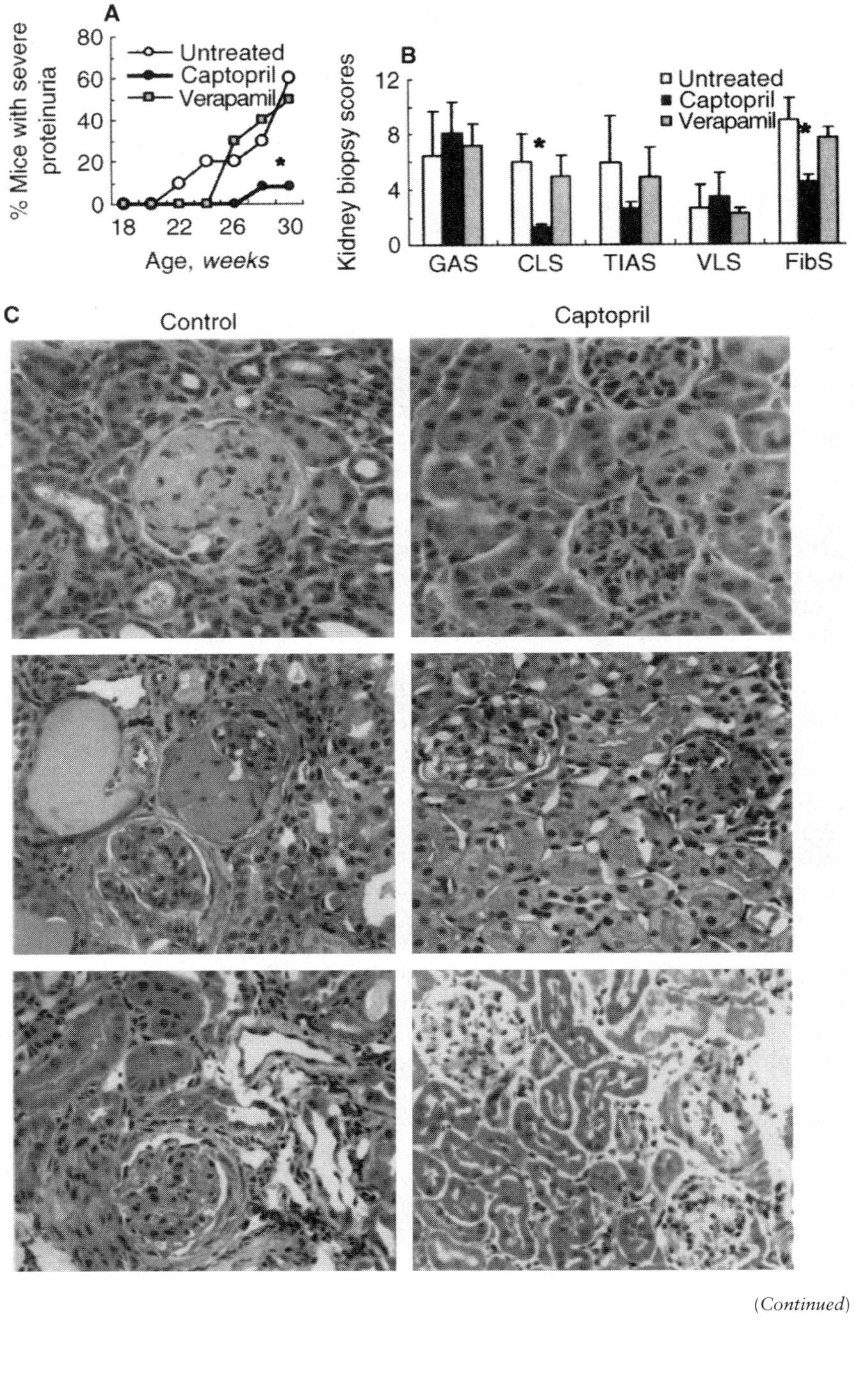

(Continued)

FIGURE 1 (cont.)

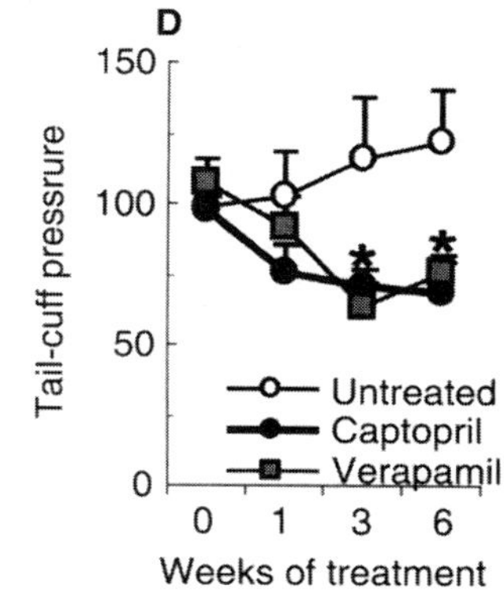

FIGURE 1.—Captopril treatment delays the onset of proteinuria and inhibits chronic lupus nephritis in BWF1 mice. Sixteen-week-old BWF1 mice were treated with captopril (n = 12), verapamil (n = 10), or left on normal drinking water (n = 10) for 14 weeks. (**A**) Mice were monitored for proteinuria by Albustix. Results are expressed as the cumulative frequency of severe proteinuria (≥3+ on two consecutive occasions). **P* < .02 captopril-treated versus verapamil-treated or untreated groups. (**B**) At 30 weeks of age, mice were sacrificed to analyze the effect of treatment on renal histology. Individual kidney biopsy scores, including glomerular activity score (GAS), chronic lesion score (CLS), tubulointerstitial activity score (TIAS), and vascular lesion score (VLS) are expressed as the mean ± SE. Immunofluorescence in glomeruli, blood vessels and tubules were scored on a scale of 0 to 3 in kidney sections stained with fluorescein isothiocyanate (FITC) antifibrinogen; the individual scores were summed to obtain a fibrinogen score (FibS). **P* < .05. (**C**) Representative renal sections stained with hematoxylin and eosin (H&E) (**upper panel**), periodic acid-Schiff (PAS) (**middle panel**), and Masson's trichrome (**lower panel**) are shown. (**D**) Blood pressure measurements are shown as the mean ± SE of the mean tail-cuff pressure on the 4th day of consecutive daily recordings. **P* < .05 to < .91 in the untreated versus captopril- or verapamil-treated mice. (Courtesy of De Albuquerque DA, Saxena V, Adams DE, et al: An ACE inhibitor reduces Th2 cytokines and TGF-β1 and TGF-β2 isoforms in murine lupus nephritis. *Kidney Int* 65:846-859, 2004. Reprinted by permission of Blackwell Science, Inc.)

► The effects of ACE inhibitors on scleroderma are well known. What is not known is what is reported in this very interesting article; that is, ACE inhibitors specifically inhibit certain TH2 cytokines. Cytokines of the anti-inflammatory varieties, which are associated with diffused proliferative glomerulonephritis, are inhibited by the ACE inhibitor used in this study, captopril. Captopril apparently has its major activities as well, inhibiting TGF-β. TGF-β is extremely important apparently in the production of proteinuria. The fact that the interleukin type 2 cytokines, such as IL-4, IL-10, and IL-13 are involved in tissue fibrosis, it makes sense that induction or use of a TH2 cytokine blocker would inhibit the fibrosis that one sees in scleroderma and also inhibit the proteinuria that one sees in lupus nephritis. This is an article well worth reading, if only for mechanisms of action of old drugs on new pathology.

R. G. Lahita, MD, PhD

Beneficial Effects of the Anti-oestrogen Tamoxifen on Systemic Lupus Erythematosus of (NZB×NZW)F1 Female Mice are Associated With Specific Reduction of IgG3 Autoantibodies

Sthoeger ZM, Zinger H, Mozes E (Kaplan Med Centre, Rehovot, Israel)

Ann Rheum Dis 62:341-346, 2003 2–7

Background.—Sex hormones have been shown to influence the immune system and to alter the course of autoimmune disorders. The effects of an estrogen antagonist, tamoxifen, on the course of mice with systemic lupus erythematosus (SLE) were investigated.

Methods.—Several groups of 8-week-old (NZB×NZW)F1 female mice were treated with tamoxifen (800 μg per mouse; twice weekly) or with double-distilled water for 4 months. The mice were evaluated monthly for the presence of autoantibodies directed against DNA and nuclear extract (NE) by enzyme-linked immunosorbent assay (ELISA). White blood cells and thrombocytes were quantified by a cell counter, and proteinuria was quantified by combistix kit. At 6 months of age, all of the mice that did not die spontaneously were killed and evaluated for the presence of glomerular immune deposits by indirect immunofluorescence assay. IgG isotypes of autoantibodies in the mouse sera and glomeruli were determined by γ-chain specific antibodies.

Results.—Treatment with tamoxifen resulted in a significant reduction in the production of antibodies directed against either NE or DNA. Reduction of antibody production against DNA occurred mainly in autoantibodies of the IgG3 isotype. In addition, tamoxifen had significant beneficial effects on the course of SLE in the (NZB×NZW)F1 mice. At 6 months old, 40% of the untreated mice died spontaneously, while all of the tamoxifen-treated mice were still alive. All of the untreated mice demonstrated severe thrombocytopenia and persistent proteinuria and had diffuse glomerular immune deposits of IgG2a and IgG3 isotypes in their kidneys. However, the tamoxifen-treated mice had a normal number of thrombocytes and only minimal proteinuria. In addition, glomerular deposits were detected in less than 40% of the tamoxifen-treated mice. These deposits were mainly of the IgG2a isotype and not of the IgG3.

Conclusions.—Tamoxifen has significant therapeutic effects on SLE in (NZB×NZW)F1 female mice. These beneficial effects apparently are associated with the specific reduction of IgG3 autoantibodies.

► Tamoxifen is an antiestrogen that has been tried in humans for the treatment of lupus erythematosus. Traditionally reported results from human testing suggest that the drug blocks the estrogen receptors but, in some cases, may act as an estrogen receptor agonist and actually stimulate the effect of estrogen on the immune system. Now, in an amazingly interesting study, these Israeli investigators show remarkable therapeutic effects of tamoxifen on lupus in (NZB×NZW) F1 female mice. The reduction that is seen in these mice includes the suppression of IgG3 antibody isotype. This isotype is of significant importance to diffuse endothelial immune deposits in this mouse strain. We all know that this is what kills this strain of mice, so we now have the use of an antiestrogen in murine lupus. What could its value be in human lupus?

R. G. Lahita, MD, PhD

Inhibition of Adjuvant Arthritis by a DNA Vaccine Encoding Human Heat Shock Protein 60

Quintana FJ, Carmi P, Mor F, et al (Weizmann Inst of Science, Rehovot, Israel)
J Immunol 169:3422-3428, 2002 2–8

Background.—Adjuvant arthritis (AA) is an autoimmune disease that is inducible in rats by immunization with heat-killed *Mycobacterium tuberculosis* (Mt). AA is characterized by peripheral joint lesions that share many, though not all, features with human RA. Mycobacterial 65-kd heat shock protein (HSP65) is a target of pathogenic T cells in AA; a T cell clone (A2b) specific for the epitope contained between amino acids 180 and 188 of HSP65 could adoptively transfer AA. The effects on AA of DNA vaccination using constructs coding for HSP65 (pHSP65) or human HSP60 (pHSP60) were investigated, with the objective of documenting the immune effects of DNA vaccination on the immune reactions to the Ags that develop at the peak of AA.

Methods.—Female Lewis rats were used in this experimental study. Groups of rats were injected with 200 µL of 10-mmol/L cardiotoxin into the quadriceps using a sterile 27-gauge syringe. The test DNA vaccine was administered 3 times at 5, 19, and 33 days after the cardiotoxin injection. AA was induced 12 days after the last injection of DNA. Blood samples were collected at day 12 after the last injection of DNA. Heat-killed Mt strain H37Ra was injected into test rats at the base of the tail with 100 µL of the Mt suspension. The day of AA induction was designated as day 0.

Results.—Both the pHSP65 and pHSP60 constructs could inhibit AA, but pHSP60 was more effective. The immune effects associated with specific DNA-induced suppression of AA were complex and included enhanced T cell proliferation to a variety of disease-associated Ags. Effective vaccination with HSP60 or HSP65 DNA had the paradoxical effect of causing upregulation of IFN-γ secretion to HSP60 and, concomitantly, to downregulation of IFN-γ secretion to the P180-188 epitope of HSP65. Variable changes in the profiles of IL-10 secretion to different Ags were also observed. However, vaccination with pHSP60 or pHSP65 was found to enhance the production of TGF-β1 to both HSP60 and HSP65 epitopes.

Conclusions.—The results are supportive of a regulatory cycle for HSP60 autoreactivity in AA and show that this control mechanism can be activated by DNA vaccination with both HSP60 and HSP65.

► This article deals with something called adjuvant-induced arthritis in susceptible rats, which is a condition produced by immunizing such rats with heat shock proteins from the *M tuberculosis* bacillus. These rats get erosive joint lesions that share many features with human RA. This article describes novel mechanisms to inhibit adjuvant-induced arthritis, and it has done so by understanding heat shock proteins. The heat shock proteins are quite an interesting group of proteins. There are both human and bacterial heat shock proteins, and the interesting aspect of this article concerns the vaccination of rats with a DNA that is a DNA from either 1 of these heat shock proteins. The differences found between the rats that were vaccinated with DNA and those who were not were significant. Effective vaccination was associated with an increased T-cell response to the specific antigen. Of course, the authors report that the effects seen were really the result of cytokine secreted by T cells that have been stimulated to react. In this particular case, the cytokines were a result of a downregulation of interferon-γ and the upregulation of IL-10 and TGF-β. These TH2 cytokines which are upregulated obviously have a markedly positive effect on adjuvant-induced arthritis. What never cease to amaze me are the various clinical conditions found in men or animals that are associated with 1 or another cytokine profile. In this case, the novel use of the DNA antigen to inhibit something as bizarre as TB-induced AA seems quite important. It may also be feasible in the human to control certain kinds of arthritis with a DNA vaccine in order to upregulate and not downregulate certain immune responses.

R. G. Lahita, MD, PhD

A Lupus-like Syndrome Develops in Mice Lacking the Ro 60-kDa Protein, a Major Lupus Autoantigen

Xue D, Shi H, Smith JD, et al (Yale Univ, New Haven, Conn)
Proc Natl Acad Sci U S A 100:7503-7508, 2003 2–9

Introduction.—Antibodies against a conserved RNA-binding protein, the Ro 60-kDa autoantigen, occur in between 24% to 60% of all patients with systemic lupus erythematosus (SLE). Anti-Ro antibodies are associated with photosensitivity and cutaneous lesions in these patients and with neonatal lupus, a disorder in which mothers with anti-Ro antibodies give birth to infants with complete congenital heart block and photosensitive skin lesions. In higher eukaryotes, the Ro protein binds small RNAs of unknown function (Y RNAs).

Since the Ro protein also binds misfolded 5S ribosomal RNA precursors, it may function in a quality-control pathway for ribosome biogenesis. Consistent with a role in the recognition or repair of intracellular damage, an orthologue of Ro in the radiation-resistant eubacterium *Deinococcus radiodurans* augments survival of this bacterium after ultraviolet irradiation. Mice lacking the Ro 60-kDa protein were created to assess the role of Ro ribonucleoproteins.

Findings.—Mice lacking the Ro autoantigen acquire an autoimmune syndrome that shares several characteristics with SLE in humans. The autoimmune syndrome in mice is characterized by anti-ribosome antibodies, anti-chromatin antibodies, and glomerulonephritis. In one strain background, $Ro^{-/-}$ mice exhibit increased sensitivity to irradiation with ultraviolet light.

Conclusion.—One function of the Ro 60-kDa protein may be protection against autoantibody development, possibly by sequestering defective ribonucleoproteins from immune surveillance. The finding that mice lacking the Ro protein are photosensitive indicates that loss of Ro function could contribute to the photosensitivity linked with anti-Ro antibodies in humans.

► Often we get the most insight into mechanisms of autoimmunity from people not directly involved in either the management of patients or the analysis of clinical signs and symptoms. Such is the case with this article written by a group of molecular biologists who are intimately involved in studying the expression of the antigen Ro. This antigen is involved in normal repair of intracellular damage within the mammalian body and even in bacteria (an orthologue) where this protein protects against radiation damage. Such is apparently the case with the mouse, since removal of this antigen results in an autoimmune disease characterized by anti-ribosome antibodies, anti-chromatin antibodies, and glomerulonephritis. The most important point of this article is that autoantibodies are again involved in the pathogenesis of disease and not just epiphenomena, as many believe.

R. G. Lahita, MD, PhD

Attenuation of Autoimmune Disease in Fas-Deficient Mice by Treatment With a Cytotoxic Benzodiazepine

Bednarski JJ, Warner RE, Rao T, et al (Univ of Michigan, Ann Arbor; Univ of California, Berkeley)

Arthritis Rheum 48:757-766, 2003 2–10

Background.—The current pharmacologic treatment for systemic lupus erythematosus (SLE) focuses on lymphocytes and includes corticosteroids, azathioprine, and cyclophosphamide. These agents are believed to induce cytotoxic responses to B and T lymphocytes, although the exact mechanism is unclear. The accompanying serious adverse effects limit the overall clinical benefit. A more selectively targeted approach to treat SLE is desirable. A novel 1,4-benzodiazepine (Bz-423) was developed and tested in mice, where it limited germinal center (GC) hyperplasia and the development of glomerulonephritis. Further study revealed it also preserves renal function and reduces nephritis when given to a strain of mice in which peripheral autoreactive T cells induce a lupuslike disease process. Normal immune mice who received Bz-423 showed no effect on lymphocyte activation, T cell–dependent delayed-type hypersensitivity (DTH), or T cell–dependent antibody production. Bz-423 was tested to determine its activity against lupuslike disease associated with defective Fas expression. Its cytotoxic activity, therapeutic potential in Fas-deficient mice, and therapeutic mode of action were examined.

Methods.—By using primary lymphocytes isolated from Fas-deficient mice (MRL/*MpJ-Fas*^{lpr} [MRL-*lpr*]), the sensitivity to Bz-423 was evaluated. Doses were given for 1 or 4 weeks, and the effects on cell survival were documented. The presence of nephritis, arthritis, antibody titers, and Th subpopulations was also determined. In vivo experiments used BALB/c mice to determine if the normal immune system is changed by Bz-423.

Results.—Bz-423 killed freshly isolated splenocytes in culture in a time-dependent and concentration-dependent manner. Although Bz-423 was effective against cells with defective Fas signaling, it showed no in vitro selectivity between MRL-*lpr* splenic lymphocyte lineages and subsets. Bz-423 selectively reduced MRL-*lpr* T cells, indicating that its in vivo effects are modulated by factors not present in the in vitro model. Mice that received 14 weeks of Bz-423 therapy developed significantly less proteinuria and had lower serum blood urea nitrogen levels than control subjects. Less histopathologic evidence of nephritis was also found (Fig 3). Normal glomerular architecture was preserved with this treatment. Although 40% of control subjects died with evidence of significant renal disease, none of those receiving Bz-423 had renal impairment. Synovitis was also significantly reduced in the treated mice, with less evidence of articular erosion or pannus formation. Normal immune function remained unimpaired when Bz-423 was given.

Conclusions.—Bz-423 was tested in MRL-*lpr* mice, which are defective in Fas-mediated activation-induced cell death. As a result, autoimmune nephritis was reduced and survival improved. Treated mice also had a blunted humoral autoimmune response but did not have alterations in their total immunoglobulin levels, and blood cell count indexes were normal. The immune response to autoantigens was reduced without altering total immunoglobulin levels or suppressing bone marrow hematopoiesis.

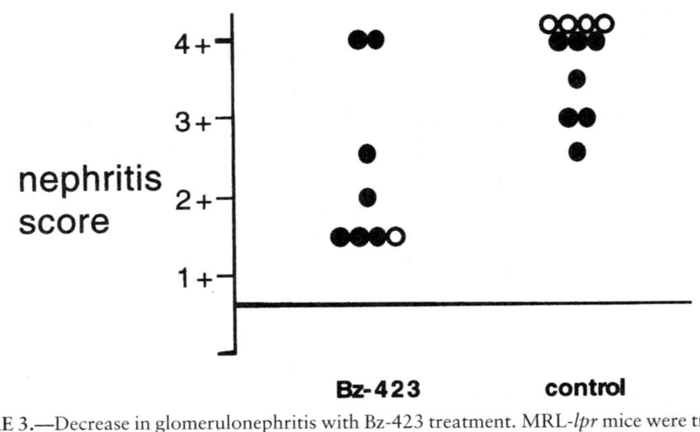

FIGURE 3.—Decrease in glomerulonephritis with Bz-423 treatment. MRL-*lpr* mice were treated for 14 weeks with Bz-423 or vehicle (*control*). At the termination of treatment period, glomerulonephritis was scored. *Open circles*, mice that died during treatment period. Histologic data were available for only 1 of the 3 Bz-423–treated mice that died during the study; however, all 3 mice had proteinuria measurements of <2+ before death, indicative of minimal glomerular disease. These animals died as a result of intraperitoneal adhesions causing bowel obstruction; the adhesions were caused by the injections. (Courtesy of Bednarski JJ, Warner RE, Rao T, et al: Attenuation of autoimmune disease in Fas-deficient mice by treatment with a cytotoxic benzodiazepine. *Arthritis Rheum* 48:757-766, 2003. Reprinted by permission of John Wiley & Sons, Inc.)

► In this study, the authors used, of all things, a benzodiazepine that promotes apoptosis in mice, specifically in Fas-deficient mice. These mice developed autoimmunity, namely SLE, in which B cells play a central role in the development and pathogenesis of the illness. The amazing thing here is that the administration of this compound to MRL-*lpr* mice reduces autoimmunity, specifically the deadly nephritis associated with the demise of the strain and the overall improvement of survival. It has always been the contention of many people that autoimmune diseases, lupuslike diseases in mice, are the result of faulty apoptosis at the organ level. In this study the benzodiazepine has very little effect on such things like total immunoglobulin and bone marrow hematopoiesis. As I read through this study, I of course thought of the general class of benzodiazepines and their widespread use in patients with and without autoimmune disease. If the data here are true, then experimental treatment of these mice with a new benzodiazepine containing natural product also affects the Th1-Th2 balance by blocking the anti-inflammatory response and I suppose shifting mice over to the Th1 response or inflammatory cytokines. All in all, this is a fascinating study that deals with a number of phenomena that cannot otherwise be explained.

R. G. Lahita, MD, PhD

Antinuclear and Other Autoantibodies

Anti-DFS70 Antibodies in 597 Healthy Hospital Workers
Watanabe A, Kodera M, Sugiura K, et al (Nagoya Univ, Japan; Social Insurance Chukyo Hosp, Nagoya, Japan; Scripps Research Inst, La Jolla, Calif; et al)
Arthritis Rheum 50:892-900, 2004 2–11

Background.—Antinuclear antibodies (ANA) are found in sera from patients with a variety of systemic autoimmune diseases and in sera from healthy persons. DFS70, which is also known as lens epithelium-derived growth factor (LEDGF), has recently been identified as a major ANA with a characteristic pattern in immunohistochemical analysis showing a nuclear distribution of dense, fine speckles (DFS) as the most common ANA in patients with atopic dermatitis. The antigen was designated DFS70, as a 70-kd protein was recognized on immunoblotting. Anti-DFS70 antibody was initially identified among ANAs from a patient with interstitial cystitis and has recently been identified among the ANAs in patients with atopic disorders. The prevalence of anti-DFS70 antibodies in a large number of healthy people was analyzed.

Methods.—The sera of 597 healthy persons working in 1 hospital (142 men, 455 women) were analyzed for ANAs and for anti-DFS70 antibodies by indirect immunofluorescence (IIF) with human laryngeal tumor cells (Hep-2) as a substrate and by immunoblotting using DFS70 recombinant protein and whole human cervical carcinoma cells (HeLa) extract.

Results.—ANAs were identified by IIF in 20% of all study subjects. Of the 597 persons evaluated, 9% were ANA positive at a serum dilution of 1:40; 4% at 1:80, 5.5% at 1:160, 1% at 1:320, and 0.3% at 1:640. There were 64 anti-DFS70 antibody-positive subjects. An unexpected finding was that this anti-DFS70 antibody-positive status represented 11% of the whole population and 54% of the ANA-positive population. The percentage of female anti-DFS70 antibody-positive subjects was 86%, compared with a percentage of 75% for female anti-DFS70 antibody-negative subjects. A decline was noted in the prevalence of antibody-positive sera with increasing age.

Conclusions.—Because anti-DFS70 antibody positivity is rare in patients with systemic autoimmune diseases, the introduction of the anti-DFS70 antibody examination as a screening test for ANA-positive persons could be used to exclude systemic autoimmune diseases, which would provide significant cost savings. This test would also be effective in identifying a subpopulation of healthy people in whom long-term follow-up might uncover other disease states, as anti-DFS70 antibodies have been demonstrated to be associated with some illnesses.

▶ This article deals with an antibody, which was looked for in a number of healthy hospital workers. There has often been the contention that autoantibodies occur in the normal population more often than we think. I think articles like this indicate that antibody positivity, though rare in systemic autoimmune disease, can be found in normal individuals. ANAs in this study were found in 20% of all individuals by IIF. Up to 30% of healthy people are after all ANA positive when HEP-2 cells are used as substrates. We have often warned about using an ANA screen to diagnose autoimmune disease. This antibody, believe it or not, which causes dense, fine speckles by IIF is called lens epithelium-derived growth factor with an initialism of LEDGF. The antibody is directed against that antigen. I have no reason to understand why this antibody would be more common than, for example, anticardiolipin antibody, except to tell you that this particular antibody causes specific immunofluorescence and it is obviously much easier to study.

R. G. Lahita, MD, PhD

Antiphospholipid Antibodies and Syndromes

Asymptomatic Avascular Necrosis in Patients With Primary Antiphospholipid Syndrome in the Absence of Corticosteroid Use: A Prospective Study by Magnetic Resonance Imaging

Tektonidou MG, Malagari K, Vlachoyiannopoulos PG, et al (Natl Univ of Athens, Greece)

Arthritis Rheum 48:732-736, 2003 2–12

Background.—In avascular necrosis (AVN) of the bone, cells in components of bone die because the blood supply is interrupted. The femoral head is the site most often affected. Often the patient remains asymptomatic or has nonspecific clinical findings. AVN is best detected by MRI. An assessment of the prevalence of AVN in patients with primary antiphospholipid syndrome (APS) and in those with systemic lupus erythematosus (SLE) with or without anticardiolipin antibodies (aCL) was undertaken.

Methods.—The 79 subjects were asymptomatic for AVN. MRI of the femoral head was performed in 30 patients with primary APS who had not taken corticosteroids, 19 SLE patients who had not taken steroids, and 30 healthy subjects matched for age and sex with the APS patients. The SLE patients were subgrouped into those who were aCL positive and those who were aCL negative.

Results.—Twenty percent of the APS patients had asymptomatic AVN, with 3 cases of intermediate bilateral AVN with a double-line sign and 3 of early uncomplicated AVN. None had abnormal findings on hip and pelvis radiography or dynamic scintigraphy. One patient had knee pain 3 months later and was found to have AVN in both knees. No changes were seen in the 6-month follow-up MRI. Unilateral bone marrow edema was the only MRI abnormality in 2 patients, but was found in a total of 4 patients. Edema had completely resolved at the 6-month assessment. Neither the SLE patients nor the healthy individuals had positive MRI findings for AVN. The mean age of the patients who had AVN was 31.2 years; the mean age of patients with APS but no AVN was 42.4 years. Patients with primary APS and AVN had livedo reticularis significantly more often than those without AVN, but no other clinical characteristics differed between the 2 groups.

Conclusions.—Asymptomatic AVN of the femoral head was seen more often in patients with primary APS than in those with SLE or healthy individuals. AVN occurred in approximately 20% of the individuals with primary APS, was seen more often in younger patients, and was associated with an increased incidence of livedo reticularis.

► This study is particularly important because it proves what has always been suspected: patients with primary APS do get AVN of major bones. In this particular study none of the patients with SLE, with or without aCL, who never received corticosteroids and none of the healthy control subjects had documented AVN. This indicates that something with regard to primary APS is important to the development of AVN. There have been isolated and sometimes anecdotal reports in the literature over a long period of time. Finally this study proves that the association is real. Undoubtedly in this population of young women with AVN there are probably many causes, among them steroid use, antiphospholipid antibodies, and other mechanisms as yet to be determined. This study is quite interesting in that it talks about a prospective study of those patients with asymptomatic AVN and primary phospholipid syndrome.

R. G. Lahita, MD, PhD

Anti–β_2-Glycoprotein I and Antiphosphatidylserine Antibodies Are Predictors of Arterial Thrombosis in Patients With Antiphospholipid Syndrome

Lopez LR, Dier KJ, Lopez D, et al (Corgenix, Westminster, Colo; Oklahoma Med Research Found, Oklahoma City)

Am J Clin Pathol 121:142-149, 2004 2–13

Background.—IgM and IgG anticardiolipin (aCL) enzyme-linked immunosorbent assays (ELISAs) are the most commonly used methods for detection of antiphospholipid antibodies, the presence of which is one of the major serologic criteria for the classification of antiphospholipid syndrome (APS). However, significant variability is seen in aCL results among clinical laboratories, and efforts by many groups to standardize the aCL assay have been unsuccessful. This lack of success in standardization is likely attributable to the heterogeneity of these antibodies, the complex nature of the interaction between cofactors and phospholipids, and the lack of participation of cardiolipin in regulation. An additional problem with APS is the low specificity of the aCL ELISA, which might result in possible misdiagnosis and unnecessary anticoagulation. The predictive value and association of 4 antiphospholipid antibodies with clinical manifestations of APS were assessed.

Methods.—The study group included 90 patients with systemic lupus erythematosus (SLE) and 100 patients with APS. The patients with APS were stratified into 3 subgroups: arterial thrombosis, venous thrombosis, and pregnancy morbidity. IgG, IgM, and IgA aCL, antiphosphatidylsterine (aPS), anti–B2-glycoprotein I (anti-B2GPI), and antiprothrombin (aPT) antibodies were determined by ELISA.

Results.—Anti-B2GPI and aPS antibodies had the strongest predictive value for APS in patients with SLE. The predictive value for APS attained 100% when 2 or more antibodies were present. Similarly, anti-B2GPI and aPS antibodies had a stronger predictive value and association for arterial thrombosis compared with that for venous thrombosis. Weak predictive value and association with pregnancy morbidity were observed in all antibodies.

Conclusions.—Anti-B2GPI antibodies have an important pathogenic role in arterial thrombosis. The results are also supportive of anti-B2GPI and aPS antibodies as providing the best diagnostic value for the laboratory assessment of APS.

► It has been very difficult to predict arterial thrombosis in patients with the APS, yet this article seems to indicate that thrombosis in such patients is easily predictable with aPS and anti-B2GPI antibodies. The study indicated that the predicted value of thrombosis was significant especially for arterial thrombosis. The predictive value of antibodies in association with pregnancy morbidity is described here and is quite important. I for one have been looking for a long time for something predicting thrombosis. I must say that after reading this article, I am no closer to being able to predict thrombosis than I was prior to reading it. I am sure the data have some significance but it is not apparent to this reviewer.

R. G. Lahita, MD, PhD

Randomized Study of Subcutaneous Low Molecular Weight Heparin Plus Aspirin Versus Intravenous Immunoglobulin in the Treatment of Recurrent Fetal Loss Associated With Antiphospholipid Antibodies

Triolo G, Ferrante A, Ciccia F, et al (Univ of Palermo, Italy)

Arthritis Rheum 48:728-731, 2003 2–14

Introduction.—Women with antiphospholipid antibodies (aPL) have a high rate of pregnancy loss and complications of premature delivery and uteroplacental insufficiency. These adverse pregnancy outcomes may be linked with poor placental perfusion caused by local thrombosis. The 2 most efficacious therapeutic regimens for treatment of women with recurrent pregnancy loss associated with aPL were compared. They are IV immunoglobulin (IVIG) and anticoagulation with low molecular weight (LMW) heparin plus low-dose aspirin.

Methods.—Forty women with recurrent abortion (minimum, 3 abortions) and repeatedly positive test results for anticardiolipin or lupus anticoagulant were randomly assigned to treatment with IVIG or LMW heparin plus low-dose aspirin. The treatment regimens were initiated when pregnancy was verified by a positive urine test. Treatment with IVIG was stopped at 31 weeks' gestation, aspirin was stopped at 34 weeks, and heparin was discontinued at week 37. The primary outcome measure was the rate of live births in the 2 treatment groups.

Results.—Characteristics of the 2 groups were similar at randomization. Women treated with LMW heparin plus low-dose aspirin had a higher incidence of live birth (84%) than those treated with IVIG (57%) (Table 2).

TABLE 2.—Major Outcomes of Pregnancy in the Study Groups

	IVIG Group	LMW Heparin Plus Low-Dose Aspirin Group	*P*
No. of pregnancies	21	19	
Live births, no. (%)	12 (57)	16 (84)	0.06*
Duration of pregnancy, mean ± SD weeks	38.3 ± 2.1	38.7 ± 2.4	0.67†
Birth weight, mean ± SD gm	3,246 ± 218	3,298 ± 236	0.46†
Preterm deliveries, no.	1	0	
Infants admitted to NICU, no.	1	0	
Congenital anomalies, no.	0	0	
Cesarean deliveries, no.	1	0	
First-trimester fetal loss, no. (%)	6 (29)	2 (11)	
Fetal loss after 13 weeks, no.	2	0	
Intrauterine death, no.	1	1	

*Fisher's exact test.
†Student's *t* test.
Abbreviations: NICU, Neonatal ICU; *IVIG*, IV immunoglobulin; *LMW*, low molecular weight; *SD*, standard deviation.

(Courtesy of Triolo G, Ferrante A, Ciccia F, et al: Randomized study of subcutaneous low molecular weight heparin plus aspirin versus intravenous immunoglobulin in the treatment of recurrent fetal loss associated with antiphospholipid antibodies. *Arthritis Rheum* 48:728-731, 2003. Reprinted by permission of John Wiley & Sons, Inc.)

Conclusion.—Treatment with LMW heparin plus low-dose aspirin is recommended as standard therapy for recurrent pregnancy loss due to aPL.

▶ There is concern about the treatment of pregnant patients with the antiphospholipid syndrome. Originally, the use of aspirin in women who had no miscarriages or any evidence of thrombosis was invalidated due to lack of effect. The outcome however in this study is fetal loss, which was present in 100% of the 383 women studied. We can now say that the efficacy of heparin (low dose) and aspirin was better than IVIG alone in the treatment of the pregnant female with documented aPL. Live births went from 83% for the aspirin and heparin group to 54% for the IVIG alone group. Treatment was safe and effective for both groups. This treatment awaits the consensus opinion of the phospholipid experts around the globe, but the data are legitimate and this should remain the standard until changes are suggested.

R. G. Lahita, MD, PhD

Clinical Aspects

Cigarette Smoking and the Risk of Systemic Lupus Erythematosus: A Meta-analysis

Costenbader KH, Kim DJ, Peerzada J, et al (Harvard Med School, Boston)
Arthritis Rheum 50:849-857, 2004 2–15

Background.—The etiology of systemic lupus erythematosus (SLE) is unknown, although genetic factors have been shown to have a role. The disease is 9 times more common in women than in men. The prevalence of SLE is apparently higher in nonwhite populations, and the severity of disease is greater. Hormonal factors have been thought to be fundamental to the development of SLE, and multiple environmental exposures have also been suggested for its development. Cigarette smoking has been causally linked to the development of autoimmune diseases, including RA, Graves' disease, and primary biliary cirrhosis. The studies conducted thus far regarding cigarette smoking and SLE have presented conflicting evidence for the role of smoking as a risk factor for development of SLE. The relationship between smoking and the development of SLE was retrospectively investigated, and a more precise estimate of this possible relationship was determined.

Methods.—A comprehensive computerized literature search was performed for all studies in all languages, using Medline and EMBASE (1966 to present) and the Cochrane Collaboration database, and hand searches were conducted of relevant bibliographies and abstracts of conference proceedings. The studies were reviewed in aggregate for heterogeneity and publication bias. The relationships of current smoking and past smoking (before the onset of SLE) to development of SLE were analyzed separately.

Results.—A total of 52 studies was identified and selected for review. Of these 52 studies, 7 case-control and 2 cohort studies were deemed appropriate for inclusion in this meta-analysis. For current smokers compared with nonsmokers, the odds ratio (OR) for development of SLE was significantly increased (OR, 1.50; 95% confidence interval [CI], 1.09-2.08). Former

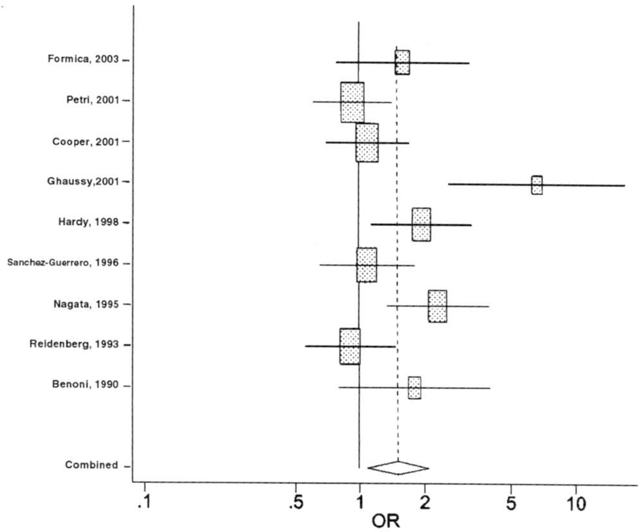

FIGURE 2.—Forest plot of the odds ratios (ORs) of systemic lupus erythematosus (SLE) developing in current smokers versus never smokers in the 7 case-control and 3 cohort studies, along with the meta-analysis summary estimate (*diamond*). The size of each box reflects the sample size (number of SLE cases) of the study, and the horizontal lines represent the 95% confidence intervals. (Courtesy of Costenbader KH, Kim DJ, Peerzada J, et al: Cigarette smoking and the risk of systemic lupus erythematosus. *Arthritis Rheum* 50:849-857, 2004. Reprinted by permission of John Wiley & Sons, Inc.)

smokers, compared with nonsmokers, did not demonstrate an increased risk of SLE (Fig 2).

Conclusions.—A small but statistically significant association between current smoking and development of SLE was identified in this meta-analysis. However, no association was observed between past smoking and development of SLE.

► Another nail in the tobacco coffin is this concise study that shows a significant association between smoking and the development of SLE. Caution is warranted in this collection of meta-analyses. Comforting are the words "previous smokers have no increased risk of developing SLE". The "N" is very small here but the data—analyzed in every statistical way—confirm the findings found in RA and smoking, and in SLE as well. Just what is it in a cigarette that "revs-up" the immune system?

R. G. Lahita, MD, PhD

Hormonal and Reproductive Risk Factors for Development of Systemic Lupus Erythematosus: Results of a Population-Based, Case-Control Study

Cooper GS, Dooley MA, Treadwell EL, et al (Natl Inst of Environmental Health Sciences, Durham, NC; Univ of North Carolina, Chapel Hill; East Carolina Univ, Greenville, NC; et al)
Arthroscopy 46:1830-1839, 2002 2–16

Introduction.—Nearly all autoimmune diseases are more common in women. The female predominance is especially strong in patients with systemic lupus erythematosus (SLE). Decreased androgen levels, increased α-hydroxylation of estradiol, and increased prolactin levels have been reported in patients with SLE. Hormonal and reproductive risk factors for SLE were examined in a population-based case-control investigation.

Methods.—A total of 240 women with SLE diagnosed between January 1, 1995, and July 31, 1999, who fulfilled the American College of Rheumatology classification criteria and 321 healthy control subjects matched by age, gender, and state were evaluated. Logistic regression was used to estimate odds ratios and 95% confidence intervals as measures of association, with adjustment for age, state, race, and education. Analyses were restricted to exposures before diagnosis.

Results.—Breast-feeding was linked to a reduced risk of developing SLE (odds ratio, 0.6; 95% confidence interval, 0.4-0.9). There was a statistically significant trend for number of babies breast fed and total weeks of breast-feeding. There were no correlations with number of pregnancies or live births. Natural menopause occurred earlier in women with subsequent development of SLE, compared to control subjects ($P < .001$). There was little correlation between SLE and current use of hormone replacement therapy or oral contraceptives and none with prior use of fertility drugs.

Conclusion.—There was little evidence that estrogen- or prolactin-associated exposures are linked with an increased use of lupus. The lower risk among women who breast fed one or more babies should be investigated further. Early natural menopause, rather than reducing the risk of SLE due to diminished estrogen exposure, may be a marker of susceptibility to the development of SLE.

► I have to place this article in the series for this year because the data refute the oft-held belief that exposure to estrogen or related compounds increases one's risk of developing SLE later in life. In fact, this study of 240 young female SLE patients shows that prolactin or estrogen exposure has little or nothing to do with the later development of SLE. Fertility drugs, estrogen contraceptives, or hormonal replacement therapy had little to do with the disease expression. Interestingly—and I have no clue as to what this means from an immunologic or endocrinologic point of view—breast-feeding decreases the risk of developing SLE. The data that would be of great interest to most rheumatologists would be the data on patients who took hormone replacement therapy or oral contraceptives after the disease was diagnosed. These data are coming, however.

R. G. Lahita, MD, PhD

Comparison of Risk Factors for Vascular Disease in the Carotid Artery and Aorta in Women With Systemic Lupus Erythematosus

Selzer F, Sutton-Tyrrell K, Fitzgerald SG, et al (Univ of Pittsburgh, Pa; Univ of Vermont, Burlington)

Arthritis Rheum 50:151-159, 2004 2–17

Background.—B-mode US and pulse-wave velocity (PWV) are used to assess atherosis and vascular stiffness, respectively, in women with systemic lupus erythematosus (SLE). Findings indicate that focal carotid plaque and intima-media wall thickness (IMT) are abnormal among women with SLE. In addition, traditional and SLE-specific risk factors for cardiovascular disease tend to be present to a higher degree in younger, premenopausal women with SLE.

Thus, SLE-related factors and aortic stiffness may contribute to the higher level of premature cardiovascular disease found in younger women with SLE. The risk factors for various stages of subclinical vascular disease in various vascular beds were assessed in 214 women with SLE who had no clinical evidence of cardiovascular disease.

Methods.—The 214 women were enrolled in the Pittsburgh Lupus Registry. Carotid plaque levels and IMT were determined by B-mode US. To measure aortic stiffness, Doppler probes collected PWV waveforms from the right carotid and femoral arteries. Other data were collected when the US evaluation was performed.

Results.—Sixty-eight patients had evidence of focal plaque. These women were significantly older, less educated, more likely to be postmenopausal, and weighed more than women who had no plaque. The median duration of SLE was longer, cumulative organ damage score was higher, SLE activity score was lower, prednisone was used for a longer period of time, and antidepressants were more likely to be taken for women with carotid plaque compared with those without. IMT values were greater for the women with plaque and their aortas were stiffer compared with those without plaque.

Women with plaque had significantly higher mean blood pressure and pulse pressure and were more likely to have hypertension. Compared with those without plaque, a greater percentage of women with plaque were taking antihypertensive medications, had higher mean total cholesterol levels and higher triglyceride levels, and showed higher median levels of the inflammatory markers C-reactive protein (CRP) and fibrinogen. Statistical analysis showed older age, higher systolic blood pressure, lower levels of albumin, and a smoking history to be independently associated with a higher plaque index, which indicated more severe plaque. Factors related to high IMT were older age, higher pulse pressure, low levels of albumin, high CRP levels, high cholesterol levels, and higher glucose levels.

The risk factors for high PWV were identified as older age, higher systolic blood pressure, higher C3 levels, lower white blood cell count, higher insulin levels, and renal disease. Women at potentially the highest risk for cardiovascular events had carotid plaque and IMT and PWV values in the highest quartile. The risk factors found in these women were older age, higher CRP levels, higher pulse pressure, lower pulse, antidepressant use, and higher fibrinogen levels.

Conclusion.—The risk factors linked to subclinical carotid plaque and IMT included the traditional cardiovascular risk factors plus CRP, which is a marker for inflammation. Subclinical aortic stiffness was linked to these traditional factors, but also to factors such as low white cell count and elevated C3 levels, which are characteristic of SLE. Both early adverse effects on vascular stiffening and later influences on wall thickening and plaque deposition caused by inflammatory-mediated processes appear to contribute to the higher rates of cardiovascular disease among women with SLE.

▶ This article talks about the risk factors associated with carotid plaques and IMT in women with SLE. The risk factors include SLE-specific variables related to immune disregulation and complement. One of the most common causes of death in SLE is accelerated atherosclerosis, which affects primarily women and is a result of chronic vascular inflammation. Women under the age of 45 years, as the article mentions, experience higher than expected cardiovascular disease, stroke, myocardial infarction, and hypertension among them.

In previous works from these authors, they used B mode US to evaluate carotid plaque and IMT among 175 selected women with SLE and noted that 40% of these women had evidence of focal carotid plaque and that their IMT was fairly substantial. The findings that higher systolic pressure, with stiffness of blood vessels, lower levels of high-density lipoproteins, and use of antidepressants and smoking were all factors that apparently affect or are risk factors for vascular disease and the carotid artery and aorta in women with SLE.

This is an extremely important article because it places other factors for vascular disease on a par that is equal to, or even in some cases higher than, cholesterol and dislipidemia, which has been thought for many years to be the mainstay of pathology with regard to coronary artery disease. It is very important to note that these factors are not necessary to the immune-mediated inflammatory process of SLE. Although present in a patient who has SLE, these factors can be of great significance and make a bad situation worse.

R. G. Lahita, MD, PhD

Patients With Rheumatoid Arthritis and Systemic Lupus Erythematosus Have Increased Renal Excretion of Mitogenic Estrogens in Relation to Endogenous Antiestrogens

Weidler C, Härle P, Schedel J, et al (Univ Med Ctr Regensburg, Germany; Schiller Univ, Jena, Germany)

J Rheumatol 31:489-494, 2004 2–18

Background.—It has been shown that women with systemic lupus erythematosus (SLE) and RA have abnormal patterns of estradiol metabolism, which may result in increased estrogenic activity. It has been suggested that

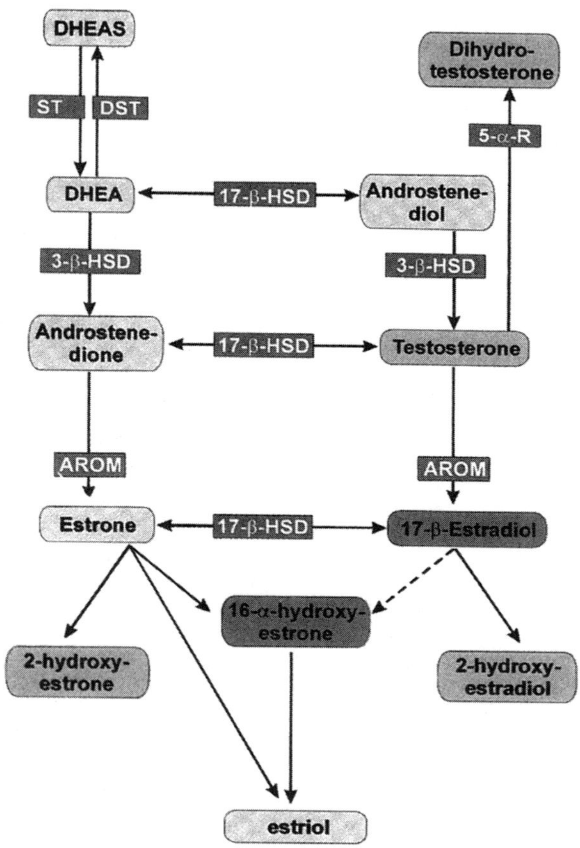

FIGURE 1.—The biosynthesis of steroid hormones. Precursor hormones such as DHEAS and DHEA can be converted to downstream androgens (androstenedione, testosterone) and estrogens (hormones below the aromatase enzyme [AROM]). The steroid hormones dihydro-testosterone, testosterone, 2-hydroxy-estrone, and 2-hydroxy-estradiol indicate supposed antiinflammatory activity. The steroid hormones 17-β-Estradiol and 16-α-hydroxy-estrone indicate supposed proinflammatory activity. *Abbreviations: DHEA*, dehydroepiandrosterone; *DHEAS*, DHEA sulfate. Enzymes: *3-β-HSD*, 3β-Hydroxysteroid dehydrogenase; *5-α-R*, 5α-reductase; *17-β-HSD*, 17β-hydroxysteroid dehydrogenase; *DT*, DHEA sulfatase; *ST*, sulfotransferase. (Courtesy of Weidler C, Härle P, Schedel J, et al: Patients with rheumatoid arthritis and systemic lupus erythematosus have increased renal excretion of mitogenic estrogens in relation to endogenous antiestrogens. *J Rheumatol* 31:489-494, 2004.)

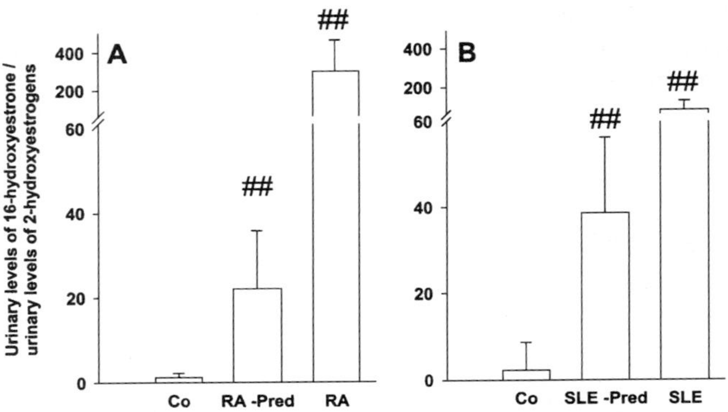

FIGURE 4.—Molar ratio of 16α-hydroxyestrone and 2-hydroxylated estrogens in patients with RA (**panel A**) and SLE (**panel B**). *Abbreviations: Co*, Healthy controls; *−Pred*, no prior prednisolone therapy. ## $P < .001$ for comparison of the respective median with control. Data are given as mean ± SEM (without unit). (Courtesy of Weidler C, Härle P, Schedel J, et al: Patients with rheumatoid arthritis and systemic lupus erythematosus have increased renal excretion of mitogenic estrogens in relation to endogenous antiestrogens. *J Rheumatol* 31:489-494, 2004.)

17β-estradiol plays a dual pro- and antiinflammatory role in these conditions, depending on its concentration or perhaps its conversion to downstream mitogenic 16α-hydroxyestrone or naturally occurring antiestrogens, such as 2-hydroxyestrone. The renal excretion of 16α-hydroxyestrone was compared with that of 2-hydroxyestrone in patients with RA and SLE and in healthy subjects.

Methods.—This prospective study included 30 patients with RA, 32 patients with SLE, and 54 healthy control subjects. Urinary levels of 16α-hydroxyestrone and 2-hydroxyestrogens were measured by enzyme immunoassay. Renal excretion was studied to estimate the time-integral of hormone production.

Results.—The urinary concentration and total urinary loss of 2-hydroxyestrogens were found to be 10 times higher in healthy subjects compared with those of patients with either SLE or RA, regardless of prior prednisolone treatment or sex (Fig 1). The urinary concentration and loss of 16α-hydroxyestrone did not differ between healthy subjects and patients with RA or SLE. No difference was noted between healthy subjects and patients with RA or SLE in the ratio of urinary 16α-hydroxyestrone. However, the ratio of urinary 16α-hydroxyestrone:2-hydroxyestrogens was more than 20 times higher in RA and SLE than in healthy subjects, regardless of prior glucocorticoid treatment or sex (Fig 4).

Conclusions.—A large shift is seen to mitogenic estrogens in relation to endogenous antiestrogens. Both steroids are converted from the precursor 17β-estradiol and estrone. The magnitude of conversion to the mitogenic 16α-hydroxyestrone is greatly upregulated in patients with RA and SLE, which is likely a contributing factor in the maintenance of the proliferative state in these diseases.

► Here is another study confirming the conversion of female hormone to very feminizing estrogens. In this article, these are called mitogenic estrogens. The latter title is derived from the effects of these estrogens on the mitogenicity of breast cancer cells. The 16 hydroxylated estrogens (16α-hydroxyestrone and estriol) are very potent—much more so than estradiol. As such, their role in the inflammatory diseases as cytokine stimulants can only be imagined, since no 16-hydroxylation data on cytokine levels exist. The key point here is that this hormonal shift is not disease specific (both SLE and RA). This hormonal pathway is of great interest to the pathogenesis of both diseases, as we can now realize.

R. G. Lahita, MD, PhD

Spontaneous Pregnancy in a Woman With Lupus and Thyroiditis Despite Imminent Premature Ovarian Failure

Le Thi Huong D, Gompel A, Wechsler B, et al (Groupe Hospitalier Pitié-Salpêtrière, Paris Cedex)

Ann Rheum Dis 63:108-109, 2004 2–19

Background.—A woman who became pregnant despite having lupus and imminent premature ovarian failure (POF) is described.

Case Report.—Woman, born in 1962, was diagnosed with Raynaud's phenomenon, photosensitivity, and subacute cutaneous lupus at the age of 15 years. She had 3 abortions before she was 28, when she was diagnosed with giant cell thyroiditis. Endometriosis was discovered 2 years later. Five years after that, at the age of 35, she showed signs of imminent POF, including polyarthritis, sustained climacteric symptoms, and an increased follicle-stimulating hormone (FSH) level (95 U/L). However, her menstrual cycles were only occasionally ovulatory, and tests were negative for antinuclear antibody, anti-dsDNA, anti-extractable nuclear antigen, and anticardiolipin. A few months later, she became spontaneously pregnant and at the age of 36, after an uneventful pregnancy, delivered a healthy baby girl.

Conclusion.—Despite lupus, hypothyroidism, endometriosis, and imminent POF, this woman became spontaneously pregnant and delivered a healthy baby.

► The article presented here is remarkable only for the fact that the patient described became pregnant after ovarian failure, in the face of hypothyroidism (giant cell thyroiditis), and systemic lupus. Any one of these could plausibly prevent her from getting pregnant. Moreover, she had an FSH greater than 40 and had not menstruated for some time. I cite this article because of the resilience of the ovary implicit in the description of this patient. She delivered a healthy baby girl despite the described findings and her apparent premature menopause. I salute this article as a tribute to the resilience of the female reproductive system.

R. G. Lahita, MD, PhD

Does Hermansky-Pudlak Syndrome Predispose to Systematic Lupus Erythematosus?

Mitsui H, Komine M, Watanabe T, et al (Univ of Tokyo)

Br J Dermatol 146:908-911, 2002 2–20

Background.—Hermansky-Pudlak syndrome (HPS) is a rare, autosomal recessive disorder that is characterized by oculocutaneous albinism, bleeding caused by a storage-pool deficiency of platelets, and lysosomal ceroid storage. The single gene responsible for this disorder is located on chromosome 10q23. Approximately 20 cases of HPS have been reported in Japan; however, among Puerto Ricans, the incidence is 1 per 1800. A case of HPS with systemic lupus erythematosus (SLE), in which a mutation was identified at codon 441 in the HPS gene (HPS1) is reported.

> *Case Report.*—Woman, 35, Japanese, whose parents were consanguineous, had oculocutaneous albinism at birth. At 26 years old, a malar rash, oral ulcers, and multiple arthritis developed. Close examination revealed serositis, nephritis, white blood cell (WBC) decrement, and positive antinuclear antibody (ANA). A diagnosis of SLE was made. The patient was treated with oral prednisolone, with the dose gradually decreased to 7.5 mg. At 34 years old, the patient was referred to the dermatology department of a university hospital because of new formation of malar ash and bulla on her extremities after exposure to the sun. The patient's hair was completely white, her entire skin was devoid of pigment, and her pupils were blue. Nail-sized scaly erythema was scattered across her nose and both cheeks. Egg-sized erythema were noted on both upper extremities, with coin-sized flaccid, bloody bullae on the erythema. Laboratory findings showed decreased WBC and platelet counts and decreased CH50 level. CT showed pulmonary fibrosis in the S6 and S3 area, which appeared as several focal low-density areas. The HPS gene mutation in this patient was analyzed in a previous report, which found 1-bp duplication of adenine at codon 441, an effect that caused a frameshift. These and other clinical and biopsy data resulted in a diagnosis of HPS complicated with bullous lupus erythematosus.

Conclusions.—The findings are indicative of the potential for a patient with Hermansky-Pudlak syndrome to be predisposed to SLE.

► On occasion I like to pick up an unusual article, and my question on the title of this article is "Does the Hermansky-Pudlak Syndrome predispose to SLE?" This syndrome is a rare autoreceptive disorder characterized by oculocutaneous albinism, bleeding caused by storage pool deficiency of platelets, and lysosomal steroid storage. Hermansky-Pudlak is a single gene disorder, and it is described here as being associated with the onset of oral ulcers and so forth. Off hand, I can't think of any pathologic connection between the onset of this condition and the onset of SLE. Since the condition lupus erythematosus is uncommon and Hermansky-Pudlak syndrome is extremely rare, the authors postulate that people with the Hermansky-Pudlak syndrome have a higher incidence of SLE. Various genes have been looked at but none have been indicated as responsible for SLE, although there is a small amount of discussion about things like albinism and photosensitivity in this syndrome as being responsible for the overproduction of apoptotic keratinocytes, which can be responsible for autoantigen exposure. All in all, it is an interesting little article on a rare syndrome and a very rare syndrome occurring together in the same patient.

R. G. Lahita, MD, PhD

Autoimmune Thyroditis During Leuprolide Acetate Treatment
Eyal O, Rose SR (Univ of Cincinnati, Ohio)
J Pediatr 144:394-396, 2004 2–21

Background.—Leuprolide acetate is a depot gonadotropin-releasing hormone (GnRH) agonist that is used to suppress puberty to ensure normal adult height in children with central precocious puberty. The case of a child who started treatment with leuprolide acetate and subsequently was diagnosed with autoimmune thyroiditis is presented.

Case Report.—Girl, 9 years, observed with menarche and central precocious puberty with rapid rate of progression. Her medical history was significant for congenital hydrocephalus and insertion of a ventriculoperitoneal shunt when she was 7 years old. The patient's family history was significant for type I diabetes mellitus and primary hypothyroidism in the patient's younger sister. Leuprolide acetate was begun at 15 mg (0.38 mg/kg) by IM injection every 28 days. At follow-up after 4 months of therapy, physical examination showed good clinical response to therapy with decreased breast firmness, decreased vaginal estrogen effect, and no further menses. At a follow-up visit after 8 months of therapy, the patient had a decreased level of energy and rapid weight gain (4 kg in 4 months). No signs suggestive of progression of puberty were identified on physical examination. Examination of the neck revealed a thyroid gland at the upper limit of normal size. Laboratory evaluation showed low T4 levels with increased thyroid-stimulating hormone (TSH). Treatment with levothyroxine 75 μg daily was initiated, with clinical improvement in energy level. Repeated laboratory evaluation was obtained after 1 month on levothyroxine and just before her next scheduled dose of leuprolide acetate, after which the levothyroxine dose was increased

TABLE 1.—Summary of Laboratory Evaluation*

Variable	Initial Visit	8 mo on Leuprolide Acetate	4 wk of Levothyroxine 75 μg	4 wk of Levothyroxine 100 μg	Normal Range (Prepubertal)
Chronologic age (y)	9.4	10			
Bone age (y)	10.5	11			
Height (cm)	140.6	143.2			
Weight (kg)	39	48.2			
TSH (μU/mL)	2.88	233.3	46.16	2.71	0.37-4.5
T_4 (μg/dL)	7.0	< 1.05	8.7	11.1	5.6-11.7
Free T_4 (ng/dL)	0.94	< 0.4	0.91	1.26	0.82-1.58
LH (mIU/mL)	2.7	9.8	6.0	2.6	<3.0
LH third generation (IU/L)			0.29		0.01-0.21
FSH (mIU/mL)	2.6	14.3	9.7	3.0	<2.5-7.8
FSH third generation (IU/L)			0.84		0.50-2.41
Estradiol (pg/mL)	14	3			5-10

*Assays were as follows: LH, FSH: ICN Diagnostics RIA (Costa Mesa, Calif); LH, FSH third generation: Quest RIA; Estradiol: Quest RIA (San Juan Capistrano, Calif); T_4, free T_4, TSH: Abbott ICMA (Abbott Park, Ill). (Courtesy of Eyal O, Rose SR: Autoimmune thyroiditis during leuprolide acetate treatment. *J Pediatr* 144:394-396. Copyright 2004 by Elsevier.)

to 100 μg daily. Laboratory data were obtained after 1 month on the higher dose and just before a scheduled leuprolide acetate dose. These data showed significant improvements in all thyroid variables and in follicle-stimulating hormone (Table). The repeated α-subunit level after 12 weeks of levothyroxine therapy was 1.8 ng/mL. The leuprolide acetate dose was unchanged throughout.

Conclusions.—This case is demonstrative of the importance of careful attention to thyroid status when GnRH agonists are given to patients who are at risk for autoimmune thyroid disease. It is also suggested that TSH levels be obtained before the initiation of GnRH agonist therapy and again at 6 to 8 months of such therapy.

► This is a very important article that describes the onset of autoimmune thyroiditis in a 9-year-old girl given a GnRH agonist to treat precocious puberty. The elevated estrogen levels are the key here, and the authors barely mention that as the possible etiology. This article reveals the intricate relationship between the immunology of the thyroid and elevated levels of sex hormones like estradiol. Intriguing is the overall effect of thyroid replacement therapy on the gonadotrophin levels. Moreover, the whole issue of TSH and α-subunit crossover with TSH and luteinizing hormone is as confusing to me as it probably is to the immune system.

R. G. Lahita, MD, PhD

Therapy

LJP 394 for the Prevention of Renal Flare in Patients With Systemic Lupus Erythematosus: Results From a Randomized, Double-Blind, Placebo-Controlled Study

Alarcón-Segovia D, and the LJP 394 Investigator Consortium (Instituto Nacional de Ciencias Médicas y Nutrición Salvado Zubirán, Mexico City; et al)

Arthritis Rheum 48:442-454, 2003 2–22

Background.—Nephritis is a major cause of morbidity and mortality in systemic lupus erythematosus (SLE). The use of immunosuppression with high-dose corticosteroids, azathioprine, methotrexate, mycophenolate mofetil, and/or cyclophosphamide is often required for management of the renal manifestations of SLE. However, the usefulness of these agents is limited by significant drug-induced toxicity. LJP 394 (abetimus sodium) was designed to halt the progression of renal disease of SLE by selectively reducing antibodies to dsDNA and their parent B cells via antigen-specific tolerance. LJP 394 is capable of crosslinking anti-dsDNA antibodies in solution or on the surface of B cells. In previous studies, it has been shown that the crosslinking of membrane immunoglobulin on the surface of naive B cells in the absence of T cells can help tolerize B cells via anergy or apoptosis. Whether LJP 394 can delay or prevent renal flare in patients with SLE and a history of renal disease was determined.

Methods.—In this 76-week double-blind, placebo-controlled study, 230 patients with SLE were randomly assigned to receive 16 weekly doses of 100 mg of LJP 394 or placebo, followed by alternating 8-week drug holidays and 12 weekly doses of 50 mg of LJP 294 or placebo. A high-affinity population of patients was identified by an assay measuring the affinity of the serum IgG fraction for the epitope of LJP 394 (80% taking LJP 394 and 90% taking placebo). Analyses were performed on both the intention-to-treat population and the high-affinity population.

Results.—Treatment with LJP 394 resulted in a decrease in antidouble-stranded DNA antibodies and a tendency toward an increase in C3 levels. In the intention-to-treat population, the time to renal flare was not significantly different between treatment groups, but the patients taking LJP 394 had a longer time to the institution of high-dose corticosteroids and/or cyclophosphamide (HDCC) and required 41% fewer treatments with HDCC. In the high-affinity population, the patients taking LJP 394 experienced a longer time to renal flare, 67% fewer renal flares, longer time to institution of HDCC, and 62% fewer HDCC treatments compared with the same variables in the placebo group. Patients with serum creatinine levels ≥ 1.5 mg/dL taking LJP 394 had 50% fewer renal flares. No renal flares were observed in the high-affinity group taking LJP 394 (Fig 5). Serious adverse events were noted in 25 (21.9%) of the 114 LJP 394-treated patients and in 34 (29.3%) of the 116 placebo-treated patients.

Conclusions.—Treatment with LJP 394 in SLE patients with high-affinity antibodies to its DNA epitope prolonged the time to renal flare, reduced the

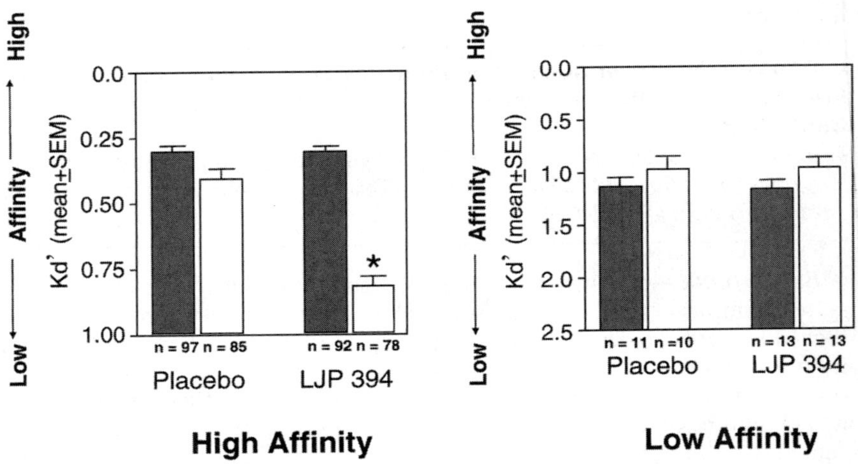

FIGURE 5.—Affinity analysis in the high- and low-affinity populations of the LJP 394-treated and the placebo-treated groups. Serum samples were evaluated at study entry (baseline; *shaded bars*) and after 4 months of treatment with LJP 394 (100 mg/week; *open bars*) or placebo. The initial affinities (*Kd'*) in the high- and low-affinity groups of both treatment cohorts were similar. There was a significant reduction in mean affinity in the high-affinity LJP 394 group after 4 months of treatment. Values are the mean and SEM. (Courtesy of Alarcón-Segovia D, Tumlin JA, Furie RA, et al: LJP 394 for the prevention of renal flare in patients with systemic lupus erythematosus: Results from a randomized, double-blind, placebo-controlled study. *Arthritis Rheum* 48:442-454, 2003. Reprinted by permission of John Wiley & Sons, Inc.)

number of renal flares, and required fewer HDCC treatments compared with the same variables for placebo.

► This article has a very-very interesting therapeutic aspect to it, and it deals with the drug LJP394, a tetrameric platform with native DNA on each of the tetrameric arms. Using antidouble-stranded DNA antibodies as a marker for systemic lupus renal disease, the authors of this article conducted a large double-blinded placebo-controlled study and were able to inhibit renal disease after injecting the tetramer. The drug has proven efficacy and was injected weekly in 100-mg amounts in about half of the participants. Initially, the data were not significant for the initial aspects of this particular study, but with time and the realization that DNA antibody affinity was a major factor in the induction of tolerance, the drug was shown to be a successful inducer of tolerance. The induction of tolerance is not easy and based on these studies, truly depends on the antibody affinity. In fact, this is a promising approach to all sorts of immune phenomena. There was a 67% reduction in renal flares in these patients and that is pretty profound. The exciting thing about these agents is that there are virtually no side effects associated with their use.

R. G. Lahita, MD, PhD

Autoimmunity

IL-1 Receptor-Associated Kinase 1 Regulates Susceptibility to Organ-Specific Autoimmunity

Deng C, Radu C, Diab A, et al (Univ of Texas, Dallas; Univ of Iowa, Iowa City)
J Immunol 170:2833-2842, 2003 2–23

Introduction.—Infection frequently precedes the development of autoimmunity. The correlation between infection with a specific pathogen and a specific autoimmune disease varies between moderately strong and very weak. This lack of correlation indicates that autoimmunity may result from the microbial activation of a generic versus a pathogen-specific host-defense response.

The Toll-like receptors, crucial to host recognition of microbial invasion, signal through a common, highly conserved pathway, activate innate immunity, and control adaptive responses. To ascertain the effect of Toll/interleukin (IL)-I signaling on the development of autoimmunity, the responses of wild-type mice and IL-1R–associated kinase 1 (IRAK1)–deficient mice to the induction of experimental autoimmune encephalomyelitis were compared.

Findings.—Both C57BL/6 and B6.IRAK1-deficient mice were immunized via MOG 35-55/CFA or MOG 35-55/CpG DNA/IFA. Wild-type mice developed severe disease. IRAK1-deficient animals were resistant to experimental autoimmune encephalomyelitis, demonstrating little or no CNS inflammation. The IRAK1-deficient T cells also exhibited impaired Th1 development, especially during disease induction, despite normal TCR signaling.

Conclusion.—It may be that IRAK1 and the Toll/IL-1 pathway have an important function in T-cell priming and demonstrate the one means through which innate immunity can control the subsequent development of autoimmunity. This may help explain the relationship between antecedent infection and the development or exacerbation of some autoimmune diseases.

► In a very cogent manner, the authors of this article provide a substantial amount of data on the possibility that multiple sclerosis could be an infectious disease. Specific mentions of some new and exciting mechanisms for immune responses constitute the bulk of this article. You will learn about Toll receptors and something called IL-1 receptor associated kinase 1 (IRAK1), which plays a major role in the establishment of a condition in animals called experimental allergic encephalomyelitis. The latter is a well-known model for multiple sclerosis, but the fact that it can only be caused in an animal with adjuvant therapy has always been an enigma.

This article takes us through the mechanisms, the possible alternatives, and the final belief that these molecules are essential to the autoimmune manifestations of possible infectious diseases (at least in rodents) like multiple sclerosis. For those of you who are prepared to spend a good deal of time analyzing bits of important data to understand new ideas in disease pathogenesis, this is your article.

R. G. Lahita, MD, PhD

The Protective Effect of 17β-Estradiol on Experimental Autoimmune Encephalomyelitis Is Mediated Through Estrogen Receptor-α

Polanczyk M, Zamora A, Subramanian S, et al (Oregon Health and Science Univ, Portland; Veterans Affairs Med Ctr, Portland, Ore; Warsaw Agricultural Univ, Poland; et al)

Am J Pathol 163:1599-1605, 2003 2–24

Background.—Autoimmune diseases, such as multiple sclerosis (MS), RA, Graves' disease, systemic lupus erythematosus (SLE), and myasthenia gravis, are sexually dimorphic, occurring more frequently in women than in men. Several factors may account for this dimorphism, but it is probable that sex-related differences in immune responsiveness and sex hormones play a significant role. It has been established that the first clinical symptoms of MS develop after the onset of puberty. It has also been determined that increased levels of sex hormones produced during pregnancy are associated with a significant reduction in the severity of MS. In addition, the clinical symptoms of MS are often exacerbated pospartum, a period that is characterized by significant alterations in sex hormone levels. Low-dose estrogen (E2) therapy has been found to significantly inhibit the clinical signs and histopathologic lesions of experimental autoimmune encephalomyelitis (EAE) and is currently being used in clinical trials for the treatment of MS. The role of intracytoplasmic estrogen receptors in mediating the suppression of EAE was investigated.

Methods.—Mice with disrupted estrogen receptor-α (*Esr1*) and -β (*Esr2*) genes were studied to determine which estrogen receptor is involved in mediating the protective effect of E2 on EAE.

Results.—The protective effect of E2 is abrogated in B6.129-*Esr1*$^{\mathrm{tm1Unc}}$ mice (*Esr1* −/−) but not in B6.129-*Esr2*$^{\mathrm{tm1Unc}}$ mice (*Esr2* −/−). This loss of E2-mediated protection from EAE in Esr1 −/− mice immunized with the encephalitogenic MOG-35-55 peptide was manifested phenotypically by the development of severe acute clinical signs and histopathologic lesions, even in the presence of moderately high serum E2 levels. A pattern that showed a lack of E2-dependent inhibition of EAE in Esr1 −/− mice was reflected in an enhanced rather than a reduced secretion of TNF-α, IFN-γ, and interleukin (IL)-6 in MOG-specific splenocytes and a lack of inhibition of message for inflammatory cytokines, chemokines, and chemokine receptors in CNS tissue.

Conclusions.—The immunomodulatory effects of E2 in EAE are dependent on *Esr1* and not *Esr2* signaling.

► This study is particularly important because it demonstrates the protective effects again of estrogen on a very interesting condition, that is, the murine model of MS, namely EAE. The authors in this article indicate that estrogen receptor-α is really the principle mediator of protection in this condition. The estrogen receptor-α is proven as the principle component involved in the pathogenesis of this condition by using mice that are either absent of estrogen receptor-α or -β. Those mice that lack the estrogen α-receptor do not respond to estrogen, and their MS-like syndrome continues to cause significant disability. At least in this disease, EAE, estrogen receptor-α plays a major role in the protection of the animals. This may give some significant insight into the effects of sex steroid hormones like 17-β estradiol on human MS.

R. G. Lahita, MD, PhD

Captopril Prevents Experimental Autoimmune Myocarditis

Godsel LM, Leon JS, Wang K, et al (Northwestern Univ, Chicago; Univ of Missouri, Kansas City)

J Immunol 171:346-352, 2003 2–25

Background.—Myocarditis treatments focus on reducing or eliminating the causative infectious agent and eliminating associated disease complications. Drugs used include diuretics, digitalis, (β-blockers and vasodilators, including angiotensin II receptor and angiotensin-converting enzyme (ACE) inhibitors. Captopril, an ACE inhibitor, is often prescribed. It can modulate chemotaxis, motility, adhesion, differentiation, activation, and cytokine and chemokine production by immune cells; ameliorate many cardiomyopathies; and decrease inflammation, calcification, and fibrosis. Its effect on experimental autoimmune myocarditis was investigated in the mouse model.

Methods.—Captopril 75 mg/L was given to A/J mice immunized with cardiac myosin or saline solution in their drinking water.

Results.—Both myosin- and saline-immunized mice had significantly higher levels of ACE than did untreated controls, so captopril was shown to effectively block the production of angiotension II by inhibiting ACE. Elevated serum ACE levels resulted when the captopril dose was increased or the treatment prolonged. The hearts of captopril-treated mice had a significant decline in the typical signs of myocarditis, specifically, hypertrophy, induration, and pallor. Reduced hypertrophy was also found through analysis of heart weight, body weight, and heart-weight–to–body-weight ratios.

These ratios in captopril-treated mice resembled the ratios in saline-immunized mice, so the reduction was attributed to the reduction in hypertrophy. The incidence and severity of myocarditis were significantly reduced by captopril, which suppressed inflammation, fibrosis, and necrosis. Captopril also significantly reduced the myosin delayed–type hypersensitivity (DTH) in mice immunized with myosin. This indicates captopril's role in influencing T cell–mediated inflammation in vivo. In assaying OVA (Sigma-Aldrich, St Louis, Mo) DTH in OVA-immunized mice that received captopril, it was shown that captopril significantly reduced OVA DTH levels, which suggests that captopril reduces inflammatory responses to self and foreign antigen, regardless of myocardial damage.

Captopril also reduced local inflammatory processes needed to induce DTH response. A local effect for captopril was shown by its ability to mediate the effects of DTH by a direct influence on T-cell function, T-cell trafficking, or generalized inflammatory suppression. Myosin- and OVA-specific antibody production was not influenced by captopril, nor did it affect antigen-specific T-cell proliferation or cytokine secretion, either in vivo or in vitro.

Conclusion.—Autoimmune myocarditis was ameliorated by the administration of captopril, which reduced cardiac hypertrophy, inflammation, necrosis, and fibrosis. Cell-mediated inflammatory responses were also reduced in vivo, but not by a direct effect on T cells. No effect was seen on either myosin- or OVA-specific antibody responses. Thus, patients who have autoimmune myocarditis may benefit from the use of captopril.

▶ This article really discusses another drug that has an effect on an autoimmune condition, which is the disease autoimmune myocarditis. Captopril is an ACE inhibitor, and these authors actually show that one can prevent autoimmune myocarditis using this drug. The mechanism is an interference of the drug with cell-mediated immunity because myosin DTH was reduced. Antibody production was not affected, but only DTH was affected, which is pretty interesting. The article also mentions that cytokines are really not affected in this particular trial.

The other thing to be learned from this article is that there are beneficial effects of captopril on human cardiomyopathy; infection-induced myocarditis; and, in the animal model, experimental autoimmune disease, primarily affecting the heart. This is quite important to understand in a condition that is not widely known among clinicians: that ACE inhibition may have a direct role on the immune system and the prevention of significant disease in a variety of models.

Interestingly, the authors conclude that the actual effect of captopril on proliferation of T cells or cytokine secretion is not important in this mechanism of action. This goes against what has been observed in other articles; however, the authors claim that their difference of results is really the effect of captopril on antigen-specific T-cell proliferation and cytokine secretion. The final conclusion of this article is that captopril reduces inflammation by decreasing cell-mediated immunity but does not affect T cells and really does not affect humoral immunity. It really is an anti-inflammatory drug in a very loose sense. This is quite an interesting pronouncement and one that clinicians should explore further.

R. G. Lahita, MD, PhD

Antigliadin Antibodies in Huntington's Disease

Bushara KO, Nance M, Gomez CM (Univ of Minnesota, Minneapolis)

Neurology 62:132-133, 2004 2–26

Introduction.—The significance of gluten sensitivity in sporadic and hereditary ataxia is not clear. The association between gluten sensitivity and Huntington disease (HD), a molecularly characterized hereditary neurodegenerative disease, was evaluated in patients with genetically confirmed HD.

Methods.—The study included 52 patients (21 women, 31 men; mean age 47.5 years) with HD. All participants underwent measurement of antigliadin antibodies (AGA), immunoglobulin (Ig) G and IgA AGA titers. The prevalence of positive AGA in patients with HD was compared with that of the general United States population.

Results.—Twenty-three (44.2%) patients had positive IgA (n = 13), IgG (n = 4), or both (n = 6) AGA (IgA or IgG AGA levels > 25 U/mL). The incidence of AGA positivity was significantly higher in patients with HD than that of the general population ($P < .00001$). No significant between-group differences were noted between AGA-positive and AGA-negative patients in age at onset (42.14 vs 36.10 years; $P = .065$), disease duration (9.09 vs 8.37 years; $P = .61$), disease stage (3.04 vs 3.13; $P = .78$), or the number of trinucleotide repeats (45.50 vs 47.75; $P = .66$). The AGA-positive and AGA-negative patients also did not differ in the prevalence of gastrointestinal symptoms ($P = .82$), prevalence of wheat intolerance ($P = .20$) or body weight (158.20 vs 161.50 lb; $P = .67$).

Conclusion.—A previously unrecognized association may exist between AGA and HD. This, along with earlier data, questions whether "gluten ataxia" is a distinct disease entity.

► HD is a neurodegenerative hereditary illness that is quite devastating. For some reason, the authors of this article decided to look at the incidence of gliadin antibodies in patients with HD, and the results indicate that some 44% of patients with HD have such antibodies. All of us have at 1 time or another seen a case of polyneuropathy with celiac disease or dermatitis herpetiformis. The ultimate diagnosis can be quite challenging, and the assessment of gliadin antibodies is not always a first thought on clinical presentation. Here we have yet another immune response that might have a role in the ultimate pathologic presentation. I for one have never seen "gluten ataxia," which the authors conclude is similar to many of the other ataxic illnesses like HD. While the results are interesting, this could be yet another epiphenomenon.

R. G. Lahita, MD, PhD

Oral Contraceptive Induced Chorea: Another Condition Associated With Anti-basal Ganglia Antibodies

Miranda M, Cardoso F, Giovannoni G, et al (Univ of Chile, Santiago; Federal Univ of Minas Gerais, Brazil; Inst of Neurology, London)

J Neurol Neurosurg Psychiatry 75:327-328, 2004 2–27

Background.—The use of oral contraceptives (OCs) is an infrequent cause of chorea. It has been proposed that the development of chorea in this setting is the result of the reactivation of Sydenham's chorea, but this antecedent is not present in some patients, whereas in other patients, the development of chorea in patients using OCs has been related to the development of other autoimmune disorders, such as systemic lupus erythematosus (Table 1). No previous studies have been reported of an association of this form of chorea with the presence of antibasal ganglia antibodies, a condition that would be supportive of an immunologic mechanism for the pathogenesis of this disorder. A case of chorea development in a patient that was triggered by the use of OCs with no definite evidence of previous Sydenham's chorea or recent streptococcal infections is reported.

Case Report.—Woman, 19, previously healthy college student, observed with abnormal facial grimacing and writhing movements of her left hand, conditions that developed insidiously and followed a stable course during a year without exacerbation or remission. The patient related no premonitory urges and could not control the movements at will. Her college performance was unaffected, and no evidence was noted of cognitive or psychiatric manifestations or obsessive-compulsive behavior. The patient reported that she had begun taking an OC 1 year earlier, which contained ciproterona 2 mg and ethinylestradiol 0.035 mg, for a menstrual irregularity. She had never been pregnant. Her family history was not relevant, and she had no previous history of rheumatic fever, or antecedent streptococcal or other infections. Her general medical examination was normal. Neurologic examination showed the presence of facial grimacing, mainly affecting the lower face, and choreiform movements of the left hand. The patient reported that the abnormal movements, though mild, adversely affected her social functioning. Laboratory evaluation, throat culture, blood work, and MRI findings were unremarkable. Western immunoblotting demonstrated the presence of antibasal antibodies and revealed reactivity against antigens of 40 and 45 kDa. These 40- and 45-kDa bands appeared to be relatively specific for the group of disorders associated with antibasal ganglia antibodies. The patient's neurologic symptoms subsided gradually 2 months after the initiation of treatment with sulpiride 300 mg daily and the withdrawal of the OC pill. Neurologic examination 2 months after cessation of sulpiride therapy yielded normal findings.

TABLE 1.—Clinical Features of Patients With Chorea Associated With the Use of Oral Contraceptives in the Last 23 Years

Reference	Patient Age (Years)	Time of Use	Duration of Chorea (Weeks)	Clinical Presentation/ Onset	Medical History	Comments
Nausieda[2]	20	12 weeks	1	Hemichorea/ insidious	Congenital cardiopathy	
	17	2 weeks	2	Bilateral/ insidious	Sydenham's chorea	
	18	8 weeks	3	Bilateral/ insidious	Sydenham's chorea	
	21	2 weeks	2	Bilateral/ insidious	Congenital cardiopathy	
	20	11 weeks	2	Hemichorea/ insidious	Purpura	Normal pregnancy
Dove[7]	20	8 months	8	Hemichorea/ insidious	Rheumatic fever	2 normal pregnancies
Greene[8]	16	2 months	8	Bilateral/ insidious	Syndenham's chorea	Chorea gravidarum
Buge[9]	26	2 months	6	Hemichorea/ insidious	None	
	23	8 years	2	Hemichorea/ insidious		Normal pregnancy
Berger[10]	21	4 years	4	Hemichorea/ insidious	None	Normal pregnancy
Vela[15]	27	Not specified	16	Hemichorea/ insidious	None	PET with FDG showed increased glucose metabolism in contralateral caudate nucleus
Present case	19	2 years	57	Hemichorea/ insidious	None	Presence of anti-basal ganglia antibodies

Abbreviations: PET, Positron emission tomography; *FDG,* ^{18}F-fluorodeoxyglucose.
Note: See original article for references.
(Courtesy of Miranda M, Cardoso F, Giovannoni G, et al: Oral contraceptive induced chorea: Another condition associated with anti-basal ganglia antibodies. *J Neurol Neurosurg Psychiatry* 75:327-328, 2004, with permission from the BMJ Publishing Group.)

Conclusions.—Chorea, triggered by the use of OCs, developed with no definite evidence of previous Sydenham's chorea or recent streptococcal infections. This patient was found to have positive antibasal ganglia antibodies, a finding that is supportive of an immunologic basis for the pathophysiologic characteristics of this chorea.

► This article is literally a 1-page review of all of the cases of OC-induced chorea. Only in this article are antibasal ganglia antibodies described in some detail. If this is the case for all such OC-induced chorea, it might be another very postinfection (with streptococci) detrimental effect of estrogens. Estrogens can stimulate the production of many different antibodies in both animals and people.

R. G. Lahita, MD, PhD

Evidence Linking Neuronal Cell Death to Autoimmunity in Alzheimer's Disease

D'Andrea MR (Johnson & Johnson Pharmaceutical Research and Development, Spring House, Pa)

Brain Res 982:19-30, 2003 2–28

Background.—Alzheimer's disease (AD) is associated with the loss of neurons and the development of amyloid plaques and cerebral amyloid angiopathy. Dysfunction of the blood-brain barrier (BBB) in patients with AD results in the extravasation of serum proteins into the brain parenchyma. Whether the anomalous presence of serum immunoglobulins (Igs) in the brain might be a cause of neuron loss in AD was investigated.

Methods.—Cortical and hippocampal postmortem brain tissues were obtained from 18 patients with sporadic AD and 13 age-matched subjects without AD. Tissue sections were incubated with antibodies to IgG, IgA, IgM, pan-Ig (which recognizes IgG, IgA, and IgM), and cleaved caspase 3 (a marker of apoptosis). Antigen expression was examined by immunohistochemical analysis. Micrographs of the stained areas were analyzed to determine the percentage of Ig immunolabeling ($^{+}$Ig for positive and $^{-}$Ig for negative immunoreactivity) in the total tissue area and to compare the distribution and characteristics of neurons positive for Ig ($^{+}$Ig-neurons) between the 2 groups.

Results.—Ig immunolabeling (IgG, IgM, and/or IgA) was significantly increased in the parenchyma of brain tissues from patients with AD compared with that of the control subjects (>50% Ig immunoreactivity in the AD tissues vs <10% in the control tissues). Ig immunolabeling in the control brains was associated only with vessels, whereas Ig immunoreactivity was present throughout the AD brain parenchyma. In both the AD and control tissues, $^{+}$Ig-neurons were much more common in areas with greater parenchymal Ig reactivity. Many $^{+}$Ig-neurons had morphologic signs of degeneration (eg, cell atrophy, dense nuclear chromatin), whereas neighboring $^{-}$Ig-neurons appeared normal. Furthermore, significantly more $^{+}$Ig-neurons in the AD tissue showed neurodegenerative changes than did $^{+}$Ig-neurons in the control tissues, and virtually all of the neurons showing degeneration were Ig positive. Some of the $^{+}$Ig-neurons with neurodegenerative changes expressed caspase 3, but caspase 3 was not seen in any of the $^{-}$Ig-neurons. In contrast, $^{+}$Ig-astrocytes appeared healthy in both AD and control tissues.

Conclusion.—Neuronal death in AD is directly linked to the presence of neuron-specific autoantibodies in the serum and to an impaired BBB. These findings suggest plasma exchange therapy to remove circulating Igs could be useful in treating AD, as could therapeutic interventions at the BBB level to restrict Ig penetration into the brain.

► Everything else has autoimmunity as its basis, so why not AD? These authors hypothesize that autoimmunity is involved in AD because they find an Ig adherence to neurons from patients with the disease. More specifically, antineuronal antibodies, perhaps like those seen in systemic lupus erythematosus (SLE), are found in the cerebral fluid and on neurons by histochemical staining, and there is putative disruption of the BBB. The article is extensive, and the photos of neurons that are stained with antibody are numerous. The author himself admits that this theory is very controversial, but he presents rather interesting data that are plausible on the surface. There are many suspected pathogenetic theories that go with this very important illness and 1 is amyloid, which would be a natural result of such immune findings. It is difficult to bring objectivity to this article since the author's data are riveting and convincing, and this reviewer is an immunologist and accepting of such data.

R. G. Lahita, MD, PhD

An Association of IgG Anti-Laminin-1 Autoantibodies With Endometriosis in Infertile Patients

Inagaki J, Sugiura-Ogasawara M, Nomizu M, et al (Okayama Univ, Japan; Nagoya City Univ, Japan; Hokkaido Univ, Sapporo, Japan; et al)
Hum Reprod 18:544-549, 2003 2–29

Background.—At least 15 different isoforms of laminin, a major basement membrane glycoprotein, have been identified. Laminin-1 appears to play important roles in embryogenesis, embryonic implantation, and placentation. Serum IgG anti-laminin-1 autoantibodies are significantly linked to recurrent first-trimester miscarriages. On the basis of this and other evidence, it is likely that anti-laminin-1 autoantibodies are responsible for reproductive failure during the early stages of pregnancy. The prevalence of IgG anti-laminin-1 autoantibodies in infertile patients was assessed to determine if the antibodies are linked with reproductive disorders during the preimplantation and peri-implantation stages specifically. Additionally, any relation between the antibodies and endometriosis was sought to determine if they operate in endometriosis-associated infertility.

Methods.—Either laparoscopy or laparotomy was performed in 68 infertile patients and 39 healthy nonpregnant women to look for IgG anti-laminin-1 antibodies. Links between the antibodies and endometriosis were assessed. Lesions of endometriosis displayed laminin-1 mRNA.

Results.—The levels of immunoglobulin G anti-laminin-1 antibodies were significantly higher in infertile patients than in the healthy nonpregnant women. Antibodies were present in 20 infertile patients and with endometriosis in 17 of 42 infertile women. No other causes of infertility were related to antibodies. Comparing women with and without endometriosis, significantly elevated levels of the antibodies were found in 42 infertile women who had endometriosis than in those without endometriosis (Fig 2). Adopting a threshold value of 1.0 U/mL yielded a diagnostic validity of antibody assay to detect endometriosis in infertile women whose sensitivity was 43%, specificity 89%, positive predictive value 86%, and negative predictive value 49%. When the severity of endometriosis was divided into 4 stages, higher stages had significantly higher levels of antibodies than stage I, which had the same level as found in patients without endometriosis. antibody

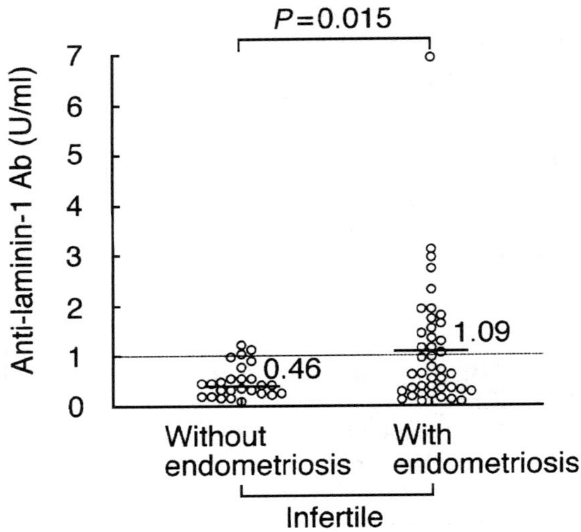

FIGURE 2.—Comparison of IgG values of anti-laminin-1 autoantibodies between infertile patients with or without endometriosis. *Dotted* and *solid* lines show threshold and mean values of the antibodies, respectively. (Courtesy of Inagaki J, Sugiura-Ogasawara M, Nomizu M, et al: An association of IgG anti-laminin-1 autoantibodies with endometriosis in infertile patients. *Hum Reprod* 18:544-549, 2003. Copyright European Society for Human Reproduction and Embryology, reproduced by permission of Oxford University Press/Human Reproduction.)

binding to intact laminin-1 molecule and to laminin-α1 chain G domain showed a good correlation, indicating that a potential epitope for the antibodies is located in the G domain. The mRNA encoding for the chains of laminin-1 was detected in tissues at all 4 stages of endometriosis.

Conclusions.—A strong association was found between the presence of anti-laminin-1 antibodies and infertility, particularly that caused by endometriosis. A specific domain, the laminin-α1 chain G domain, was identified by the antibodies. Ninety percent of endometriotic lesions had laminin mRNA present. Thus, an assessment of IgG anti-laminin-1 autoantibodies may prove of value in diagnosing and treating endometriosis.

▶ Patients with endometriosis are characteristically infertile. We have always thought that endometriosis is an autoimmune disease. In this particular study the association of an autoantibody against laminin-1, a major basement membrane glycoprotein consisting of 3 different subunits, was described in a large number of patients with endometriosis. As the authors state, this may be an early test to look at a noninvasive means of diagnosing endometriosis. More importantly, this report indicates that endometriosis itself is a disease in which the immune system is intimately involved. These antibodies are associated with infertility, and we all know that endometriosis is a major source of infertility for young women. The authors detected laminin mRNA in 90% of endometriotic lesions. One can only wonder what relationship this antibody has with endometriosis, explanted uterine cells that grow with abandon in patients with a variety of autoimmune diseases, as well as of and by itself a cause of infertility. The authors hypothesized in an original way that these endometrial cells developed after the adhesion, proliferation, and migration of these endometrial implants was affected by immune mechanisms. And this hypothesis cannot be rejected. I suppose the laminins are important here because they are involved in an adhesion process. This is a very interesting study that brings reproductive immunology to the forefront with specific autoantibodies that are directed against specific molecules involved in cellular implantation, indicating that endometriosis can be autoimmune on several fronts.

R. G. Lahita, MD, PhD

High Prevalence of Autoimmune Thyroid Disease in Pulmonary Arterial Hypertension

Chu JW, Kao PN, Faul JL, et al (Stanford Univ, Calif)

Chest 122:1668-1673, 2002 2–30

Background.—Hyperthyroidism, hypothyroidism, and thyroglobulin antibodies have all been described in patients with pulmonary arterial hypertension (PAH). All 3 of these are autoimmune thyroid diseases (AITDs) and share immunogenetic features, which suggests that an immune system dysfunction may be the link between PAH and thyroid disease. This association was investigated by determination of the prevalence of thyroid disease in patients with PAH.

Methods.—The research subjects were 63 adults (10 men and 53 women; mean age, 47 years) with PAH (sustained pulmonary artery systolic pressure, >25 mm Hg). Research subjects were tested to detect thyroid gland dysfunction (goiter, levels of thyrotropin and free thyroxine) and immune system dysfunction (antibodies to thyroglobulin and thyroid peroxidase). They were also questioned to identify any first-degree relatives with AITD.

Results.—Almost half of these patients with PAH—31, or 49%—had AITD. This included 16 of 24 patients (67%) with idiopathic PAH, 4 of 6 patients (67%) with anorexigen-associated PAH, 5 of 13 patients (38%) with PAH associated with connective tissue disease, 4 of 11 patients (36%) with PAH associated with drug abuse, and 2 of 6 patients (33%) with PAH associated with liver disease. Of these 31 patients, 13 (42%) had already had a diagnosis of AITD; however, 8 (58%) were given a diagnosis during the study, and half of these (9 patients, or 50%) required pharmacologic treatment. No temporal relationship between the onset of PAH and the diagnosis of AITD could be identified. Half the patients (16 [51.6%], including 8 patients with AITD) had 24 first-degree relatives being treated for either Graves' disease or Hashimoto's disease.

Conclusion.—About half of these patients with PAH had concomitant AITD, and about half had first-degree relatives with AITD. These findings suggest PAH and AITD may be linked by a common immunogenetic susceptibility. Understanding this association may enable more effective diagnosis and treatment of AITD and PAH. The data also support testing patients with PAH for occult thyroid dysfunction.

► The association of AITD with PAH is another mystery of rheumatology and medicine. The suggestion that the thyroid disease caused the PAH or that the PAH caused the thyroid disease is not tenable. However, the association of thyroid pathology with many autoimmune disorders strongly suggests that this PAH is indeed autoimmune. The point made in the article, namely that the thyroid disease can exacerbate the PAH, is a good one. The suggestion of an immunogenetic link between the 2 diseases is not tenable. As with the other connective tissue diseases, this link to the thyroid is quite remarkable and totally unexplained.

R. G. Lahita, MD, PhD

Complement Activation by Direct C4 Binding to Thyroperoxidase in Hashimoto's Thyroiditis

Blanchin S, Estienne V, Durand-Gorde J-M, et al (Université de la Méditerranée, Marseille, France)

Endocrinology 144:5422-5429, 2003 2–31

Introduction.—Biosynthesis of thyroid hormones is an oxidative process that produces reactive oxygen species. It involves thyroperoxidase (TPO), one of the primary autoantigens involved in autoimmune thyroid diseases. A large N-terminal myeloperoxidase-like module, followed by a complement control protein (CCP)–like module and an epidermal growth factor–like module, comprises the ectodomain of TPO.

The presence of these 2 additional gene modules indicates that they may have some crucial and previously unsuspected role in thyroid function. The CCP module is a constituent of the molecule involved in the activation of C4 complement compound. The possibility that C4 could bind to TPO and activate the complement pathway in autoimmune conditions was examined.

Findings.—Thyroperoxidase via its CCP module directly activated complement without any intervention by immunoglobulin. It may be that this additional complement pathway needs the production of reactive oxygen species and especially hydroxyl radicals that aggregate TPO and oxidize methionines of C4. In patients with Hashimoto's thyroiditis (HD), thyrocytes overexpress C4 and all of the downstream components of the complement pathway.

Conclusion.—It appears that evaluating this complement pathway would provide an excellent means for achieving a better understanding of the etiology of other degenerative diseases.

► I have always believed that HD has some importance to the manifestations of diseases like lupus and fibromyalgia. These are 2 entities where this manifestation is commonly found. Some have even suggested that the incidence of HD in these diseases can approximate 60%. Many women, moreover, with aches, pains, and weight gain eventually have nothing but a weakly positive antinuclear antibody and HD as their major clinical manifestation. We have also been taught not to do anything about the HD since it often resolves on its own, especially if the thyroid-stimulating hormone is normal.

Now this article describes the direct activation by TPO of a major component of complement (C4). When you read this article, you will also wonder about this association, which has little clinical relevance at this time but could result in some startling associations and significance for the overall disease processes. The article is written from the endocrine perspective and not the rheumatologic one. This makes it even more interesting.

R. G. Lahita, MD, PhD

Thalidomide Inhibits Tumor Necrosis Factor-α Production and Antigen Presentation by Langerhans Cells

Deng L, Ding W, Granstein RD (Cornell Univ, New York)

J Invest Dermatol 121:1060-1065, 2003 2–32

Background.—Many inflammatory and autoimmune disorders, such as erythema nodosum leprous, Behçet's syndrome, discoid lupus erythematosus, and Crohn's disease, respond to thalidomide. Its anti-inflammatory effects are attributed to its inhibition of tumor necrosis factor-α (TNF-α) production by monocytes and its stimulation of interleukin (IL)-12 production. Epidermal Langerhans cells (LCs) are antigen-presenting cells important in the local immune response. Whether thalidomide affects TNF-α production and antigen presentation by LCs was investigated.

Methods.—Cell lines derived from female BALB/c (XS52) and A/J (XS106A) mice were enriched to serve as surrogates for LCs. To examine the effects of thalidomide on TNF-α production, LCs were treated with thalidomide at various concentrations, then stimulated with lipopolysaccharide (LPS). The concentration of TNF-α in supernatants collected at various times was measured by enzyme-linked immunosorbent assay (ELISA). In addition, fresh epidermal LCs were purified via incubation with anti-Ia antibody and goat anti-mouse IgG, then pretreated with thalidomide, stimulated with LPS, and assayed. To examine the mechanism by which thalidomide inhibits TNF-α production, XS52 cells were pretreated with thalidomide or dimethyl sulfoxide (DMSO) (control), then stained to identify dead cells. In addition, TNF-α mRNA levels in XS106A cells before and after thalidomide treatment were analyzed by Northern blot analysis. To examine the effects of thalidomide on antigen presentation by LCs, cells were pretreated with thalidomide or DMSO, then incubated with chicken ovalbumin (cOVA). Cells were washed to remove cOVA and thalidomide, then incubated with T-T hybridoma DO11.1 cells. These supernatants were incubated with CTLL-2 cells, and the IL-2 content of the supernatant was assayed. In addition, purified LCs were treated by thalidomide, keyhole limpet hemocyanin (KLH), or DMSO, then incu-

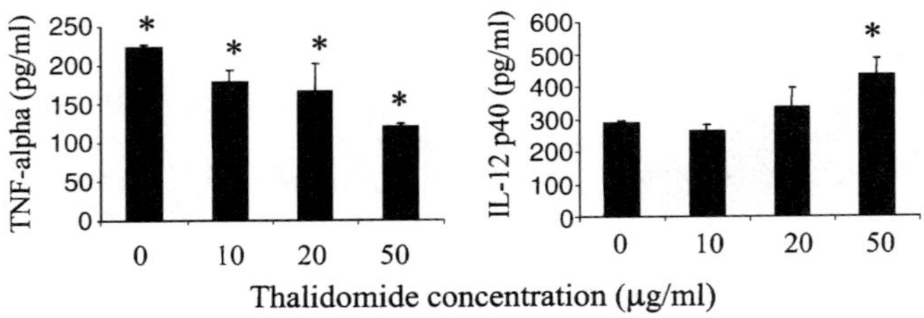

FIGURE 3.—Inhibition of TNF-α production and increase of IL-12 production by thalidomide in LPS-stimulated XS52 cells at low concentrations. A total of 3×10^5 cells were treated with thalidomide at various concentrations (10, 20, or 50 μg/mL) or DMSO for 12 hours. Supernatants were taken out at 9 hours after LPS stimulation. Data represent the concentration of TNF-α and IL-12 p40 subunit in the supernatants, expressed as averages ± SD from triplicates in one experiment. $^*P < .05$ for no thalidomide vs thalidomide. *Abbreviations: TNF*, Tumor necrosis factor; *IL*, interleukin; *LPS*, lipopolysaccharide; *DMSO*, dimethyl sulfoxide. (Courtesy of Deng L, Ding W, Granstein RD: Thalidomide inhibits tumor necrosis factor-α production and antigen presentation by Langerhans cells. *J Invest Dermatol* 121: 1060-1065, 2003. Reprinted by permission of Blackwell Publishing.)

bated with HDK-1 cells, and interferon-γ (INF-γ) production by HDK-1 cells was assayed by ELISA.

Results.—Thalidomide inhibited TNF-α production in a dose-dependent fashion, both in cultured cells and in fresh epidermal LCs. Thalidomide also significantly increased IL-12 p40 subunit levels (Fig 3). Staining revealed thalidomide did not increase the proportion of dead cells compared with that of DMSO, indicating thalidomide's lack of toxic effect. However thalidomide did dramatically decrease TNF-α mRNA levels in XS106A cells. Thalidomide also inhibited antigen presentation by LCs, as thalidomide pretreatment significantly decreased the ability of LCs to stimulate DO11.1 cells and the ability of HDK-1 cells to produce (INF-γ).

Conclusion.—Thalidomide inhibits TNF-α production by LCs and the ability of these LCs to present antigen to a responsive Th1 clone. These actions may be at least partly responsible for the immunomodulatory affects of this agent.

► This very important article deals with the overall effects that the drug thalidomide has on immune function. We have been using this drug for the past year with care and selection. It has proven itself excellent for skin lesions related to lupus and even some conditions not related to the dermatologic manifestations of the disease. This article tells us why. After all, thalidomide is 1 drug that apparently is a sedative and had horrendous effects when given to expectant mothers back in the 1950s. This drug alone was responsible for the careful review and approval of most therapeutic agents by the Food and Drug Administration. Its use is limited by the side effects of neuropathy and its potential for teratogenicity. We now know through this article that thalidomide lowers TNF-α and also interferes with antigen presentation by epidermal Langerhans cells. Who would have thought?

R. G. Lahita, MD, PhD

3 Vasculitis, Systemic Rheumatic Diseases, and Other Related Disorders

Introduction

I understand that the Chinese tradition is to dedicate each year to an animal. It appears that the vasculitis literature this year has followed the Chinese tradition and dedicated itself to one beastly disorder—giant cell arteritis (GCA). Oh, to be sure there are important articles on other forms of vasculitis. But this was an especially important year for GCA. Can you name a medication other than prednisone that reduces the chance of blindness or stroke in patients with GCA? What is the risk of developing a stroke or blindness in patients with GCA? How frequent is large artery disease in these patients? Does large artery disease affect patient mortality? This year you can find the answers to these important questions in the pages that follow.

David B. Hellmann, MD

Lead Article

Low-Dose Aspirin and Prevention of Cranial Ischemic Complications in Giant Cell Arteritis

Nesher G, Berkun Y, Mates M, et al (Shaare Zedek Med Ctr, Jerusalem, Israel; Bikur Holim Hosp, Jerusalem, Israel; Hadassah Med Orgainization, Jerusalem, Israel; et al)

Arthritis Rheum 50:1332-1337, 2004 3–1

Background.—Cranial ischemic complications, including cerebrovascular accidents (CVAs) and acute visual loss, are among the major causes of morbidity in patients with giant cell arteritis (GCA). The effects of low-dose aspirin treatment on the incidence of cranial ischemic complications in GCA were investigated.

TABLE 1.—Characteristics of Aspirin-Treated and Nonaspirin-Treated Patients With GCA at the Time of Diagnosis*

Characteristic	Aspirin (n = 36)	No Aspirin (n = 139)	*P*
Age, mean ± SD years	76.1 ± 7.5	73.5 ± 8.7	0.11
Female:male ratio	1.4	1.8	0.57
Headache	27 (75)	105 (76)	1.00
Systemic symptoms	25 (69)	73 (53)	0.09
Jaw claudication	6 (17)	25 (18)	1.00
Polymyalgia rheumatica	14 (39)	49 (35)	0.70
Symptom duration, weeks	6.5 ± 5.8	6.1 ± 6.6	0.22
Erythrocyte sedimentation rate, mm/hour	102 ± 27	103 ± 27	0.84
Platelet count, $10^3/\mu l$	459 ± 154	448 ± 159	0.70
Hemoglobin, gm/dl	11.3 ± 1.5	11.2 ± 1.5	0.71
Positive temporal artery biopsy	34 (94)	118 (85)	0.17
Cerebrovascular risk factors	14 (38.9)	28 (20)	0.03
Cranial ischemic complications	3 (8)	40 (29)	0.01

*Except where indicated otherwise, values are the number (%). Systemic symptoms include fever, anorexia, and weight loss. Cerebrovascular risk factors include hypertension, hyperlipidemia, or diabetes. Cranial ischemic complications include cerebrovascular accidents and visual loss due to anterior ischemic optic neuropathy or central retinal artery occlusion.

(Courtesy of Nesher G, Berkum Y, Mates M, et al: Low-dose aspirin and prevention of cranial ischemic complications in giant cell arteritis. *Arthritis Rheum* 50:1332-1337, 2004. Reprinted by permission of John Wiley & Sons, Inc.)

Methods.—The charts of 175 consecutive patients with GCA diagnosed between 1980 and 2000 were analyzed. Data on 166 patients followed up for 3 months or more were also analyzed.

Findings.—At the time of GCA diagnosis, 21% of the patients had already been taking aspirin, 100 mg/d for ischemic heart disease. The aspirin-treated and nonaspirin-treated groups were comparable in mean patient age, male-to-female ratio, duration of GCA-related symptoms, headache rates, systemic symptoms, and jaw claudication (Table 1). Mean erythrocyte sedimentation rate, hemoglobin count, and platelet count were also comparable in the 2 groups. However, cerebrovascular risk factors occurred in 38.9% of

TABLE 2.—CICs at the Time of GCA Diagnosis in 175 Patients*

	Type of CIC: Visual Loss (n = 32)	CVA (n = 13)
No. (%) of patients with other GCA symptoms prior to CICs	11 (34)	10 (77)
Mean duration (range) of other GCA symptoms prior to CICs, weeks	3 (0-28)	6 (0-24)
No. (%) of patients with premonitory amaurosis fugax or TIA	7 (22)	3 (23)
No. (%) of patients receiving aspirin treatment	2 (6)	1 (8)

*Two patients had a CVA and vision loss simultaneously (within 24 hours).

Abbreviations: CICs, Cranial ischemic complications; *TIA*, transient ischemic attack.

(Courtesy of Nesher G, Berkun Y, Mates M, et al: Low-dose aspirin and prevention of cranial ischemic complications in giant cell arteritis. *Arthritis Rheum* 50:1332-1337, 2004. Reprinted by permission of John Wiley & Sons, Inc.)

the aspirin-treated group and in only 20% of the nonaspirin-treated group. Cranial ischemic complications were diagnosed in 43 patients at their initial evaluation (Table 2). These included 30 patients with acute visual loss, 11 with CVAs, and 2 with both conditions. Only 8% of the aspirin-treated group had cranial ischemic complications, compared with 29% of the nonaspirin-treated group. Despite steroid treatment, cranial ischemic complications occurred in 14 of the 166 patients with a 3-month or longer follow-up. Cranial ischemic complications developed in only 3% of patients given aspirin, compared with 13% of those given prednisone only.

Conclusions.—Clinicians should consider adding low-dose aspirin to steroid therapy in patients with GCA, at least for those presenting with GCA-related cranial ischemic complications. This strategy can minimize the chances of further cranial ischemic complications.

► I believe this is an important study that will change the treatment of GCA: Standard treatment for GCA should now include prednisone AND low-dose aspirin. The addition of low-dose aspirin reduces the risk of ischemic complications from GCA nearly 5-fold, both at presentation (Table 1) and during follow-up (Table 2).

D. B. Hellmann, MD

Systemic Vasculitis

Vβ-Restricted T Cell Adherence to Endothelial Cells: A Mechanism for Superantigen-dependent Vascular Injury

Brogan PA, Shah V, Klein N, et al (Inst of Child Health, London)
Arthritis Rheum 50:589-597, 2004 3–2

Background.—Superantigens may play a role in the etiopathogenesis of several autoimmune diseases. The best case can be made currently for Kawasaki disease (KD), in which T cells infiltrating the walls of coronary arterial aneurysms and the intestinal mucosa have a skewed T-cell V_β repertoire, with more cells expressing $V_\beta 2$. Even with this evidence, the debate over conventional antigens versus superantigens in KD continues. The potential for endothelial cells to operate as superantigen-presenting cells for T cells and for such an interaction to produce activation of endothelial cells and injury was investigated.

Methods.—Purified T cells and the superantigens staphylococcal enterotoxin B or toxic shock syndrome toxin 1 were cultured with class II major histocompatibility complex (MHC)–positive human umbilical vein endothelial cells (HUVECs) for 4 hours. Fluorescence-conjugated monoclonal antibodies were used to stain the HUVECs and T cells, which were then assessed by flow cytometric analysis. The observations included V_β-restricted T cell adherence to the endothelial cell monolayer, V_β-restricted T-cell activation, surface expression of endothelial cell activation markers, and the generation of endothelial microparticles.

Results.—HUVECs pretreated with recombinant interferon-γ were the only ones able to present superantigen to T cells, yielding V_β-specific CD4 and CD8 upregulation of CD69 on the T cells adhering to the HUVEC monolayer. Both CD4V_β2 and CD8V_β2 were activated with toxic shock syndrome toxin 1 (Fig 1). With staphylococcal enterotoxin B, CD4V_β3, CD4V_β5.1, CD4V_β12, CD8V_β3, and CD8V_β12 were activated.

Nonadherent T cells showed no upregulation of CD69. Upregulation of the expression of intercellular adhesion molecule 1, E-selectin, and vascular cell adhesion molecule 1 occurred on the class II MHC-positive HUVECs after being exposed to superantigen in the presence of T cells. Endothelial microparticle release increased from activated HUVECs. This generation occurred early and was greater than the release seen in response to tumor necrosis factor–α.

Conclusion.—By using endothelial cells as a superantigen-presenting cell for T lymphocytes, superantigens may initiate and maintain vascular injury. As a result, many T cells become activated directly on the endothelial surface. This mechanism could explain why there are upregulated cell adhesion molecules on endothelial cells in most vasculitis syndromes and why the skewed V_β T-cell infiltrate persists in lesions observed in patients with KD. It was also shown that CD8 lymphocytes are activated and adhere to endothelial cells in a V_β-restricted manner in response to superantigens. This activation and adherence depend on the presence of superantigen-presenting cells

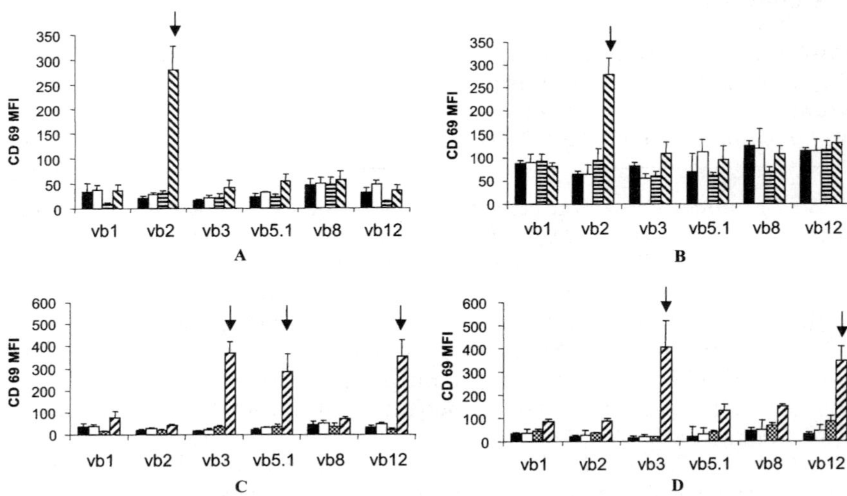

FIGURE 1.—V_β-specific CD4 (**A** and **C**) and CD8 (**B** and **D**) T-lymphocyte activation within the adherent population of T cells. Class II major histocompatibility complex (MHC)–positive human umbilical vein endothelial cells (HUVECs) were co-cultured with T cells in the presence of toxic shock syndrome toxin 1 (TSST-1) (**A** and **B**) or staphylococcal enterotoxin B (SEB) (**C** and **D**). Coculture with TSST-1 results in upregulation of CD69 on CD4V_β2+ and CD8V_β2+ cells. Co-culture with SEB resulted in upregulation of CD69 on CD4V_β3, CD4V_β5.1, and CD4V_β12, as well as CD8V_β3 and CD8V_β12. Values are the mean and SEM of 4 experiments. *Solid bars* show class II MHC-negative HUVECs and T cells; *open bars*, class II MHC-positive HUVECs and T cells; *horizontal-striped bars* (**A** and **B**) or *shaded bars* (**C** and **D**), class II MHC-negative HUVECs, T cells, and either TSST-1 (*horizontal-striped bars*) or SEB (*shaded bars*); *diagonal-striped bars*, class II MHC-positive HUVECs, T cells, and either TSST-1 or SEB. *Arrow indicates P < .05. Abbreviation: MFI*, Median fluorescence index. (Courtesy of Brogan PA, Shah V, Klein N, et al: V_β-restricted T cell adherence to endothelial cells: A mechanism for superantigen-dependent vascular injury. *Arthritis Rheum* 50:589-597, 2004. Reprinted by permission of John Wiley & Sons, Inc.)

that express class II MHC. The endothelial response outlined could be a marker of or contributor to the propagation of vascular injury in such systemic vasculitides as KD.

► How might superantigens cause certain forms of vasculitis (especially KD)? The authors of this study address that question, showing in vitro that endothelial cells have the capacity to present superantigen to T cells (Fig 1).

D. B. Hellmann, MD

Polyarteritis Nodosa Presenting as Acute Leg Ischemia

Héron E, Fiessinger J-N, Guillevin L (CHNO des Quinze-Vingts, Paris; Hôpital Européen Georges Pompidou, Paris; Hôpital Avicenne, Bobigny, France)

J Rheumatol 30:1344-1346, 2003 3–3

Background.—Polyarteritis nodosa (PAN) is a systemic vasculitis involving exclusively small and medium-size arteries, which causes vessel stenoses, thromboses, and microaneurysms. Reports of limb ischemia have been exceptional in this vasculitis, despite the systemic distribution of arterial lesions. Presented was an unusual case of PAN in diffuse visceral and peripheral arterial lesions seen as acute leg ischemia in a patient who was otherwise in good health.

Case Report.—Woman, 33, an Afro-Caribbean, was seen in the emergency department of a French hospital with sudden coldness and paresthesia of the right foot. She had a history of arterial hypertension which had been discovered in 1988; it was complicated by malignant hypertension in 1992. The patient was otherwise healthy.

Arterial thromboembolism was clinically suspected, and IV heparin was administered. Standard laboratory test results were normal. Aorto-arteriography showed diffuse vascular abnormalities sparing the large arteries (Fig 1). A diagnosis of PAN was strongly suspected on the basis of imaging studies because of the size of the involved arteries and the presence of multiple aneurysms. Angiography and US imaging showed multiple microaneurysmal and thrombotic lesions, most notably in the kidneys and the 4 extremities.

Cutaneous biopsy was performed, and necrotizing angiitis was demonstrated. The patient was successfully treated with corticosteroids for 1 year, beginning with a dose of 1 mg/kg/d of prednisone. The leg ischemia improved gradually after the development of collaterals. After 6 months, the patient was able to walk 1 km without plantar claudication. At 1 year, her walking distance was not limited at normal speed. The appearance and size of the tibial microaneurysms on US scans has not changed.

Conclusion.—There are 3 notable findings in this case: the unusual presentation of the patient, the absence of constitutional symptoms despite the

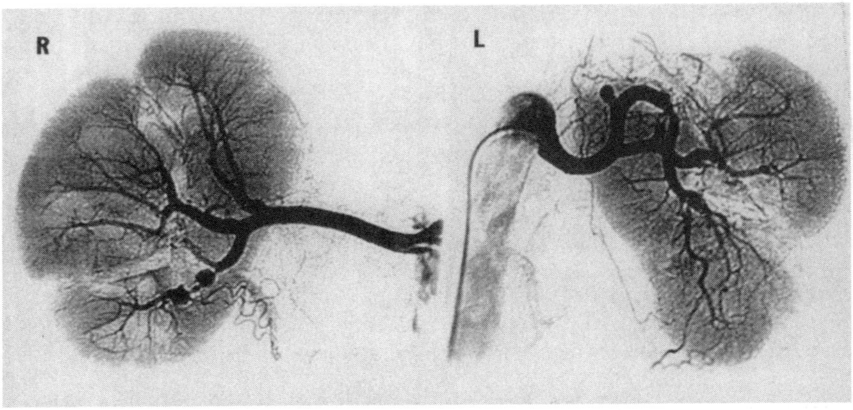

FIGURE 1.—Renal arteriography showing microaneurysms, stenoses, and segmental branch occlusions involving the right and left renal artery beds, with hypoperfused parenchymal areas (mainly right kidney) and renal infarcts (mainly left kidney). (Courtesy of Héron E, Fiessinger J-N, Guillevin L: Polyarteritis nodosa presenting as acute leg ischemia. *J Rheumatol* 30:1344-1346, 2003.)

diffuse distribution of vascular lesions, and the good visualization of peripheral microaneurysms by US. This case demonstrates a potential diagnostic application for US of the limbs in PAN.

► For years I have been teaching my students that PAN typically presents over weeks or months. Acute onset of PAN is very unusual. But, as emphasized by this case report, abrupt onset of PAN can occur (Fig 1).

D. B. Hellmann, MD

Regression of Abdominal Visceral Aneurysms in Polyarteritis Nodosa: CT Findings

Tarhan NC, Coskun M, Kayahan EM, et al (Baskent Univ, Ankara, Turkey)
AJR 180:1617-1619, 2003 3–4

Background.—Polyarteritis nodosa is a rare systemic necrotizing vasculitis that affects small and medium-size arteries. Gastrointestinal involvement is common and occurs in up to 50% of patients. Other sites that may be affected include the kidneys, heart, liver, pancreas, muscles, spleen, CNS, and skin. The aneurysms may rupture, and this rupture is most often observed in renal and mesenteric vessels. The early diagnosis of polyarteritis nodosa is important for prognosis.

There have been reports of regression of associated aneurysms after combined medical treatment with steroids and immunosuppressant drugs. To date, angiography has been required for detection of the small aneurysmal dilatations. A case of polyarteritis nodosa was described in which multidetector CT (MDCT) demonstrated small intact aneurysms of the hepatic, gas-

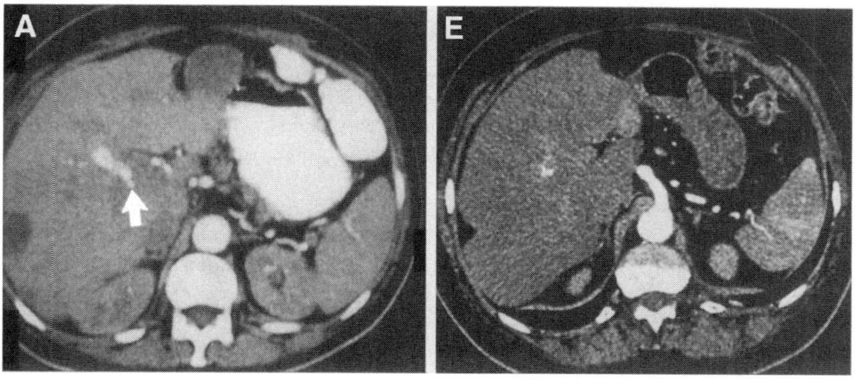

FIGURE 1.—A, In 58-year-old man with polyarteritis nodosa, contrast-enhanced arterial phase axial multidetector CT (MDCT) image shows multiple aneurysms in liver parenchyma. The smallest aneurysm has a diameter of 3 mm (*arrow*). E, Five months later, follow-up contrast-enhanced arterial phase MDCT image shows that aneurysms previously detected in the liver and pancreas are no longer present. (Courtesy of Tarhan NC, Coskun M, Kayahan EM, et al: Regression of abdominal visceral aneurysms in polyarteritis nodosa: CT findings. *AJR* 180:1617-1619, 2003. Reprinted with permission from the American Journal of Roentgenology.)

troduodenal, and pancraeaticoduodenal arteries as well as intraparenchymal hematomas caused by spontaneous rupture.

Case Report.—Man, 58, who had recently been given a diagnosis of necrotizing vasculitis as a result of polyarteritis nodosa at another medical center, was referred to the study hospital for additional evaluation. MDCT was performed before IV contrast administration and during the arterial, portal, and delayed phases after contrast injection. The arterial phase images showed multiple strongly enhanced nodular structures in various segments of the liver, with the highest number in the central part of the medial segment of the left lobe (Fig 1). MDCT also showed multiple nodular lesions in the liver parenchyma.

The patient was given a diagnosis of polyarteritis nodosa on the basis of clinical and imaging findings, and a combination of corticosteroid and immunosuppressive treatment was prescribed. Follow-up abdominal MDCT performed 5 months after the patient was first admitted to the study center showed significant regression of all the aneurysms previously detected in the liver. Lesions in the liver and pancreas were also reduced.

Conclusion.—In a patient with polyarteritis nodosa, MDCT showed aneurysms of the hepatic, pancreatic, and renal artery and lesions inside these organs caused by either aneurysm rupture or thrombosis. MDCT also confirmed the patient's excellent response to treatment. These results demonstrated that MDCT can be used as a noninvasive imaging technique for the diagnosis of small aneurysms in patients with suspected polyarteritis nodosa and for follow-up of these patients after treatment.

► I included this case report because it demonstrates 2 useful points. First, CT angiography can detect the microaneurysms of polyarteritis (Fig 1A). Second, the microaneurysms can heal with treatment (Fig 1E).

D. B. Hellmann, MD

Cerebral Amyloid Angiopathy Associated With Primary Angiitis of the Central Nervous System: Report of 2 Cases and Review of the Literature

Schwab P, Lidov HGW, Schwartz RB, et al (Brigham and Women's Hosp, Boston)

Arthritis Rheum 49:421-427, 2003 3–5

Introduction.—Cerebral amyloid angiopathy (CAA) is a frequently observed pathologic entity in the elderly characterized by β-4 ("senile") amyloid deposition in the media of small- to medium-sized cortical and leptomeningeal arteries. Reported are the clinical presentation, radiographic characteristics, brain biopsy results, and treatment courses of 2 patients with CAA.

Case 1.—A 74-year-old man was seen for evaluation of seizure and growing right temporal lesion. Two months earlier, he had a generalized tonic-clonic seizure. A CT scan of the brain revealed a small right temporal lesion that may have been caused by trauma associated with the seizure. A repeat CT performed 1 month later after he had a second seizure showed an increase in the size of the lesion noted previously, along with possible meningeal enhancement. He had a 1-month history of difficulty with both short-term and long-term memory, diminished sense of balance, behavioral changes, and headaches. An MRI investigation of his brain showed diffuse leptomeningeal enhancement bilaterally with reduced signal in the adjacent tissues, indicating edema (Fig 1). Because of concern for carcinomatous meningitis, a temporal lobe biopsy was performed. Small- to medium-sized blood vessels in both the leptomeninges and brain parenchyma showed marked perivascular inflammatory cuffs; in some instances, true vasculitis was seen. Scattered microhemorrhages of various ages were adjacent to or around the blood vessels. The inflammatory infiltrate composed predominantly of CD68-positive immunoreactive macrophages and of a sparse lymphocytic component. Walls of the involved blood vessels had a thick hyaline appearance. Immunohistochemistry for β-amyloid demonstrated strong reactivity in the blood vessel walls. At 1-year follow-up after treatment with steroids, he had returned to his baseline cognitive level, although occasionally displayed lapses in judgment. There were no further seizures.

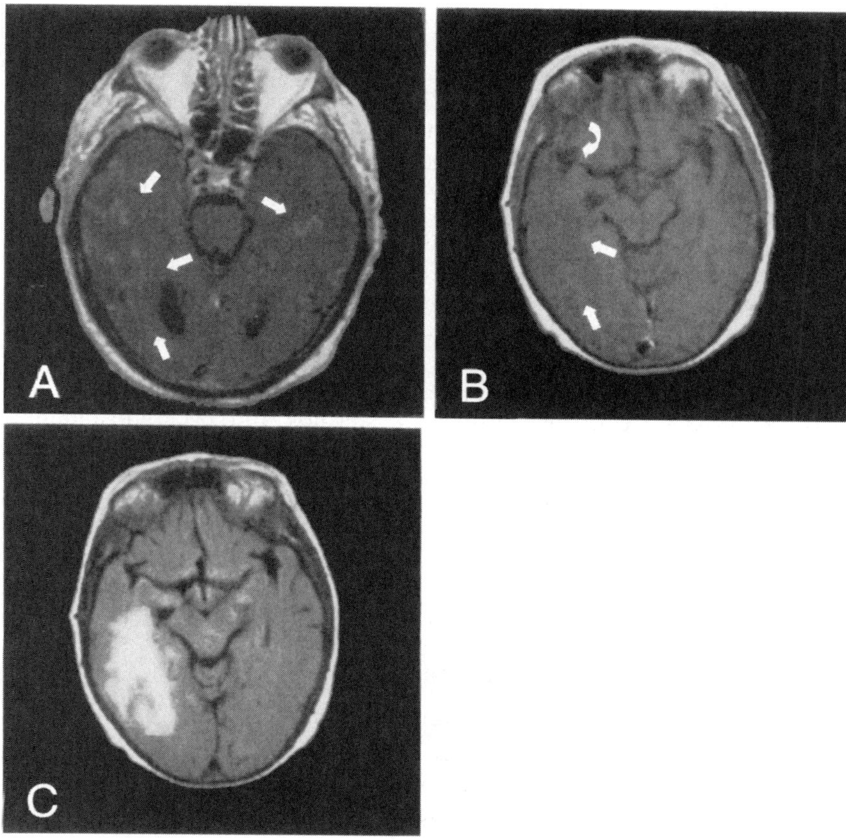

FIGURE 1.—MRI of brain of patients FK and MB. **A**, MRI of FK. Axial T1-weighted image (repetition time [TR]/echo time [TE]: 500 ms/30 ms) obtained through temporal lobes shows diffuse leptomeningeal enhancement (*arrows*) bilaterally, with decreased signal in adjacent tissues, indicating edema. **B**, MRI of MB. Axial T1-weighted image [TR/TE: 500 ms/30 ms) obtained through temporal lobes shows slight leptomeningeal enhancement in posterior lobe (*arrows*). Decreased signal in adjacent tissues indicates edema. There is mild mass effect of brain, resulting in mild entrapment of right temporal horn (*curved arrow*). C, MRI of MB. Axial fluid-attenuated inversion recovery (FLAIR) images (8002 ms/133 ms [eff]) obtained through temporal lobes show diffuse edema in white matter of right temporal lobe. (Courtesy of Schwab P, Lidov HGW, Schwartz RB, et al: Cerebral amyloid angiopathy associated with primary angiitis of the central nervous system: Report of 2 cases and review of the literature. *Arthritis Rheum* 49:421-427, 2003. Reprinted by permission of John Wiley & Sons, Inc.)

Case 2.—A 70-year-old woman was admitted for assessment of a transient episode of confusion and a right temporal mass. She began having daily bitemporal headaches 7 months earlier. An MRI of the brain showed a slightly enhancing T2-bright infiltrative lesion in the right temporal lobe with mild mass effect (Fig 1). Biopsy of the brain showed mild to moderate inflammation consisting of lymphocytes and CD68-positive macrophages in the perivascular spaces and in walls of medium-size vessels. She improved with dexamethasone treatment and was discharged home. She was readmitted 4 weeks later while taking 30 mg of prednisone for treatment of fevers up to 105°F and rigors. Thorough evaluation revealed no cause. The fever persisted despite treatment with broad-spectrum antibiotics. An MRI showed recurrence of the infiltrative mass of the posterior temporal lobe with confluent peripheral enhancement. A craniotomy was performed. Only small amounts of underlying cortical parenchyma was observed and were necrotic, indicating ischemic injury. Even in the presence of inflammation, β-amyloid immunoreactive vessels could still be observed. She was discharged on daily prednisone (1 mg/kg per day) with a plan for a very slow taper. At 18-month follow-up, she was living semi-independently, had developed short-term memory deficits, and continued to take a moderate dose of prednisone.

Conclusion.—Treatment with corticosteroids and cyclophosphamide used alone or in combination seem to be effective in the treatment of CAA/primary angiitis of the CNS. Given their risk for potentially fatal infectious complications, their use should be individualized and based on severity of presentation and close follow-up.

► This report is instructive because it reminds us that CAA can occur with primary angiitis of the CNS (PACNS). One should consider the possibility of CAA/PACNS in patients who have features of PACNS but are older (both of these patients were in their 70s) and have diffuse white matter changes on MRI.

D. B. Hellmann, MD

Positive Classic Antineutrophil Cytoplasmic Antibody (C-ANCA) Titer at Switch to Azathioprine Therapy Associated With Relapse in Proteinase 3–Related Vasculitis

Slot MC, Cohen Tervaert JW, Boomsma MM, et al (Univ Hosp Maastricht, The Netherlands; Univ Hosp Groningen, The Netherlands)

Arthritis Rheum 51:269-273, 2004 3–6

Background.—Cyclophosphamide treatment is lifesaving in many patients with small-vessel vasculitides, it is also associated with severe morbidity and mortality in the short and long term. Disease-free survival in patients with antineutrophil cytoplasmic antibody (ANCA)-associated small-vessel vasculitis (AAV) given cyclophosphamide only or switched to azathioprine after 3 months of full remission while taking cyclophosphamide was determined.

Methods.—One hundred twenty-eight patients who received a diagnosis of AAV between 1990 and 2000 at 1 center were included in the analysis. Between 1990 and 1996, patients were given cyclophosphamide only. Between 1997 and 2000, patients were switched to azathioprine after 3 months of remission with cyclophosphamide. All patients were followed up for at least 12 months.

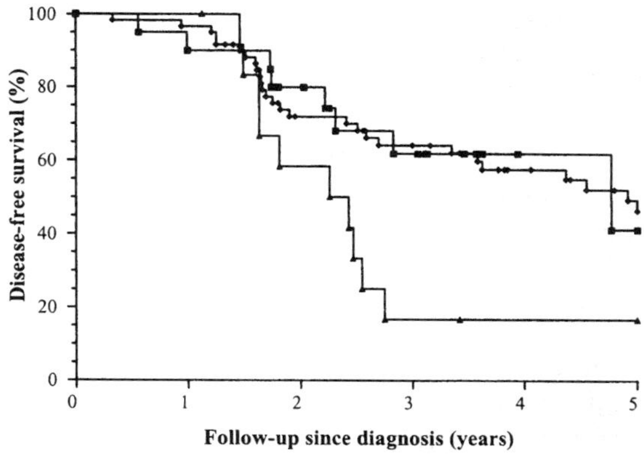

FIGURE 3.—Disease-free survival in 93 patients diagnosed with proteinase 3 (PR3)-antineutrophil cytoplasmic antibody (ANCA)-associated vasculitis, according to treatment arm: patients positive for ANCA at treatment switch to azathioprine (▲); patients negative for ANCA at switch (■); patients treated with cyclophosphamide only (*filled diamond*). (Courtesy of Slot MC, Cohen Tervaert JW, Boomsma MM, et al: Positive classic antineutrophile cytoplasmic antibody (C-ANCA) titer at switch to azathioprine therapy associated with relapse in proteinase 3–related vasculitis. *Arthritis Rheum* 51:269-273, 2004. Reprinted by permission of John Wiley & Sons, Inc.)

Findings.—Forty-one percent of the patients relapsed. Thirty-four percent of the total group had been switched to azathioprine treatment. In the cyclophosphamide group, disease-free survival was 76% at 2 years and 65% at 4 years. In the azathioprine group, these rates were 76% and 51%, respectively. Among 33 patients with proteinase 3 (PR3) classic ANXA (C-ANCA)-associated vasculitis switched to azathioprine, a positive C-ANCA titer at the time of the treatment switch correlated significantly with relapse. Among patients with a negative ANCA titer at the time of the switch, disease-free survival was 80% at 2 years and 62% at 4 years, identical to those for patients given cyclophosphamide only. In patients ANCA-positive at the time of the switch, disease-free survival was only 58% at 2 years and 17% at 4 years (Fig 3).

Conclusions.—These findings call into question the safety of switching cyclophosphamide to azathioprine in ANCA-positive patients with PR3 AAV. It is unclear whether alternative treatment regimens can prevent relapses in this patient population. It appears that C-ANCA response during remission induction and early follow-up may be a useful tool for risk-adjusted treatment regimens.

► C-ANCA status after 3 months of cyclophosphamide therapy predicts who will do well when azathioprine is substituted for cyclophosphamide. Patients who are C-ANCA positive at 3 months are 2.6 times more likely to flare on azathioprine than C-ANCA negative patients (Fig 3).

D. B. Hellmann, MD

Mycophenolate Mofetil for Remission Maintenance in the Treatment of Wegener's Granulomatosis

Langford CA, Talar-Williams C, Sneller MC (NIH, Bethesda, Md)

Arthritis Rheum 51:278-283, 2004 3–7

Background.—Mycophenolate mofetil (MMF) has been somewhat successful in the treatment of several autoimmune diseases. One group of patients with active Wegener's granulomatosis (WG) treated with MMF instead of daily cyclophosphamide (CYC) for remission maintenance was described.

Methods.—Fourteen patients were treated for active WG with the use of a standardized regimen of CYC and glucocorticoids to induce remission and MMF for remission maintenance. Predetermined definitions based on clinical characteristics and pathologic, laboratory, and radiographic findings were used to assess outcomes.

Findings.—All patients achieved remission at a median of 3 months (Table 2). Median time to glucocorticoid discontinuation was 8 months. None of the patients died during treatment. Forty-three percent of the patients experienced a relapse at a median of 10 months after achieving remission. The patients tolerated MMF well, with no one withdrawing because of medication toxicity.

Conclusions.—The use of CYC and glucocorticoids to induce remission and MMF for remission maintenance in patients with WG was well tolerated. However, disease relapses occurred in almost half the patients.

► The search for the Holy Grail continues (with apologies to fans of *The Da Vinci Code*)! Researchers have long been on a crusade to find the drug that can produce sustained remission in WG with minimal toxicity. Unfortunately,

TABLE 2.—Clinical Response of 14 Wegener's Granulomatosis Patients Treated With a Cyclophosphamide and Glucocorticoid Induction and Mycophenolate Mofetil Remission-Maintenance Regimen

Response	Result
Surviving, no. (%)	14 (100)
Achieving remission, no. (%)	14 (100)
Relapse after achieving remission, no. (%)	6 (43)
Time to remission, median (range) months	3 (1-7)
Time to tapering to alternate-day prednisone, median (range) months	4 (3-8)
Time discontinuation of prednisone, median (range) months	8 (6-24)
Time from remission to relapse in 6 patients, median (range) months	10 (1-25)
Time off prednisone before relapse in 6 patients, median (range) months	5 (1-9)

(Courtesy of Langford CA, Talar-Williams C, Sneller MC: Mycophenolate mofetil for remission maintenance in the treatment of Wegener's granulomatosis. *Arthritis Rheum* 51:278-283, 2004. Reprinted by permission of John Wiley & Sons, Inc.)

MMF does not fit the bill. Although it is relatively well tolerated, it is ineffective (Table 2).

D. B. Hellmann, MD

Polymyalgia Rheumatica and Giant Cell and Takayasu's Arteritis

Endothelial Nitric Oxide Synthase Gene Polymorphisms in Giant Cell Arteritis

Salvarani C, Casali B, Nicoli D, et al (Arcispedale S Maria Nuova, Reggio Emilia, Italy)

Arthritis Rheum 48:3219-3223, 2003 3–8

Background.—The pathogenesis and clinical expression of giant cell arteritis (GCA) may involve the genetically determined downregulation of nitric oxide (NO) release. The basal release of NO by the endothelium mediates local vasodilation, antagonizes platelet aggregation, and inhibits the proliferation of vascular smooth muscle cells, as well as platelet and leukocyte adhesion. These events may play a role in promoting the vessel wall damage noted in GCA. The roles of the Glu/Asp^{298} polymorphism in exon 7 and the 4a/b polymorphism in intron 4 of the endothelial NO synthase (eNOS) gene were evaluated in relation to susceptibility to and clinical expression of GCA.

Methods.—Genotyping by polymerase chain reaction and allele-specific oligonucleotide techniques for eNOS polymorphisms in exon 7 and intron 4 was performed in 91 consecutive patients with biopsy-proved GCA and 133 population-based control subjects from the same area of Italy. The presence or absence of ischemic complications (visual loss and/or jaw claudication and/or aortic arch syndrome) provided the criterion for dividing patients into 2 groups.

Results.—Patients who had ischemic complications had GCA at a much older age than those without these developments. Patients with ischemic complications also had scalp tenderness significantly more often than patients without these complications. The distribution of the Glu/Asp^{298} genotype was significantly different between patients with GCA and control subjects (Table 2). The difference in the allele distribution was related to a reduction in the frequency of Glu/Glu homozygosity in GCA patients in comparison to control subjects.

Patients with GCA had a higher frequency of Glu/Asp heterozygosity. Control subjects had allele Asp^{298} significantly less frequently than GCA patients. Among the GCA patients, there were significantly more carriers of the Asp^{298} allele than among control subjects. No difference in the distribution of allele and genotype frequencies was noted between groups for the 4a/b polymorphism. No association was found between the eNOS 4a/b or Glu/Asp^{298} polymorphisms and GCA clinical presentation.

Conclusion.—An association was found between the Asp^{298} polymorphism of the eNOS gene and GCA. Thus, individuals may be genetically predisposed to this condition. Drugs that improve endothelial function—

TABLE 2.—Frequencies of the Alleles, Genotypes, and Carriage Rates of Glu/Asp^{298} and the Variable Number Tandem Repeat a/b in Patients with Giant Cell Arteritis and Controls*

Variable	Control Subjects (n = 133)	GCA Patients (n = 91)	*P*†	GCA Patients With Ischemic Complications (n = 52)	GCA Patients Without Ischemic Complications (n = 39)	*P*‡
Alleles						
Asp	101/266 (38.0)	89/182 (48.9)	0.02	50/104 (48.1)	39/78 (50.0)	NS
Glu	165/266 (62.0)	93/182 (51.1)		54/104 (51.9)	38/78 (50.0)	
4b	221/266 (83.1)	142/182 (78.0)	NS	80/104 (76.9)	62/78 (79.5)	NS
4a	45/266 (16.9)	40/182 (22.0)		24/104 (23.1)	16/78 (20.5)	
Genotypes						
Asp/Asp	19/133 (14.3)	13/91 (14.3)		8/52 (15.4)	5/39 (12.8)	
Asp/Glu	63/133 (47.4)	63/91 (69.2)	0.001	34/52 (65.4)	29/39 (74.4)	NS
Glu/Glu	51/133 (38.3)	15/91 (16.5)		10/52 (19.2)	5/39 (12.8)	
4b/b	92/133 (69.2)	57/91 (62.6)		33/52 (63.5)	24/39 (61.5)	
4b/a	37/133 (27.8)	28/91 (30.8)	NS	14/52 (26.9)	14/39 (35.9)	NS
4a/a	4/133 (3.0)	6/91 (6.6)		5/52 (9.6)	1/39 (2.6)	
Carriage rate						
Asp/Asp + Glu/Asp	81/133 (60.9)	76/91 (83.5)	0.0001	42/52 (80.8)	34/39 (87.2)	NS
Glu/Glu	52/133 (39.1)	15/91 (16.5)		10/52 (19.2)	5/39 (12.8)	
4b/b + 4b/a	129/133 (97.0)	85/91 (93.4)	NS	47/52 (90.4)	38/39 (97.4)	NS
4a/a	4/133 (3.0)	6/91 (6.6)		5/52 (9.6)	1/39 (2.6)	

*Ischemic complications comprised visual loss or jaw claudication and/or aortic arch syndrome.
†Comparison between patients with giant cell arteritis and control subjects. The corrected *P* values for each significant difference are 0.04, 0.003, and 0.0002, respectively.
‡Comparison between patients with giant cell arteritis with ischemic complications and those without ischemic complications.
Abbreviation: GCA, Giant cell arteritis.
(Courtesy of Salvarani C, Casali B, Nicoli D, et al: Endothelial nitric oxide synthase gene polymorphisms in giant cell arteritis. *Arthritis Rheum* 48:3219-3223, 2003. Reprinted by permission of John Wiley & Sons, Inc.)

especially those that upregulate eNOS expression and increase NO production—may be therapeutically valuable for GCA patients.

► Yesterday I saw a patient with newly diagnosed temporal arteritis who asked "Why me?" I didn't have a great answer for him. Today, after reading this article, I have a better one.

Epidemiologic studies have shown that age is the single greatest factor for developing temporal arteritis. Ethnicity, climate, and HLA-DR antigens also influence the risk of developing temporal arteritis.[1] The current study was spurred by the observation that NO synthesis plays a critical role in maintaining the health of blood vessels. It is NO that mediates vasodilation, prevents platelet aggregation, and inhibits adhesion of white cells and platelets. Could genetically determined downregulation of NO production render a person more liable to develop temporal arteritis?

The answer to this intriguing question is "Yes." People with certain polymorphisms of NO genes are about 3 times more likely to develop temporal arteritis (Table 2). I'll call my patient back and tell him NO could be part of the answer.

D. B. Hellmann, MD

Reference

1. Levine SM, Hellmann DB: Giant cell arteritis. *Curr Opin Rheumatol* 14:3-10, 2002.

Reappraisal of the Epidemiology of Giant Cell Arteritis in Olmstead County, Minnesota, Over a Fifty-Year Period

Salvarani C, Crowson CS, O'Fallon WM, et al (Arcispedale S Maria Nuova, Reggio Emilia, Italy; Mayo Clinic, Rochester, Minn)

Arthritis Rheum 51:264-268, 2004 3–9

Background.—Giant cell arteritis (GCA), a vasculitis of large and medium vessels, occurs in persons older than 50 years, its incidence increasing with age. The cause of GCA is not known, yet a regular cyclic pattern has been observed, suggesting that an environmental cause, especially as infectious agent, may play a role in its pathogenesis. Time trends in the incidence of and survival associated with GCA were investigated in Olmsted County, Minn, during a 50-year period.

Methods.—The unified record system at the Mayo Clinic was used to identify all incident cases of GCA diagnosed initially between 1950 and 1999. Estimated incidence rates were adjusted to the 1980 US white population for sex and age. Survival rates were also determined and compared with expected survival rates in the population.

Findings.—During the 50-year study period, 173 incident cases of GCA occurred. Seventy-nine percent of the patients were women. Mean age at diagnosis was 74.8 years. Overall, the age- and sex-adjusted incidence per 100,000 persons aged 50 years and older was 18.8. The incidence was 24.4 among women and 10.3 among men. Incidence rates significantly increased during the study period, a progressive increase evident between 1950 and 1979. Subsequently, there were no substantial increases in incidence rates. A cyclic pattern of annual incidence rates was noted, including 6 peak periods. Survival among persons with GCA did not differ from that expected in the population.

Conclusions.—During the first 3 decades of this study GCA incidence increased, and then remained stable over the last 20 years. However, the cyclic pattern of annual incidence rates observed previously was evident during the entire 50-year period. Overall survival among patients with GCA was comparable with that in the general population.

► The take-home messages from this Mayo Clinic study are as follows: (1) GCA develops in about 1 of 5000 adults over the age of 50 years each year; (2) women have GCA develop more often than men; and (3) over the last 50 years, the incidence of GCA has increased (though having plateaued in the last 2 decades).

D. B. Hellmann, MD

Risk Factors for Cranial Ischemic Complications in Giant Cell Arthritis

Nesher G, Berkun Y, Mates M, et al (Shaare-Zedek Med Ctr, Jerusalem; Bikur-Cholim Hosp, Jerusalem; et al)

Medicine 83:114-122, 2004 3–10

Introduction.—Cranial ischemic complications (CICs) are frequently among the initial manifestations of giant cell arteritis (GCA), but develop in some patients at a later stage of the disease. Similarly, cerebrovascular accidents (CVAs) may be a primary manifestation of GCA or develop soon after the patient has started steroid therapy. The charts of patients with GCA were reviewed to identify risk factors for CICs, both at the time of diagnosis of GCA and during follow-up.

Methods.—Admission data were available for 175 patients and follow-up data for 166 patients with GCA confirmed by biopsy specimen or fulfilling the American College of Rheumatology criteria. Those CICs considered to be GCA related developed either within 2 weeks of diagnosis or were associated with other GCA-related manifestations or acute-phase reactions. Multivariate analysis tested the associations between CICs and patient and disease variables.

Results.—Forty-two of 175 patients (24.6%) had CICs at the time of GCA diagnosis; 32 experienced acute loss of vision and 13 had CVAs. Among patients with vision loss, only 34.4% had GCA symptoms unrelated to the eyes at the time of diagnosis. Most (77%) patients with CVAs, however, had other GCA-related symptoms at diagnosis. Risk factors for CICs at time of diagnosis included transient cerebro-ophthalmic ischemic episodes (COIEs, odds ratio [OR] 4.3) and male sex (OR 2.5). The presence of systemic symptoms and aspirin use were both associated with a reduced risk (OR 0.3) of CIC at diagnosis (Table 1). New CICs appeared in 8.4% of pa-

TABLE 1.—Variables Associated With CIC at Presentation in 175 GCA Patients

Categorical variables (univariate analysis)	No.	CIC (%)	OR	95% CI	*P* Value
Sex					
Female	110	19.1	1		
Male	65	33.8	2.17	1.08-4.4	0.045
Headache					
No	43	32.6	1		
Yes	132	22.0	0.58	0.27-1.3	0.22
Systemic symptoms*					
No	77	36.4	1		
Yes	98	15.3	0.32	0.15-0.65	0.002
Jaw claudication					
No	144	21.5	1		
Yes	31	38.7	2.30	1.01-5.2	0.06
PMR					
No	112	29.5	1		
Yes	63	15.9	0.45	0.21-0.99	0.047
TA biopsy					
Negative	23	34.8	1		
Positive	152	23.0	0.56	0.22-1.4	0.3
Cardiovascular risk†					
No	133	25.6	1		
Yes	42	21.4	0.79	0.35-1.8	0.68
Low-dose aspirin					
No	139	28.8	1		
Yes	36	8.3	0.23	0.07-0.8	0.01
Transient COIE					
No	142	18.3	1		
Yes	33	51.5	4.7	2.1-10.6	0.0002
Numeric variables (univariate analysis)					
	CIC (n = 43)	No CIC (n = 132)	*P* Value		
Age (yr)	75.3 ± 9.5	73.6 ± 8.12	0.26		
ESR (mm/h)	105.9 ± 22.2	102.1 ± 28.4	0.43		
Platelets (× 10^3/μL)	445.2 ± 94.5	451.8 ± 173.2	0.75		
Hemoglobin (g/dL)	11.4 ± 1.4	11.2 ± 1.5	0.58		
Statistically significant variables following multivariate analysis					
	OR	95% CI	*P* Value		
Transient COIE	4.3	1.8-10.3	0.001		
Male sex	2.5	1.1-5.4	0.02		
Systemic symptoms	0.3	0.1-0.6	0.002		
Aspirin use	0.3	0.08-1.02	0.06		

*Fatigue, fever, or anorexia.

†Diabetes mellitus, hypertension, or hyperlipidemia.

Abbreviations: CIC, Cranial ischemic complications (stroke or loss of vision); *COIE*, cerebro-ophthalmic ischemic episode (transient ischemic attack, amaurosis fugax, transient diplopia, or visual hallucinations); *ESR*, erythrocyte sedimentation rate; *PMR*, polymyalgia rheumatica; *TA*, temporal artery.

(Courtesy of Nesher G, Berkun Y, Mates M, et al: Risk factors for cranial ischemic complications in giant cell arteritis. *Medicine* 93(2):114-122, 2004.)

tients with GCA during follow-up and were associated with the presence of CICs at diagnosis (OR 5.6) and the development of transient COIEs during follow-up (OR 14.8). A protective factor for new CICs was low-dose aspirin use (OR 0.2).

Conclusion.—Findings in both this patient series and a review of the literature suggest that in patients with GCA, transient COIEs and a lack of systemic symptoms increase the risk of CICs at diagnosis. Risk factors for subsequent development of CICs were CICs at the time of diagnosis and late-developing transient COIEs.

▶ These authors remind us that even today CICs of GCA occur frequently: nearly 25% of patients present with CIC and another 8% experience CIC during follow-up. Men with jaw claudication are at greatest risk (Table 1). Being female, having systemic symptoms, and taking aspirin reduce the risk of CIC (Table 1).

D. B. Hellmann, MD

Incidence and Predictors of Large-Artery Complication (Aortic Aneurysm, Aortic Dissection, and/or Large-Artery Stenosis) in Patients With Giant Cell Arteritis: A Population-Based Study Over 50 Years

Nuenninghoff DM, Hunder GG, Christianson TJH, et al (Mayo Clinic, Rochester, Minn)

Arthritis Rheum 48:3522-3531, 2003 3–11

Introduction.—Previous research indicates that patients with giant cell arteritis (GCA) are at significantly increased risk for the development of a thoracic or aortic aneurysm. In addition, large-artery stenosis in GCA can lead to intermittent claudication in the arms or to ischemic neurologic symptoms. Factors predictive of large-artery complications in patients with GCA were identified.

Methods.—The cohort included all residents of Olmsted County, Minn, in whom GCA was first diagnosed between January 1, 1950, and December 31, 1999. A total of 168 patients were identified, all but 2 of whom fulfilled the 1990 American College of Rheumatology classification criteria for GCA. All patients were assessed for proven (by imaging studies, surgery, or autopsy) large-artery complications.

Results.—There were 46 incident cases (27% of the cohort) of any large-artery complication, including 30 of aortic aneurysm and/or aortic dissection (Fig 1). Eighteen of these cases involved the thoracic aorta and were the

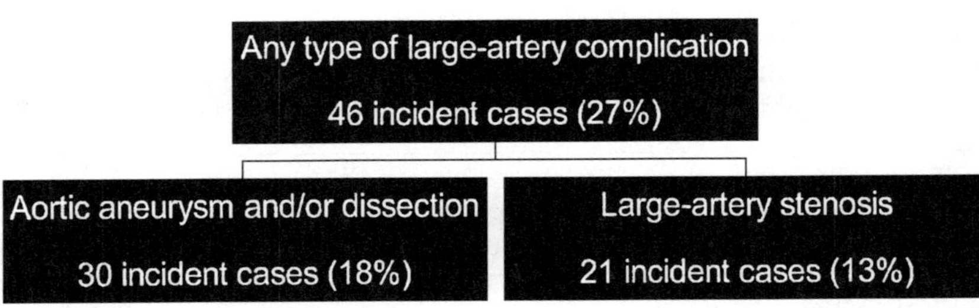

FIGURE 1.—Incidence of large-artery complications in patients with GCA. Five patients had both incident aortic aneurysm and/or dissection and incident large-artery stenosis affecting the cervical arteries. (Courtesy of Nuenninghoff DM, Hunder GG, Christianson TJH, et al: Incidence and predictors of large-artery complications (aortic aneurysm, aortic dissection, and/or large-artery stenosis) in patients with giant cell arteritis: A population-based study over 50 years. *Arthritis Rheum* 48:3522-3531, 2003. Reprinted by permission of John Wiley & Sons, Inc.)

cause of death of 7 patients. There were 16 cases of abdominal aortic aneurysm (4 patients had both incident thoracic aortic aneurysm and abdominal aortic aneurysm). Incident large-artery stenosis was identified in 21 (13%) cases, 15 of which were cervical artery stenosis. Six patients had subclavial/axillary/brachial artery stenosis and 1 had iliac/femoral artery stenosis attributable to GCA. Both hyperlipidemia and coronary artery disease were significantly associated with the development of aortic aneurysm and/or dissection in patients with GCA. Cranial symptoms and a higher erythrocyte sedimentation rate were negatively associated with the development of large-artery stenosis.

Conclusion.—A substantial proportion (27%) of these patients with GCA had also been diagnosed with aortic aneurysm and/or dissection or large-artery stenosis. Thoracic artery dissection appears to be an early complication of GCA, whereas thoracic aortic aneurysm is usually detected later. Patients with GCA should be examined carefully for the known predictive factors of large-artery complications.

► Wow! Large-artery involvement in GCA occurs more commonly than I thought (Fig 1). According to this Mayo Clinic investigation, some form of large-artery disease develops in about 1 of every 4 patients. More specifically, about 1 in 5 patients have aortic aneurysm or aortic dissection develop. Nearly 1 in 7 patients with GCA have stenosis of the subclavian, vertebral, basilar, or carotid arteries develop. When you and I see patients with GCA we should take great care in palpating pulses and listening for bruits or pathologic murmurs (especially that of aortic regurgitation).

D. B. Hellmann, MD

Mortality of Large-Artery Complication (Aortic Aneurysm, Aortic Dissection, and/or Large-Artery Stenosis) in Patients With Giant Cell Arteritis: A Population-Based Study Over 50 Years

Nuenninghoff DM, Hunder GG, Christianson TJH, et al (Mayo Clinic, Rochester, Minn)

Arthritis Rheum 48:3532-3537, 2003 3–12

Introduction.—Patients with giant cell arteritis (GCA) are at risk for large-artery complications, and these complications may be associated with increased mortality. Previous studies that examined the mortality of GCA have yielded conflicting results, however. Survival in patients with GCA and with or without large-artery complications (aortic aneurysm, aortic dissection, and large-artery stenosis) was examined.

Methods.—Patients were 168 residents of Olmsted County, Minn, in whom GCA was first diagnosed between January 1, 1950, and December 31, 1999. Records from the Mayo Clinic and the Olmsted Medical Group were reviewed by a single investigator, with a second investigator examining 10% of records for validation of data abstraction. Incident large-artery complication was defined as a complication detected within 1 year before or at any time after the diagnosis of GCA.

Results.—For the combined group of 46 patients (27%) with any kind of large-artery complication, survival did not differ when compared with the 122 patients without such a complication or with the general population of white individuals living in Minnesota. But survival was markedly increased in the 9 patients in whom thoracic artery dissection developed. The survival of patients in the subgroups of subclavian/axillary/brachial artery stenosis, iliac/femoral artery stenosis, and abdominal aortic dissection could not be statistically assessed because of their small numbers. Results were similar for the entire, 5-decade cohort and for the more recent, 2-decade cohort.

Conclusion.—Patients with GCA had similar survival rates irrespective of the presence or absence of any large-artery complication. But as expected, and consistent with previous studies, the subgroup of patients with thoracic aortic dissection had significantly decreased survival. In contrast to other studies, sex was not predictive of any type of large-artery complication.

► I conclude that large-artery disease, other than aortic dissection, causes morbidity but not mortality.

D. B. Hellmann, MD

Visual Deterioration in Giant Cell Arteritis Patients While on High Doses of Corticosteroid Therapy

Hayreh SS, Zimmerman B (Univ of Iowa, Iowa City)
Ophthalmology 110:1204-1215, 2003 3–13

Background.—Visual loss is the most devastating complication of giant cell arteritis (GCA). The incidence and extent of visual deterioration in patients with GCA taking high doses of systemic corticosteroids in the early stages of treatment were reported, along with factors influencing outcomes and the relative efficacy of IV and oral corticosteroid treatment.

Methods.—One hundred forty-four patients with biopsy-confirmed GCA were included in the study. Ninety-one patients initially had visual loss and 53 did not. The patients were followed up while taking megadoses of systemic corticosteroids for 2 weeks or longer. Steroid therapy was not tapered until both erythrocyte sedimentation rate and C-reactive protein were at their lowest stable concentrations.

Findings.—In the first 5 days of treatment, only 9 of the 91 patients who initially had visual loss (in a total of 11 eyes) had further deterioration in 1 or both eyes. None of the 53 patients without initial visual loss had visual deterioration in the beginning stages of megadose treatment. Visual deterioration occurred in 13% of patients receiving IV steroids compared with 3% of those receiving steroids orally.

Conclusions.—In most patients with GCA, early megadoses of steroid therapy prevent further visual loss. When further visual deterioration did occur, it began within 5 days of treatment initiation. IV megadose steroid therapy did not appear to be more effective than oral therapy in preventing visual deterioration.

► Somehow I had picked up during my fellowship the belief that initiating high-dose prednisone completely prevented new loss of vision in GCA. I was wrong. This and other studies show that prednisone reduces but does not eliminate the risk of visual loss. The greatest risk of new visual loss is in patients who have already experienced some visual loss and who are in the first week of treatment.

D. B. Hellmann, MD

Takayasu's Arteritis: Vascular Interventions and Outcomes

Liang P, Tan-Ong M, Hoffman GS (Cleveland Clinic Found, Ohio)

J Rheumatol 31:102-106, 2004 3–14

Background.—Many studies have shown good short-term results after surgery for Takayasu's arteritis (TA). Long-term results after endovascular revascularization, however, are unknown. The Cleveland Clinic Foundation's 21-year experience with outcomes after vascular intervention for TA were reviewed.

Methods.—The medical records of 20 patients (1 male and 19 females, 5-49 years of age) who underwent revascularization to treat TA between 1979 and 2001 were reviewed. The primary outcome was the patency of vessels after the intervention, as assessed by repeat invasive angiography or MR angiography.

Results.—These 20 patients underwent 62 revascularization procedures, including 38 bypass grafts, 7 patch angioplasties (with or without endarterectomy), 2 endarterectomies, 7 stent implantations, and 8 percutaneous transluminal angioplasties. Follow-up data were available for 52 of the 62 procedures (84%). Of these 52 evaluable patients, 23 (42.3%) were associated with restenosis, occlusion, or the need for revascularization. This included 11 of 31 (35.0%) bypass grafts, including 1 patient who developed thrombosis in all 3 grafted vessels less than 24 hours after surgery.

Four of 6 (75.0%) patch angioplasties were associated with unsatisfactory results, as were 3 of 7 (42.9%) percutaneous transluminal angioplasties and 5 of 7 (41.4%) stent implantations. The only endarterectomy that could be followed up has remained patent for 96 months since the procedure. None of the revascularization procedures was associated with death.

Conclusion.—Revascularization procedures are associated with a high failure rate in patients with TA. These results suggest that an open surgical approach with bypass grafting provides better long-term patency, whereas patch angioplasty and percutaneous endovascular procedures (particularly stents) carry a higher risk of restenosis or occlusion in this population. Although the reasons for this high rate of revascularization are unclear, inflammation at the graft site may play a role in graft failure in patients with TA.

► I find these results on vascular intervention in TA from the Cleveland Clinic to be very sobering: Restenosis or occlusion occurs frequently. The worst experience was with stents (only 2/7 long-term successes) and the best with surgical bypass grafts (20/31 successes).

D. B. Hellmann, MD

Hypertension and Elevated ESR as Diagnostic Features of Takayasu Arteritis in Children

Fieldston E, Albert D, Finkel T (Children's Hosp, Philadelphia; Univ of Pennsylvania, Philadelphia)

J Clin Rheumatol 9:156-163, 2003 3–15

Background.—Takayasu arthritis (TA) is a rare, chronic, inflammatory disease of the aorta and its branches. It is thought to progress from a systemic inflammatory disease of arteries to an occlusive ischemic disease resulting from progressive fibrotic narrowing of the affected blood vessels. The clinical features of TA are the result of limb and organ ischemia and generalized, nonspecific symptoms common in inflammatory disorders. TA was at first thought to be exclusively an Asian disease but is now known to occur throughout the world.

Delay in diagnosis is a common problem for adults and children. Although early manifestations are nonspecific, the clinical features that result in diagnosis often appear suddenly and are related to vascular involvement. Hypertension, normally rare in children, and an elevated erythrocyte sedimentation rate are found in most patients with TA. The hypothesis that these features could be used as markers for clinical suspicion of TA was tested.

Methods.—A total of 190 children and adolescents with TA (all seen before 18 years of age) were retrospectively evaluated with the use of local records and the literature to identify signs and symptoms associated with TA that could be used to educate clinicians as to when to suspect TA and to provide a screening tool for the disease.

Results.—Hypertension and elevated erythrocyte sedimentation rate were found in most patients with TA, with a sensitivity for this combination of 67% in the study group (Fig 4). When information from literature sources was included, the sensitivity was 65% for this combination of markers.

Conclusion.—The combination of hypertension and elevated erythrocyte sedimentation rate in children should warrant further screening for TA, particularly in children with systemic complaints. The physical examination of these patients should focus on abnormalities of the pulse. Additional evaluation should include extensive imaging of the vascular system.

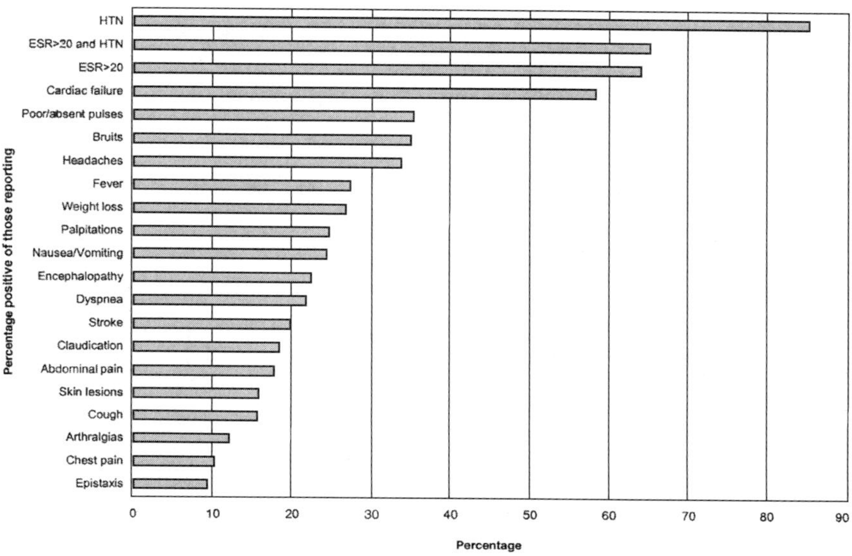

FIGURE 4.—Signs and symptoms reported (n = 30-190). *Abbreviations: HTN*, Hypertension; *ESR*, erythrocyte sedimentation rate. (Courtesy of Fieldston E, Albert D, Finkel T: Hypertension and elevated ESR as diagnostic features of Takayasu arteritis in children. *J Clin Rheumatol* 9:156-163, 2003.)

▶ Hypertension is rare in children but extremely common in patients with TA presenting before the age of 18 (Fig 4).

D. B. Hellmann, MD

Myopathies

Interstitial Lung Disease, a Common Manifestation of Newly Diagnosed Polymyositis and Dermatomyositis

Fathi M, Dastmalchi M, Rasmussen E, et al (Karolinska Hosp, Stockholm)
Ann Rheum Dis 63:297-301, 2004 3–16

Background.—Interstitial lung disease (ILD) is serious lung complication of polymyositis and dermatomyositis. The prevalence of ILD was estimated and predictors identified in patients with newly diagnosed polymyositis and dermatomyositis.

Methods.—In this prospective study, 26 consecutive patients with newly diagnosed polymyositis and dermatomyositis, regardless of clinical symptoms of pulmonary disease, were investigated with chest radiography, high-resolution CT, pulmonary function tests, and biochemical and connective tissue diseases, or antibody profile indicating other connective tissue diseases were excluded.

Results.—Of the 26 patients with newly diagnosed disease between March 1998 and September 2000, 17 patients were included in this study. ILD was identified in 65% of patients and was more common in men than in women (Table 2). Arthritis and the occurrence of anti-Jo-1 antibodies were

TABLE 2.—Clinical Data, Laboratory Data, Chest Radiograph, High-Resolution CT, and Lung Function Variables at Diagnosis of Polymyositis and Dermatomyositis

Case	Sex	Age (Years)	Diagnosis	Symptoms (months)	(CK) (μkat/l)	Jo-1	Respiratory Symptoms	Smoking	X Ray	HRCT	Spirometry (% Predicted) VC	TLC	TLCO	ILD
1	M	60	PM	9	>76.8	+	C+D	Never	1	1	77	74	61	+
2	M	49	PM	5	76.8	+	D	Current	1	1	70	75	65	+
3	F	64	PM	1	31.6	+	D	Never	0	0	68	62	NA	+
4	F	65	PM	2	47	+	C+D	Former	2	2	71	66	58	+
5	F	42	PM	10	9.5	–	C+D	Former	2	2	63	67	59	+
6	M	67	PM	3	61.3	–	–	Former	0	1	NA	NA	NA	+
7	M	58	PM	2	>76.8	–	C	Current	1	NA	NA	NA	NA	+
8	F	41	DM	1	6.3	–	C	Current	1	1	NA	NA	NA	+
9	M	64	DM	1	>76.8	–	–	Never	2	2	86	85	76	+
10	M	51	DM	1	37.7	–	–	Current	1	1	53	71	54	+
11	F	71	DM	1	>76.7	–	D	NA	0	1	109	119	64	+
12	F	53	PM	24	15	–	C+D	Never	0	0	92	100	60	–
13	F	51	PM	12	5	–	D	Former	0	0	135	134	48	–
14	F	54	DM	6	6.7	–	D	Never	0	0	NA	NA	NA	–
15	F	65	DM	10	>76.5	–	D	Never	0	NA	91	98	81	–
16	F	80	DM	3	20.7	–	–	Former	0	0	NA	NA	NA	–
17	F	49	DM	2	11.4	–	–	Former	0	0	NA	NA	NA	–

Abbreviations: CK, Creatine kinase; *C*, cough; *D*, dyspnea; *HRCT*, high-resolution CT; *VC*, vital capacity; *TLC*, total lung capacity; *TLCO*, carbon monoxide transfer factor; *NA*, not assessed.

(Courtesy of Fathi M, Dastmalchi M, Rasmussen E, et al: Interstitial lung disease, a common manifestation of newly diagnosed polymyositis and dermatomyositis. *Ann Rheum Dis* 63:297-301, 2004, copyright BMJ Publishing Group.)

TABLE 3.—Characteristics of Patients With Polymyositis and Dermatomyositis With or Without ILD

Characteristics	ILD Present (n = 11)	ILD Absent (n = 6)	*P* Value
Sex (male/female)	6/5	0/6	<0.05
Age (years), mean (SD)	57.5 (10.2)	58.7 (11.8)	NS
Time since onset of PM/DM (months) mean (SD)	3.3 (3.3)	9.5 (8.1)	<0.05
PM diagnosis, No (%)	7 (64)	2 (33)	NS
Symptoms, No (%)			
Arthritis	5 (45)	0 (0)	<0.05
Cough	5 (45)	1 (17)	NS
Dyspnoea	6 (55)	4 (67)	NS
Cough or dyspnoea	8 (73)	4 (67)	NS
Raynaud's phenomenon	2 (18)	1 (17)	NS
Dysphagia	3 (27)	2 (33)	NS
Swollen hands	3 (27)	0 (0)	NS
Laboratory tests, No (%)			
RF	6 (55)	1 (17)	NS
ANA	4 (36)	5 (83)	NS
Anti-Ro/SSA	5 (45)	1 (17)	NS
Anti-Jo-1	4 (36)	0 (0)	<0.05
Raised CK	11 (100)	6 (100)	NS
Raised ALT	8 (80)*	4 (67)	NS
Raised AST	11 (100)*	6 (100)	NS
Lung function (% predicted) mean (SD)			
VC	74.6 (16.9)†	106.0 (25.1)‡	<0.05
TLC	77.4 (18.2)†	110.7 (20.2)‡	<0.05
TLCO	62.4 (7.0)†	63.0 (16.7)‡	NS

*Data available for 10 patients.
†Data available for 8 patients.
‡Data available for 3 patients.
Abbreviations: RF, Rheumatoid factor; *ANA*, antinuclear antibodies; *Jo-1*, histidyl-tRNA synthetase; *CK*, creatine kinase; *ALT*, alanine aminotransferase; *AST*, aspartate aminotransferase; *VC*, vital capacity; *TLC*, total lung capacity; *TLCO*, carbon monoxide transfer factor.
(Courtesy of Fathi M, Dastmalchi M, Rasmussen E, et al: Interstitial lung disease, a common manifestation of newly diagnosed polymyositis and dermatomyositis. *Ann Rheum Dis* 63:297-301, 2004, copyright BMJ Publishing Group.)

found more often in patients with ILD than in those without ILD (Table 3). No statistically significant association was found between respiratory symptoms, other serologic or laboratory variables, and ILD.

Conclusions.—It would appear from these findings that ILD is a common early manifestation in patients with polymyositis and dermatomyositis and is not always related to clinical symptoms. Chest radiography, high-resolution CT, pulmonary function tests, and analysis of anti-Jo-1 antibodies should be included in the initial investigation of patients with myositis, regardless of respiratory symptoms.

► This is a detailed survey of 17 sequential patients with idiopathic polymyositis and dermatomyositis identified at a single Swedish referral center. By using pulmonary function testing and high-resolution CT, 11 (65%) had objective signs of ILD. Subclinical disease occurred in 18%. There was a strong relationship with clinical evidence of arthritis and with the serologic feature of anti-Jo-1 positivity.

The data here speak for themselves. ILD appears to be an intrinsic feature of inflammatory myopathy and should be sought in all such patients. It is likely an important influence on long-term outcome and would appear to be crucial toward the determination of initial choice of therapy.

J. R. Seibold, MD

Sjögren's Syndrome

Etanercept in the Treatment of Patients With Primary Sjögren's Syndrome: A Pilot Study

Zandbelt MM, de Wilde PCM, van Damme PA, et al (Univ Med Ctr St Radboud, Nijmegen, The Netherlands)
J Rheumatol 31:96-101, 2004 3–17

Background.—In Sjögren's syndrome (SS), a chronic exocrinopathy, sicca signs and nonspecific systemic manifestations—such as moderate to severe fatigue, arthralgia, myalgia, and intermittent fever—are characteristic. Objective input into the diagnosis includes the presence of anti-SSA or anti-SSB autoantibodies and minor salivary gland biopsy that reveals a lymphocyte focus score (LFS) of less than 1. No effective treatment is currently available. Disease-modifying antirheumatic drugs that are effective in treating other rheumatic diseases are unsuccessful in treating SS.

Treatment with infliximab, a monoclonal chimeric antitumor necrosis factor (TNF)-α antibody, reduced sicca signs and fatigue in some patients. Etanercept is a soluble fully human TNF-α-p75–receptor fusion protein with actions similar to those of infliximab. The potential local and systemic therapeutic effects accompanying the use of etanercept for patients with SS were investigated.

Methods.—Etanercept 25 mg was administered subcutaneously to 15 patients with well-defined primary SS twice a week for 12 weeks. Follow-up evaluations were conducted after 18 and 24 weeks. Patients were assessed by means of the Multidimensional Fatigue Inventory questionnaire, serologic monitoring, salivary flow tests, Schirmer test, rose bengal cornea staining, and tear film breakup time. At baseline and at the end of the 12-week period, patients had a sublabial minor salivary gland biopsy with assessment of LFS and percentage of immunoglobulin A–containing plasma cells.

Results.—Four of the 15 patients had persistently decreased fatigue. The Multidimensional Fatigue Inventory and visual analogue scale scores also reflected this finding. Patients who had a clinical response had a decrease in the mean score on the general fatigue scale from 16.8 to 8.0. Their scores on the physical fatigue scale fell from 16.2 to 10.0; the maximum effect was noted at the eighth week. Three of 4 responders had a decline in erythrocyte sedimentation rate levels and immunoglonbulin M rheumatoid factor levels with etanercept therapy. However, no substantial improvement was found in salivary or lachrymal gland function.

Low to extremely low salivary flow scores were maintained throughout the study. Tear film breakup time and rose bengal staining also showed no alterations. After etanercept therapy, LFS scores tended to decrease, but the change was not significant. Patients did not experience any adverse events, although 1 patient temporarily suspended etanercept treatment because of a prolonged episode of parotitis.

Conclusion.—Neither salivary nor lacrimal function improved with etanercept treatment, but a small group of patients reported markedly reduced fatigue and reduced erythrocyte sedimentation rate levels while they received etanercept. This indicates a possible systemic response. Decreased LFS scores were noted, but there was no significant alteration in minor salivary gland biopsy results. Etanercept was well tolerated and safe.

► This article is basically a negative study that shows that this TH2 disease, which we called Sjögren's syndrome is not amenable to treatment with TNF inhibitor, specifically etanercept. The authors gave a 12-week treatment of etanercept twice weekly, for reasons that escape this reviewer, to patients with SS. They looked to see if the symptoms and other clinical signs could be reduced. Predictably, the effects of TNF inhibition in a TH2 disease would be negative and, in fact, here it was negative.

The authors do say however that severe fatigue seemed to be ameliorated in patients who were on this biweekly injection regimen. Knowing full well the effects of etanercept in other diseases as being so salubrious, I am not likely to put patients on TNFα inhibition to overcome fatigue, a common symptom among all patients. The placebo effect found here could be significant.

R. G. Lahita, MD, PhD

Recurrent Transverse Myelitis Associates With Anti-Ro (SSA) Autoantibodies

Hummers LK, Krishnan C, Casciola-Rosen L, et al (Johns Hopkins Univ, Baltimore, Md)

Neurology 62:147-149, 2004 3–18

Background.—Transverse myelitis (TM) is a rare inflammatory disorder of the spinal cord that can be idiopathic or associated with a specific disease such as systemic lupus erythematosus (SLE), Sjögren syndrome, and antiphospholipid antibody syndrome. TM is typically monophasic, but recurrent TM develops in some patients with no identifiable associated disease. An index case was reported that indicated an association between anti-Ro antibodies and recurrent TM, which suggests that the mechanism of spinal cord injury may be autoimmune in nature.

Case Report.—Man, 65, African American, had a past history of hypertension and depression. This patient was admitted with a week of worsening bilateral lower-extremity weakness and urinary incontinence. MRI findings on admission were consistent with acute thoracic TM. Examination of the CSF showed a mildly increased protein level and leukocytosis without oligoclonal bands. The patient had a history of prior episodes of TM and bilateral optic neuritis. The patient was diagnosed with idiopathic TM. Laboratory studies were significant only for a positive antinuclear antibody and positive anti-Ro antibodies. On the basis of this case and others, a case-control study was performed to investigate the association of recurrent idiopathic TM with anti-Ro antibodies.

Results.—During the study, 13 cases were identified. The mean age of the cases at onset was 51.5 years, compared with 45.1 years in the control group. Most of the cases were women (85% vs 50% controls). Anti-Ro antibodies were detected by either Western immunoblotting or immunoprecipitation in 10 of the 13 cases and in 4 of the 12 control subjects.

Conclusions.—An association was noted between recurrent TM and anti-Ro autoantibodies, a finding that is supportive of the pathologic importance of an autoimmune process in recurrent TM.

► This in an unusual article for several reasons; first, anti Ro-antibodies have never been associated with TM. TM is an unusual condition with an insidious onset and horrendous pathologic potential and effects. The association of antiphospholipid antibodies with TM is suspected and known. I would not say that it is well known, but the finding of anti-Ro antibodies in TM makes one think of the proclivity of such antibodies for the Purkinje fibers of the heart and in some studies for the brain. This article brings forth a single reported case of anti-Ro antibodies on nervous tissue in the spine and the resulting TM.

R. G. Lahita, MD, PhD

Other Systemic and Immunologic Diseases

Auricular Chondritis in NOD.DQ8.Aβo ($A^{g7-/-}$) Transgenic Mice Resembles Human Relapsing Polychondritis

Taneja V, Griffiths M, Behrens M, et al (Mayo Clinic, Rochester, Minn; Univ of Utah, Salt Lake City)

J Clin Invest 112:1843-1850, 2003 3–19

Background.—Relapsing polychondritis (RP) is a multisystem autoimmune disease characterized by destruction of cartilaginous tissues and the development of auricular chondritis. The cause of RP has not been identified, although type II collagen (CII) appears to play a role. Many autoimmune diseases in humans are associated with HLA-DQ8 (DQA1*0301/DQB1*0302). Transgenic mice lacking endogenous HLA class II (Aβo) but expressing DQ8 were generated, and the response to immunization with various collagens was assessed.

Methods.—The *DQ8* transgene was injected into (CBA/JX B10.M) F_2 mice and backcrossed onto a B10.M background. These mice were mated with Aβo mice, which were then mated with NOD mice. Subsequent

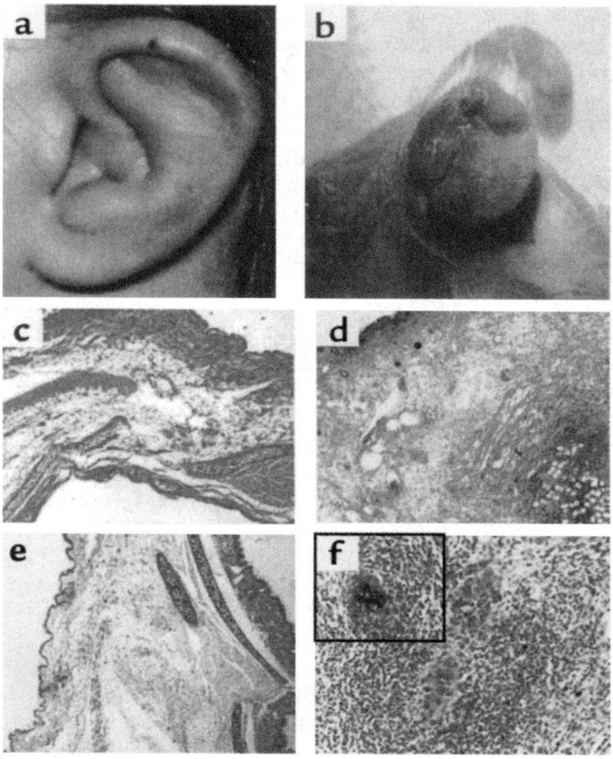

FIGURE 1.—Swelling and edema with a shrunken ear as observed in a human ear (**a**) and an affected mouse (**b**) with auricular chondritis. Hematoxylin & eosin-stained section of a normal (**c**) and a chondritic ear (**d**) of NOD.DQ8 transgenic mice showing massive infiltration of cells in the chondritic ear. Toludine blue staining of a normal ear (**e**) and a chondritic ear (**f**) showing destruction of cartilage in the latter, with residual cartilage seen among infiltrates as shown within the boxed area (magnification ×200). Micrographs are ×59 magnification. (Courtesy of Taneja V, Griffiths M, Behrens M, et al: Auricular chondritis in NOD.DQ8.Aβo ($A^{g7-/-}$ transgenic mice resembles human relapsing polychondritis. *J Clin Invest* 112:1843-1850, 2003. Reproduced from The Journal of Clinical Investigation. Reproduced by permission of the publisher via Copyright Clearance Center.)

matings (10 generations) produced DQ8 ($A^{g7-/-}$) mice with an NOD background (NOD.DQ8) and congenic DQ8 B10.M Aβo mice (B10.DQ8). The expression of antibodies specific to T cell receptor Vβ chain molecules was analyzed by flow cytometry. To examine the disease response to collagen, chick CII and bovine type IX collagen (CIX) were injected into the transgenic mice and their negative litter mates to try to induce arthritis. To examine histopathologic changes, animals were killed after the onset of auricular chondritis and arthritis, and tissues from the outer ears, paws, and other organs were stained. In addition, chondritis ear specimens were prepared for staining with antimouse antibodies specific for CD4, CD8, B220, Mac-1, and CD69. To assess in-vitro T- cell proliferation, transgenic mice, negative litter mates, and NOD mice were immunized with CII, CIX, and type XI collagen (CXI).

Results.—None of the B10.DQ8 mice, NOD mice, or negative litter mates showed any clinical or histologic evidence of auricular chondritis after immunization with chick CII. However, after chick CII immunization, 85% of the NOD.DQ8 mice had polychondritis and bilateral auricular chondritis with features similar to those of human RP (Fig 1). Both of the transgenic strains showed polyarthritis. NOD.DQ8 mice, but not B10.DQ8 mice, also had disease in the trachea, the perivascular region of the lungs, and the salivary glands; this type of involvement is characteristic of RP in humans. In vitro, both NOD.DQ8 and B10.DQ8 mice mounted a similar CII-specific response, but while NOD-DQ8 mice also mounted a strong response to CIX, B10.DQ8 mice did not. Both transgenic mice lines had anti-CII IgG antibodies after immunization, but the response was significantly higher in NOD-DQ8 mice. However, only NOD.DQ8 mice had antibodies to anti-CIX. After immunization with bovine CIX, all NOD.DQ8 mice had auricular chondritis, while none of the B10.DQ8 mice or the negative litter mates did. Compared with those of B10/DQ8 mice, NOD.DQ8 mice had more activated cells ($CD4^{+}CD44^{hi}CD62L^{lo}$), but fewer regulatory cells ($CD4^{+}CD152^{+}CD25^{+}$).

Conclusion.—NOD.DQ8 mice provide an experimental model for studying RP in humans. The susceptibility of these mice for the development of auricular chondritis is linked to the presence of collagen (CIX).

► One rather bizarre disease is RP. An animal model for this illness has been a long-time coming, and it is now here with an NOD mouse that is transgenic and gets, of all things, an auricular chondritis identical to human RP. The mice also get polyarthropathy, and the pathology greatly resembles the histologic picture found in humans with RP. This model is accomplished by the injection of type II collagen. The mice have to be transgenic for HLA-DQ8 which is the haplotype for the human disease. This article is very clever since the NOD mouse has no endogenous class II molecules. If you want elegance, this is an article that will have you amazed and not likely to forget the pathogenetic mechanisms involved in this rare disease.

R. G. Lahita, MD, PhD

Treatment of Corticosteroid-Responsive Autoimmune Inner Ear Disease With Methotrexate: A Randomized Controlled Trial

Harris JP, Weisman MH, Derebery JM, et al (Univ of California, San Diego; Cedars Sinai Med Ctr, Los Angeles; House Ear Inst, Los Angeles; et al)

JAMA 290:1875-1883, 2003 3–20

Background.—Rapidly progressing, bilateral, asymmetric inner ear dysfunction is considered to be an autoimmune disease, autoimmune inner ear disease (AIED) and can be successfully treated with high-dose corticosteroids. Methotrexate is often used to treat autoimmune disease, but has not been evaluated by a controlled, randomized clinical trial for use in patients with AIED. This prospective, multicenter, double-blind, placebo-controlled study was performed to analyze the efficacy of long-term methotrexate treatment for the maintenance of initial hearing improvement in patients with AIED.

Study Design.—The study group consisted of 98 adult patients with AIED who were prescribed a 1-month open-label regimen of 60 mg/day prednisone. Responders were offered a chance to be randomized into the methorexate trial. Of the responders, 67 patients were randomized to receive maintenance treatment with either methotrexate or placebo, during and after prednisone taper. Patients were followed for 1 year with regular audiometric examinations. The primary endpoint was progression of hearing loss.

Findings.—During the 1-year maintenance period, hearing loss reoccurred in 80% of the methotrexate group and 93.5% of the placebo group. This difference was not statistically significant.

Conclusions.—Methotrexate does not appear to be effective in maintaining hearing improvement achieved with high-dose corticosteroid treatment in patients with autoimmune inner ear disease.

► It's curious that methotrexate is so effective in rheumatoid arthritis but apparently less so for other inflammatory/immunologic conditions such as AIED (as in this study), lupus, temporal arteritis, and probably inflammatory bowel disease. There must be significant differences in pathophysiology of these disorders and mechanisms of drug effect that are not yet clear.

R. S. Panush, MD

Successful Treatment of Multicentric Reticulohistiocytosis With Alendronate: Evidence for a Direct Effect of Bisphosphonate on Histiocytes

Gotc H, Inaba M, Kobayashi K, et al (Osaka City Univ, Japan; Sankyo Co Ltd, Tokyo, Japan)

Arthritis Rheum 48:3538-3541, 2003 3–21

Introduction.—Specific treatment for multicentric reticulohistiocytosis has yet to be established. Histologically, the cutaneous and synovial lesions of this disorder reveal infiltration of multinucleated giant cells and histiocytes of monocyte or macrophage origin. A report of a patient with multicentric reticulohistiocytosis who was successfully treated with alendronate is described.

> *Case Report.*—Japanese woman, 44, with severe nodular erythematous skin lesions and arthritis mutilans was admitted for treatment of multicentric reticulohistiocytosis. Skin and synovial biopsies showed heavy infiltration with tartrate-resistant acid phosphate-positive histiocytes and multinucleated giant cells. Immunohistochemical analysis revealed that some of the mononuclear cells in the skin were positive for the receptor activator of necrosis factor-κB ligand (RANKL). The arthritis and skin nodules improved and remis-

sion was achieved with alendronate 10 mg administered once a week IV for the first 6 weeks, then once a month thereafter. She remained in remission at follow-up more than 2 years after initiation of treatment with alendronate.

Conclusion.—Osteoclast-like multinucleated giant cells differentiate locally in the skin from infiltrating histiocytes with the help of RANKL-positive stromal cells. Alendronate acts directly on monocyte or macrophage lineage in humans. It is recommended that alendronate be added to the list of drugs for treatment of multicentric reticulohistiocytosis.

► I have seen 4 cases of multicentric reticulohistiocytosis in my career, which spans well over 3 decades. All responded to daily oral cyclophosphamide, which is the standard of care for this often mutilating disease. As is true for the use of cyclophosphamide in other rheumatic diseases, the agent was introduced out of desperation and by default; nothing else seemed to work and the clinical setting could countenance a highly toxic agent. In the case of rheumatoid arthritis, the empirical use of cyclophosphamide was soon to lose its rationale once the dismal risk/benefit ratio was discerned first in a randomized controlled trial (RCT) and then in general experience. In the case of systemic lupus erythematosus, others persist in its use, whereas I am convinced that its risk/benefit ratio is no more appealing than for RA. The RCTs demonstrate marginal effect, if any, and the clinical experience is underwhelming. We all use it for Wegener's granulomatosis because the clinical experience is so positive that RCTs inducing remission with alternatives are difficult to justify in the fulminant presentation. Multicentric reticulohistiocytosis is too rare to imagine any cohort study would be feasible. Fortunately, it is seldom fulminant in presentation. Fortunately, these investigators from Japan had open and supple minds. I hope they're on to something.

N. M. Hadler, MD

4 Systemic Sclerosis and Related Disorders

Introduction

The past year has been one of incremental progress and consolidation of gains in our understanding of the pathogenesis of scleroderma, our ability to measure clinical outcomes, and, ultimately, our ability to treat these patients better.

In the realm of treatment, virtually all of the activity has been in the area of pulmonary hypertension. The private sector has *finally* become involved in drug development although the overall circumstances deserve reflection. There are three FDA licensed therapies for scleroderma (Flolan, Tracleer, and Remodulin) and all are approved for the complication of pulmonary hypertension. This syndrome is increasingly recognized as the leading cause of death and late disease morbidity and occurs either as an isolated pulmonary vasculopathy, usually in later stages of limited scleroderma, or as a component of respiratory failure in scleroderma interstitial lung disease, seen in both limited and diffuse scleroderma.

The lowest cost of these therapies is the oral dual endothelin antagonist, Tracleer, which is marketed at around US$40,000 per year. The parenteral prostacyclins, Flolan and Remodulin, cost several times more. This is a very simple market dynamic. Private sector profit is possible in scleroderma but only at very high costs per prescription. It should come as no surprise that many other candidate treatments for pulmonary hypertension are in development including sildenafil; the selective endothelin A receptor antagonists sitaxsentan and ambrisentan; inhaled prostacyclins including iloprost and treprostinil; and novel approaches such as inhaled VIP (vasoactive intestinal peptide). Around 20,000 U.S. scleroderma patients have pulmonary hypertension and at some point it is probable that most all patients will be on an appropriate therapy or therapies and that the market will become saturated. At some point, the delicate and somewhat bizarre finances of this critically important area will be much changed.

The burden remains on the practicing rheumatologist who must consider and recognize the syndrome and make appropriate referral for definitive diagnosis and treatment. The cardiopulmonary testing is beyond the average rheumatologist and too frequently the appropriate level of cardiology and pulmonary referral expertise is lacking. The situation is one of the ignorant leading the disinterested.

Nonetheless, this is a glimpse at the future of scleroderma therapy. Imagine an agent that halted fibrotic features of disease including skin, lung and vascular. What level of clinical impact could be achieved and how much might it ultimately cost? At the time of this edition, the U.S. scleroderma community is poised to embark on the most ambitious and most expensive interventional trial in the history of scleroderma – a prospective randomized comparison of immunoablation with stem cell-based immune reconstitution versus monthly moderate dose IV cyclophosphamide. What magnitude of effect will we accept as indicative of acceptable benefit compared to costs and treatment-related morbidities?

These vexing issues can be resolved through better science. If we truly understood pathogenesis, highly focused therapies might quickly follow. One only need consider rheumatoid arthritis and the revolution in patient outcomes associated with the highly specific approach of TNF–trapping strategies. Is there an etanercept-like agent for scleroderma? Will it be an effective method of modulating transforming growth factor-β? As the reader peruses the selections for this edition of YEAR BOOK, confusion is expected (although not desired). Much of the growth characteristics and synthetic repertoire of scleroderma fibroblasts seem clearly attributable to the effects of TGF-β, yet novel work suggests that this effect is not extrinsic (too much cytokine) but rather intrinsic related to underexpression of Smad 7 (inefficient counter-regulatory feedback). Results from different laboratories stand in stark disagreement in this area yet one can only feel that we are getting closer to a precise understanding of the salient underlying biologic events.

All rheumatologists must remain "students" of scleroderma. The field is evolving both in terms of scientific understanding and in the nuances and subtleties of management.

James R. Seibold, MD

Immunogenetics and Pathophysiology

Quantification of Maternal Microchimerism by HLA-Specific Real-Time Polymerase Chain Reaction: Studies of Healthy Women and Women With Scleroderma

Lambert NC, Erickson TD, Yan Z, et al (Fred Hutchinson Cancer Research Ctr, Seattle; Univ of California, Los Angeles; Univ of Washington, Seattle)
Arthritis Rheum 50:906-914, 2004 4–1

Introduction.—Microchimerism (Mc), originating from bidirectional fetal-maternal cell traffic during pregnancy, has recently been observed in healthy adults and in patients with scleroderma (systemic sclerosis [SSc]). The incidence and quantitative levels of maternal Mc (MMc) was evaluated in healthy female controls and women with SSc.

TABLE 1.—Frequency of MMc in Healthy Women and Women With SSc

	No. (%) Positive	Odds Ratio	95% CI	*P* vs. Controls
Model with all probands				
Controls	7/32 (21.9)			
Cases	13/18 (72.2)	9.3	2.5-35	0.001
Model excluding probands with transfusions				
Controls	7/31 (22.6)			
Cases	9/14 (64.3)	6.2	1.6-25	0.01

Abbreviations: MMc, Maternal microchimerism; *SSc,* systemic sclerosis.

(Courtesy of Lambert NC, Erickson TD, Yan Z, et al: Quantification of maternal microchimerism by HLA-specific real-time polymerase chain reaction: Studies of healthy women and women with scleroderma. *Arthritis Rheum* 50:906-914, 2004. Reprinted by permission of John Wiley & Sons, Inc.)

Methods.—HLA-specific primers and fluorogenic probes were used in real-time quantitative polymerase chain reaction assays to identify and quantify MMc by targeting noninherited, nonshared HLA sequences. DNA-based HLA typing was performed in 67 proband-mother pairs and in all children if the proband was parous. Statistical analysis was restricted to 50 proband-mother pairs (including 32 healthy women and 18 women with SSc) in whom MMc was able to be distinguished from potential fetal Mc.

Results.—MMc in peripheral blood mononuclear cells was more common in women with SSc versus controls (72% vs 22%; odds ratio, 9.3; *P* = .001) (Table 1). Levels of MMc, expressed as the genome equivalent of maternal cells per million (gEq/mil), were not significantly different (0.68.6 gEq/mil in patients with SSc; 0.54.5 in healthy female controls) (Table 2). In additional trials, positivity for MMc was shown in a bone marrow aspirate from a patient in whom peripheral blood was negative for MMc on 4 occasions. Tissue from a subsequent autopsy in this patient had MMc levels of 757 and 1489 gEq/mil in the lung and heart, respectively.

TABLE 2.—Levels of MMc in Healthy Women and Women With SSc

	No. of Subjects/ Observations	gEq/mil Host Cells, Median (Range)	*P* vs. Controls
Model with all probands			
Controls	32/34	0 (0-54.5)	
Cases	18/24	0.71 (0-68.6)	0.056
Model excluding probands with transfusions			
Controls	31/33	0 (0-54.5)	
Cases	14/20	0 (0-34.5)	0.18

Abbreviations: MMc, maternal microchimerism; *SSc,* systemic sclerosis; *gEg/mil,* genome equivalent per million.

(Courtesy of Lambert NC, Erickson TD, Yan Z, et al: Quantification of maternal microchimerism by HLA-specific real-time polymerase chain reaction: Studies of healthy women and women with scleroderma. *Arthritis Rheum* 50:906-914, 2004. Reprinted by permission of John Wiley & Sons, Inc.)

Conclusion.—MMc is not a rare finding in the peripheral blood of healthy adults. Its incidence is greater in patients with SSc. It may be present in bone marrow and disease-affected tissue, yet absent in peripheral blood.

▶ A provocative theory of pathogenesis of scleroderma has been the suggestion of a "graft versus host" mechanism stimulated by development of an engrafted fetal immune system stemming from pregnancy. Various studies have suggested that the persistence of fetal cells is both more frequent and at a higher level in women with scleroderma, although not all studies have supported this contention. HLA homology between parents is held to be an important cofactor in fetal stem cell expression in maternal circulation, ie, normally implanted cells more likely to persist.

This ambitious study used sophisticated and highly sensitive techniques to investigate the frequency and quantitative levels of MMc. The principal findings were that women with scleroderma were more likely to have MMc in peripheral blood in comparison with healthy controls (72% vs 22%, $P = .001$) but quantitatively, there was no difference in genome equivalent maternal cells per million between the 2 groups.

These interesting data extend recognition of persistence of fetal cells beyond identification of male chromosomal material. This phenomenon may be underestimated in women with scleroderma who are frequently receiving immunosuppressant medications. The fundamental question remains one of determining whether the evidence of fetal Mc in scleroderma is an epiphenomenon of the breakdown of immune tolerance or an actual pathogenic pathway to disease.

J. R. Seibold, MD

Systemic and Cell Type-Specific Gene Expression Patterns in Scleroderma Skin

Whitfield ML, Finlay DR, Murray JI, et al (Univ of California, San Francisco; Stanford Univ, Calif)

Proc Natl Acad Sci U S A 100:12319-12324, 2003 4–2

Background.—Gene expression studies of individuals with scleroderma have been performed in an effort to better understand the disease and in the hope of finding molecular markers for the disease. Gene expression patterns were characterized in skin biopsies from patients with systemic sclerosis (SSc) with diffuse scleroderma by using DNA microarrays.

Methods.—DNA microarrays representing more than 12,000 human genes were used. Four patients (2 men and 2 women) underwent 2 sets of biopsies, and 4 normal control subjects underwent the same number of biopsies. All the biopsies, with 1 exception, were performed in identical locations (forearms and backs). One patient underwent forearm biopsy only.

Results.—Consistent differences were found in the patterns of gene expression between skin biopsies from patients with scleroderma and those from normal, unaffected control subjects. The biopsies from affected patients showed nearly indistinguishable patterns of gene expression in clinically affected and clinically unaffected tissue, even though these were clearly distinguishable from the patterns found in similar tissue from unaffected individuals. Genes that are characteristically expressed in endothelial cells, B lymphocytes, and fibroblasts showed differential expression between patients with scleroderma and normal biopsies. Immunohistochemical analysis of lymphocyte populations in skin biopsies from scleroderma patients suggested that the B lymphocyte signature observed in the arrays used in this study is from CD20+ B cells.

Conclusions.—These findings support the view that scleroderma has systemic manifestations that affect multiple cell types and suggest genes that could be used as potential markers for scleroderma.

► Gene expression patterns were examined in 4 patients with systemic sclerosis compared with normal control subjects. Interestingly, comparisons were also performed between clinically involved and uninvolved skin.

DNA microarrays, including more than 12,000 genes, were utilized and thus multiple abnormalities and comparisons were expected. In agreement with other similar investigations, there was evidence of gene expression characteristic of fibroblasts and endothelial cells. Surprisingly, there was strong evidence of B-cell gene expression with subsequent study suggesting a signature compatible with CD20+ B cells. Results from unaffected and affected skin were essentially indistinguishable.

This powerful methodology permits detailed examination of a wide range of secondary tissue events. Perhaps most instructive is the marked similarity between uninvolved and involved skin. Past studies utilizing routine histopathology have suggested the same phenomenon, as have studies of specific markers of endothelial injury, immune activation, and matrix activation. The "myth of uninvolved skin" grows ever more complex and suggests that either our clinical measures of disease are woefully inadequate or that there are site by site differences in gene regulation that may confer therapeutic advantage.

J. R. Seibold, MD

The TNF-863A Allele Strongly Associates With Anticentromere Antibody Positivity in Scleroderma

Sato H, Lagan AL, Alexopoulou C, et al (Royal Brompton Hosp, London; Univ of Oxford, England; Royal Free Hosp, London)

Arthritis Rheum 50:558-564, 2004 4–3

Background.—Scleroderma is characterized by the presence of the predominant but almost mutually exclusive antibodies: anticentromere antibody (ACA), antitopoisomerase antibody, and anti–RNA polymerase antibody. ACA is a marker for pulmonary vascular disease in patients with scleroderma. The mechanisms underlying this association may be important to the development of more focused approaches to treatment. Tumor necrosis factor (TNF) polymorphisms were investigated in scleroderma, with the goal of determining whether TNF polymorphisms would be a stronger marker for ACA than class II major histocompatibility complex (MHC).

Methods.—The study subjects were 214 unrelated white scleroderma patients and 354 healthy control subjects in the United Kingdom. All subjects were investigated for 5 TNF promoter region polymorphisms by sequence-specific polymerase chain reaction.

Results.—An NF-κB binding site polymorphism known to be functionally relevant in the TNF promoter region was identified in 51.8% of patients with ACA and in 16.3% of patients without ACA. Haplotype mapping demonstrated that this was a primary TNF association that could explain the previous weak links between ACA production and class II MHC alleles. In contrast to the ACA findings, HLA class II (particularly DRB1*11) appeared to be primary in that it could explain the weaker TNF association with antitopoisomerase production. In addition, a separate TNF haplotype was found to be associated with scleroderma, although at a much lower level of significance.

Conclusions.—These findings may be important for both the directional pathogenesis of scleroderma progression and the treatment of scleroderma with anti-TNF agents.

► A unique feature of scleroderma is the high specificity of the disease-related autoantibodies, including antitopoisomerases, anti–RNA polymerases, and the anticentromere antibodies. Past work has suggested that these autoantigens are selectively released during a cell death mediated by hypoxemia-reperfusion conditions.

This large study investigated 214 scleroderma patients from the United Kingdom for 5 TNF promoter region polymorphisms by sequence-specific polymerase chain reaction and compared results to 354 nonscleroderma control subjects.

An NF-κB biding site polymorphism (TNF-863A) was present in 52% of patients with serum anticentromere antibody but in only 16% of patients with other serologic reactivities (P = .00002). This relationship is the strongest non-MHC genetic marker so far described in this disease

The authors speculate that scleroderma is not an inherently genetic disease but that host factors have a strong influence on the manner in which the disease progresses once established.

J. R. Seibold, MD

Disruption of Transforming Growth Factor β Signaling and Profibrotic Responses in Normal Skin Fibroblasts by Peroxisome Proliferator–Activated Receptor γ

Ghosh AK, Bhattacharyya S, Lakos G, et al (Univ of Illinois, Chicago)
Arthritis Rheum 50:1305-1318, 2004 4–4

Background.—Collagen synthesis and myofibroblast transdifferentiation in fibroblasts is stimulated in fibroblasts by transforming growth factor β

(TGFβ) through the Smad intracellular signal transduction pathway. TGFβ-mediated fibroblast activation is the hallmark of scleroderma and related fibrotic conditions; it is thought that disruption of the intracellular TGFβ/Smad signaling may represent a novel approach to controlling fibrosis. The nuclear hormone receptor peroxisome proliferator-activated receptor γ (PPARγ) may have a role in the modulation of inflammatory and fibrotic responses. The expression of PPARγ in normal skin fibroblasts and its effect on TGFβ-induced cellular responses were investigated.

Methods.—The expression and activity of PPARγ in normal dermal fibroblasts were examined by Northern and Western blot analyses, immunocytochemistry, flow cytometry, and transient transfections with reporter constructs. These methods were also used to evaluate the effects of PPARγ activation by naturally occurring and synthetic ligands on collagen synthesis and α-smooth muscle actin (α-SMA) expression. The modulation of Smad-mediated transcriptional responses was investigated by transient transfection assays with wild-type and dominant-negative PPARγ expression constructs.

Results.—Quiescent normal skin fibroblasts showed expression and full function of the PPARγ receptor. Although ligand activation of cellular PPARγ resulted in modest suppression of basal collagen gene expression, it

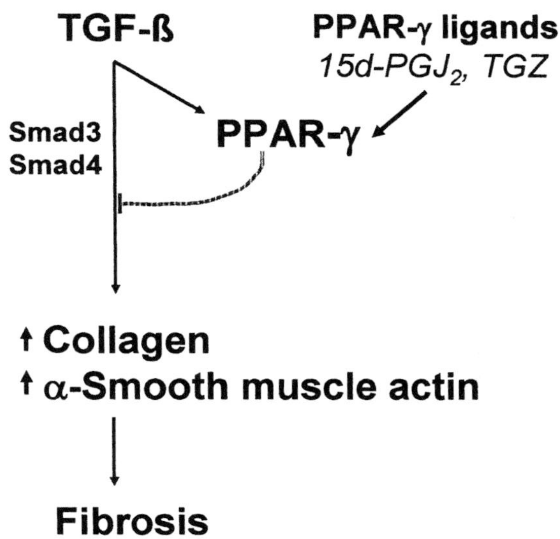

FIGURE 8.—Regulation of TGFβ-induced responses in fibroblasts by PPARγ. Through activation of intracellular Smad signal transduction pathway, TGFβ stimulates collagen synthesis, α-SMA expression, and myofibroblast transdifferentiation of resident fibroblasts in skin. These responses contribute to tissue fibrosis. Naturally occurring endogenous ligands or synthetic pharmacologic agonists activate cellular PPARγ, resulting in disruption of TGFβ/Smad signal transduction and blocking of profibrotic responses. Expression of PPARγ is enhanced on fibroblasts by TGFβ, thereby sensitizing them to antifibrotic effects of ligands. Activation of PPARγ may represent an effective antifibrotic intervention strategy. *Abbreviations: 15d-PGJ$_2$*, 15-deoxy-$\delta^{12,14}$-prostaglandin J$_2$; *TGZ*, troglitazone. (Courtesy of Ghosh AK, Bhattacharyya S, Lakos G, et al: Disruption of transforming growth factor β signaling and profibrotic responses in normal skin fibroblasts by peroxisome proliferator–activated receptor γ. *Arthritis Rheum* 50:1305-1318, 2004. Reprinted by permission of John Wiley & Sons, Inc.)

abrogated TGFβ-induced stimulation in a concentration-dependent manner. This response was mimicked by the overexpression of PPARγ in fibroblasts and was blocked by a selective antagonist of PPARγ signaling or by transfection of fibroblasts with dominant-negative PPARγ constructs (Fig 8). In addition, PPARγ ligands were found to abrogate TGFβ-induced expression of α-SMA. The stimulation Smad-dependent transcriptional responses by TGFβ was suppressed PPARγ despite the absence of a consensus PPARγ-response element in the targeted promoters. Protein expression of cellular Smad3 or Smad7 was not affected by ligand-induced activation of fibroblast PPARγ.

Conclusions.—It would appear from these findings that PPARγ may have a physiologic role in the regulation of the fibrotic response in normal fibroblasts by abrogating the TGFγ-induced stimulation of collagen gene expression, myofibroblast transdifferentiation, and Smad-dependent promoter activity. It is also suggested that PPARγ activation by pharmacologic agonists may be a novel approach to the control of fibrosis in scleroderma.

▶ Increasing amounts of data point to a crucial role of TGFβ as the key modulator of increased collagen synthesis and myofibroblast transdifferentiation in the pathogenesis of systemic sclerosis. It remains unclear if this represents an extrinsic excess of TGFβ or an intrinsic dysregulation of Smad intracellular signal transduction.

There does appear to be sufficient information at hand to justify therapeutic strategies aimed as interfering with TGFβ effects. These might include "trapping" strategies with monoclonal antibody or with free receptor, specific receptor antagonists, or amplification of endogenous counterregulatory influences.

PPARγ is constitutively expressed in normal fibroblasts. This novel work demonstrated significant abrogation of TGFβ-induced fibroblast stimulation and in a dose-dependent manner. PPARγ agonists such as troglitazone analogues might represent novel future approaches to scleroderma therapy.

J. R. Seibold, MD

Angiotensin II Induces Connective Tissue Growth Factor Gene Expression via Calcineurin-Dependent Pathways

Finckenberg P, Inkinen K, Ahonen J, et al (Univ of Helsinki; Humboldt Univ of Berlin; Max Delbrück Ctr for Molecular Medicine, Berlin)

Am J Pathol 163:355-366, 2003 4–5

Background.—Connective tissue growth factor (CTGF) has been implicated in the extracellular matrix synthesis. The mechanisms of CTGF action at the cellular level are poorly understood, but evidence from previous studies has demonstrated that adhesion of endothelial cells, platelets, and fibroblasts to CTGF is mediated through integrin receptors. The renin-angiotensin system (RAS) is also a component in the regulation of collagen synthesis, and previous studies have suggested that angiotensin II (Ang II) is a promoter of collagen synthesis and a regulator of collagen degradation. Whether CTGF is a mediator of the profibrotic effects of Ang II in the heart and kidneys was determined, and the role of calcineurin-dependent pathways in CTGF gene regulation was investigated

Methods.—The study was conducted using 3- to 4-week-old male dTGR and age-matched normotensive Sprague Dawley rats harboring human renin and angiotensinogen genes. The temporal expression of CTGF mRNA in the heart and kidney was investigated in 4 groups of rats: dTGR control, dTGR plus cyclosporine A (CsA), dTGR plus everolimus (SDZ RAD), and an SD control group. An additional dTGR group was treated with valsartan and used as a second control group.

Results.—In transgenic rats harboring human renin and angiotensinogen genes, Ang II induced an age-dependent increase in myocardial CTGF expression. This increase was 3.5-fold greater than in normotensive Sprague-Dawley rats. The overexpression of CTGF was closely correlated with the Ang II-induced increase in blood pressure. CTGF mRNA and protein were found predominantly in areas with leukocyte infiltration, myocardial, and vascular lesions and colocalized with $TGF\beta_1$, collagen I, and collagen III mRNA expressions. No expression of CTGF mRNA was found in the right ventricle or pulmonary arteries. The blockade of calcineurin activity by cyclosporine A completely normalized Ang II-induced CTGF overexpression in the heart and kidney, suppressed the inflammatory response, and mitigated Ang II-induced cell proliferation and apoptosis.

Conclusions.—CTGF mediates Ang II-induced fibrosis in the heart and kidneys via blood pressure and calcineurin-dependent pathways.

▶ There are diverse data linking angiotensin to a fundamental role in the fibroproliferative features of scleroderma. These data include past reports of elevated tissue angiotensin-converting enzyme (ACE); overexpression of Ang-II receptors; and unconfirmed reports of "disease-modifying" effects of ACE inhibitors.

This novel work suggests the underlying mechanism: Ang-II induces CTGF, which has been long implicated as a key driver of tissue fibrosis in scleroderma, most notably, skin and lung. This action is calcineurin phosphatase-dependent—the system inhibited by cyclosporine and tacrolimus. Ang II induces CTGF expression in myocardium and vascular tissues, although not in pulmonary circulation.

J. R. Seibold, MD

Expression and Regulation of Intracellular SMAD Signaling in Scleroderma Skin Fibroblasts

Mori Y, Chen S-J, Varga J (Univ of Illinois, Chicago)

Arthritis Rheum 48:1964-1978, 2003 4–6

Introduction.—Scleroderma is depicted by excessive synthesis and accumulation of matrix proteins in lesional tissues. Transforming growth factor β (TGFβ) has an important role in the pathogenesis of fibrosis by inducing and sustaining activation of fibroblasts. The underlying mechanisms are not well understood. The expression and function of SMADs, recently characterized intracellular effectors of TGFβ signaling, were analyzed in scleroderma fibroblasts.

Methods.—Primary dermal fibroblasts from 14 patients with scleroderma and from 4 healthy adult controls were evaluated. Northern analysis was used to ascertain the expression of endogenous SMAD messenger RNA (mRNA). Western analysis was used to discern SMAD protein expression (Fig 3). Intracellular compartmentalization of cellular SMAD proteins in the presence and absence of TGFβ was assessed via antibody-mediated immunofluorescence confocal microscopy. The influence of TGFβ blockade on SMAD subcellular distribution was ascertained with the use of anti-TGFβ antibodies, along with a dominant-negative TGFβ receptor type II (TGFβRII) vector to disturb TGFβ responses. The SMAD-regulated luciferase reporter expression was investigated to determine the potential

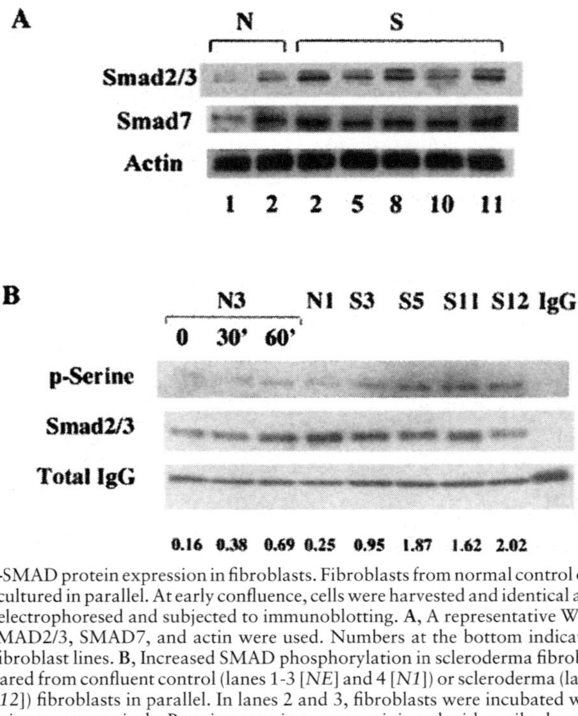

FIGURE 3.—SMAD protein expression in fibroblasts. Fibroblasts from normal control or lesional scleroderma skin were cultured in parallel. At early confluence, cells were harvested and identical amounts of whole cell lysates were electrophoresed and subjected to immunoblotting. **A**, A representative Western blot. Antibodies against SMAD2/3, SMAD7, and actin were used. Numbers at the bottom indicate control (*N*) or scleroderma (*S*) fibroblast lines. **B**, Increased SMAD phosphorylation in scleroderma fibroblasts. Whole cell lysates were prepared from confluent control (lanes 1-3 [*NE*] and 4 [*N1*]) or scleroderma (lanes 5 [*S3*], 6 [*S5*], 7 [*S11*], and 8 [*S12*]) fibroblasts in parallel. In lanes 2 and 3, fibroblasts were incubated with TGFβ for 30 minutes and 60 minutes, respectively. Proteins were immunoprecipitated with antibody against SMAD2/3. The complexes were electrophoresed through sodium dodecyl sulfate-polyacrylamide gel, followed by immunoblotting with antiphosphoserine antibody (*p-Serine*). Whole cell lysates were analyzed by immunoblotting for IgG. A representative blot is shown. Numbers at the bottom indicate the ratio of phospho-SMAD2/3 to total SMAD2/3 in each lane, determined by quantitating the signal intensities by densitometry and normalizing results to IgG to correct for small variations in protein loading and transfer. (Courtesy of Mori Y, Chen-S-J, Varga J: Expression and regulation of intracellular SMAD signaling in scleroderma skin fibroblasts. *Arthritis Rheum* 48:1964-1978, 2003. Reprinted by permission of John Wiley & Sons, Inc.)

functional significance of activation and nuclear accumulation of endogenous SMADs in scleroderma fibroblasts.

Results.—Protein and mRNA levels of SMAD3 and not of SMAD4 or SMAD7 were variably elevated in scleroderma fibroblasts versus control fibroblasts. In contrast to control fibroblasts, which demonstrated predominately cytoplasmic localization of SMAD3/4 in the absence of exogenous TGFβ, fibroblasts SMAD3 and SMAD4 in scleroderma consistently demonstrated elevated nuclear localization. Phosphorylated SMAD2/3 was also increased, indicating activation of the SMAD pathway in scleroderma fibroblasts. Blockade of autocrine TGFβ signaling with antibodies or by expression of dominant-negative TGFβRII was unable to normalize SMAD subcellular distribution, indicating that elevated nuclear SMAD import was caused by alterations downstream of the TGFβ receptors. The activity of a SMAD-responsive minimal promoter-receptor construct was augmented in transiently transfected scleroderma fibroblasts.

Conclusion.—This is the first report to show the apparently ligand-independent constitutive activation of the intracellular TGFβ/SMAD signaling axis in scleroderma fibroblasts. It may be that SMAD signaling contributes to the characteristic phenotype of scleroderma fibroblasts and has a role in the pathogenesis of fibrosis.

▶ This work should be considered carefully in parallel with the report by Asano and coworkers (Abstract 4–7). In this work, SMAD 3 protein and mRNA were elevated in scleroderma fibroblasts and were consistently localized to the cell nucleus as opposed to the cytoplasmic localization in normal human fibroblasts. SMAD 4 and SMAD 7 levels were comparable between scleroderma and controls.

Blockade of TGFβ with antibody and with the use of the dominant-negative TGFβRII failed to normalize SMAD intracellular distribution.

This work supports an intrinsic derangement of downstream effects of TGFβ receptor interaction but does not confirm that intrinsic alteration in SMAD 7 levels is either basal or inducible. It is possible that chronic overexposure to TGFβ or induction of increased surface receptors as well as nonsignaling receptor surrogates, eg, endoglin, lead to an as yet poorly characterized intracellular biologic derangement.

The basis for the widely disparate findings cannot be elucidated from the current reports.

J. R. Seibold, MD

Impaired Smad7-Smurf–Mediated Negative Regulation of TGF-β Signaling in Scleroderma Fibroblasts

Asano Y, Ihn H, Yamane K, et al (Univ of Tokyo)

J Clin Invest 113:253-264, 2004 4–7

Introduction.—The primary effect of transforming growth factor-β1 (TGF-β1) on mesenchymal cells is its stimulation of extracellular matrix

(ECM) synthesis. Prior reports suggest significance of the autocrine TGF-β loop in the pathogenesis of scleroderma. Smad7 and Smurfs, both important molecules in the negative regulation of TGF-β signaling, were examined to further understand the autocrine TGF-β loop in scleroderma.

Findings.—Scleroderma fibroblasts demonstrated increased Smad7 level versus normal fibroblasts in vivo and in vitro. Smad7 constitutively created a complex with the TGF-β receptors. The inhibitory effect of Smad7 on the promoter activity of human α2(i) collagen and 3TP-lux was completely impaired in scleroderma fibroblasts. The protein stability of TGF-β receptor type I was significantly increased in scleroderma fibroblasts versus normal fibroblasts. No significant difference was seen between Smurf1 and Smurf2 levels between normal and scleroderma fibroblasts. The transiently overexpressed Smurf1 and/or Smurf2 did not impact TGF-β receptor type I protein levels in scleroderma fibroblasts. Anti-Smad7 Ab precipitated Smurf1 and Smurf2 at identifiable levels in normal fibroblasts treated with TGF-β 1 and not in untreated normal fibroblasts.

Conclusion.—The impaired Smad7-Smurf–mediated inhibitory effect on TGF-β signaling may contribute to preserving the autocrine TGF-β loop in scleroderma fibroblasts. This is the first known report regarding a disturbed negative regulation of TGF-β signaling in fibrotic disorders.

► A variety of data support the hypothesis that TGF-β is the key cytokine operative in the fibroproliferative features of scleroderma. Divergent information suggests increased production or altered behavior of a single nucleotide polymorphic variant of TGF. Other work suggests increased presentation to fibroblast receptors perhaps influenced by altered storage on a defective fibrillin platform. A novel hypothesis was advanced last year with evidence of defective Smad7 processing. Smad7 is ordinarily induced by TGF-β/receptor interaction with results in impaired phosphorylation of Smad3/4 and enhanced degradation of TGF-β receptor. The argument becomes one of extrinsic versus intrinsic fibroblast derangement.

This work found overexpression of Smad7 in scleroderma fibroblasts—evidence in support of a normal pathway of feedback regulation. However, Smad7 was found to constitutively form a complex with TGF-β receptor and have minimal inhibitory effect on procollagen transcription. Of great interest was the inability of Smurf 1 and Smurf 2, either alone or with TGF-β, in scleroderma-derived fibroblasts, to increase TGF-β1.

Impaired Smad7 mediated inhibition of TGF-β effects appears to be a consistent finding in scleroderma but appears also to be intrinsically linked to Smad7-Smurf interaction. This is a novel report of impaired negative regulation.

J. R. Seibold, MD

Persistent Down-Regulation of Fli1, a Suppressor of Collagen Transcription, in Fibrotic Scleroderma Skin

Kubo M, Czuwara-Ladykowska J, Moussa O, et al (Med Univ of South Carolina, Charleston; Warsaw Med Academy, Poland)

Am J Pathol 163:571-581, 2003 4–8

Introduction.—The turnover of collagen type I, the primary component of human dermis, is tightly regulated under normal physiologic conditions. Very little is understood concerning regulatory mechanisms that control this process. Fli1, a transcription factor that inhibits collagen gene transcription by an Sp 1-dependent pathway, is a member of the Ets family of transcription factors and has roles in hematopoiesis, embryonic development, and vasculogenesis. The specific role(s) of the Ets factors in the maintenance of collagen level homeostasis in healthy skin and their possible role in fibroproliferative disorders, including systemic scleroderma (SSc), have yet to be sufficiently examined. The specificity of Fli1 as an inhibitor of collagen gene expression in dermal fibroblasts was assessed in vitro and in human skin in vivo, along with whether Fli1 has a role in the abnormal collagen deposition characteristic of SSc skin.

Methods.—Skin biopsies from 25 patients with diffuse cutaneous SSc and 21 healthy volunteers underwent examination by immunohistochemistry, collagen mRNA measurements by in situ hybridization, cell cultures, construction of Ets1 adenovirus and Fli1 adenovirus, procollagen analysis, Western blot, and analysis of MEFs.

Results.—It appears that Fli1 is a physiologic negative regulator of collagen gene expression in dermal fibroblasts in vitro and in human skin in vivo. This finding was supported by the analyses of mouse embryonic fibroblasts from Fli1$^{-/-}$, Fli1$^{+/-}$, and Fli1$^{+/+}$ mice. In cultured human and mouse fibroblasts, Fli1 expression levels were inversely associated with the collagen type I expression levels. These in vitro observations were confirmed in vivo. In healthy human skin, Fli1 protein was expressed in both fibroblasts and endothelial cells. Significantly, absence of Fli1 expression in individual fibroblasts was linked with elevated collagen synthesis. In contrast to healthy skin, Fli1 protein was consistently missing from fibroblasts and significantly decreased in endothelial cells in clinically involved scleroderma skin, which is associated with enhanced collagen synthesis in synthetic sclerosis skin.

► A hallmark of SSc is overexpression of extracellular matrix, including collagen. A variety of data link this to an extrinsic response of myofibroblast differentiation and migration away from their normal perivascular locations. This is clearly overly simplistic in that the normal homeostasis of collagen in health is a complex, highly regulated process.

Fli1 is a transcription factor that inhibits collagen gene transcription by an Sp1-dependent pathway. It is a member of the Ets transcription family, which in turn plays a fundamental role in hematopoiesis, embryonic development, and vasculogenesis.

In a variety of interrelated experiments, Fli1 was found to be consistently absent to reduced in both endothelium and fibroblasts from clinically affected skin obtained from patients with SSc. These observations are consistent with positive regulation of Fli1 by TNFβ and negative regulation by TGFβ.

These data strongly suggest that prolonged absence of Fli1 in SSc tissue has a direct relationship with the process of fibrosis. Dysregulation of Fli1 transcription may be secondary but in turn offers a novel approach to future manipulation of SSc fibroblast biology.

J. R. Seibold, MD

Systemic Sclerosis Th2 Cells Inhibit Collagen Production by Dermal Fibroblasts Via Membrane-Associated Tumor Necrosis Factor α

Chizzolini C, Parel Y, De Luca C, et al (Geneva Univ, Switzerland; Univ of Basel, Switzerland; Lund Univ, Sweden)

Arthritis Rheum 48:2593-2604, 2003 4–9

Background.—In scleroderma or systemic sclerosis (SSc), organs that are undergoing fibrotic changes become infiltrated with T cells. It is hypothesized that these T cells then take part in dysregulating the production of collagen by fibroblasts. Whether these infiltrating T cells seen in early SSc belong to a specific functional subset and can dysregulate collagen production was explored.

Methods.—The distribution and production of interferon-γ (IFN-γ) in T cell lines generated from the skin of patients with SSc were assessed by a 4-color cytometric analysis. The T-cell clones generated were investigated for an ability to modulate collagen and matrix metalloproteinase 1 (MMP-1) production by fibroblasts taken from patients with SSc and from unaffected persons. The T-cell mediators of fibroblast modulation were identified by using neutralizing reagents.

Results.—Four subsets of the SSc skin–derived T cells were identified with respect to the expression of CD4 and CD8. The most abundant were single-positive CD4 and single-positive CD8 T cells. Nineteen of the 20 cell lines had sizable numbers of CD4+,CD8+ double-positive cells and 16 of 20 had a few CD4−,CD8− double-negative cells. The production of IFNγ and interleukin-4 (IL-4) was significantly higher for the SSc skin–derived T cells than for control subjects. There were dramatic differences depending on the subset analyzed. Thus, T cells that infiltrate the skin of persons with early-stage SSc proved heterogeneous regarding CD4 and CD8 and are ready to produce high levels of IL-4. All SSc skin–derived T cells were able to inhibit collagen production by SSc and normal fibroblasts. Activated Th1 and Th2 plasma cell membranes were both able to inhibit control fibroblasts, but Th2 membranes could not inhibit collagen production by SSc fibroblasts. SSc fibroblasts were resistant to inhibition by Th1 cells. Thus, T cells, whether Th1 or Th2 in functional phenotype, deliver inhibitory signals to dermal fibroblasts. Tumor necrosis factor α (TNFα) and IFNγ were both involved in the contact-dependent inhibition of collagen production by Th1 cells (Fig 4).

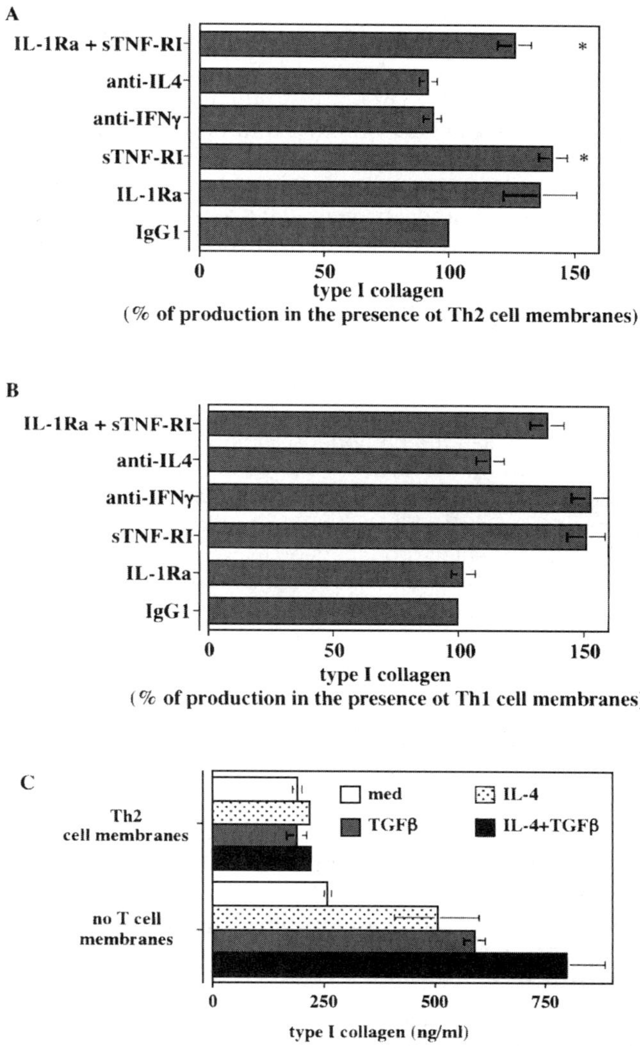

FIGURE 4.—Th2 cell contact–dependent inhibition of collagen production is mediated by TNFα and is dominant on profibrotic cytokines. Control fibroblasts were cultured in the presence of 20 μL of T-cell membrane preparations equivalent to 8 × 10^5 cells from 3 Th2 clones (**A** and **C**) and from 1 representative Th1 clone (**B**). Blocking reagents (**A** and **B**) or profibrotic cytokines (**C**) were added to fibroblast cultures 30 minutes before the addition of T-cell membranes. The N-terminal type I procollagen propeptide was assessed in 48-hour culture supernatants. Bars show the mean ± SEM (**A** and **C**) and the mean ± SD (**B**). *Abbreviations: IL-1Ra,* Interleukin-1 receptor antagonist; *sTNF-RI,* soluble TNF receptor I; *med,* medium. (Courtesy of Chizzolini C, Parel Y, De Luca C, et al: Systemic sclerosis Th2 cells inhibit collagen production by dermal fibroblasts via membrane-associated tumor necrosis factor α. *Arthritis Rheum* 48:2593-2604, 2003. Reprinted by permission of John Wiley & Sons, Inc.)

Collagen production was greatly enhanced by IL-4 and transforming growth factor β (TGFβ), but the Th2 cell membrane's inhibitory effect was more potent than the effect of these factors alone or in combination. Both Th1 and Th2 cells were able to potently inhibit collagen production when T cells were activated by CD3 crosslinking. Inhibition was reversed by TNFα blockade mediated by Th2 cell clones. IL-4, IFNγ, and IL-1 neutralization was not effective in these situations. Enhanced MMP-1 production was induced by living Th2 cells and Th1 cells. Th2 cells were able to influence the steady-state levels of type 1 collagen and MMP-1 in a way reflective of protein production.

Conclusions.—Type 1 collagen synthesis by dermal fibroblasts is reduced by Th2 cells even with the production of IL-4. This occurs because of the dominant effect of TNFα. Thus, treatments for SSc based on TNFα blockade to control fibrosis are most likely not advisable.

► The role of the T cell in the pathogenesis of SSc remains controversial. In this study, 4-color cytometric analysis was used to characterize T-cell populations generated from skin samples of SSc patients. Past data have suggested a Th2 dominance in SSc skin and in peripheral blood. CD4+ T cells predominate over CD8+ and are high producers on INFγ.

This study demonstrated T cells preferentially producing IL-4. Cloned CD4+ cells demonstrated a paradoxic contact-dependent inhibition of fibroblast collagen production. Data suggest that TNFα was the key mediator of this effect and was clearly dominant over the profibrotic effects of IL-4 produced by these same cells.

These data argue strongly against an approach to therapy of SSc with the various available TNFα trapping agents.

J. R. Seibold, MD

Insights Into the Molecular Mechanism of Chronic Fibrosis: The Role of Connective Tissue Growth Factor in Scleroderma

Leask A, Denton CP, Abraham DJ (Univ College London)

J Invest Dermatol 122:1-6, 2004 4–10

Background.—Systemic sclerosis (SSc) is a connective tissue disease that affects both the skin and internal organs. It can be fatal, and no treatment has yet proved effective, in part because the cause of the disorder remains a mystery. The development of effective treatment strategies depends on an understanding of normal wound healing processes and how they can become disrupted and produce rampant scarring and fibrosis. The cysteine-rich matricellular protein connective tissue growth factor (CTGF) is a member of the CCN family of proteins but is not normally expressed in dermal fibroblasts. The role of CTGF as a marker and mediator of the fibrotic phenotype of scleroderma was reviewed.

CTGF Function and Receptors.—Functions of CTGF include promoting fibroblast proliferation, matrix production, the formation of granulation tissue, and cell adhesion and migration for a number of cell types. Recombinant CTGF has been thought to induce chondrocyte differentiation and proliferation through p38 and mitogen-activated protein kinase, respectively, as well as angiogenesis. These roles have been supported by the findings from animal studies. No specific receptor for CTGF has been identified. Many activities are promoted through the binding of integrins and cell surface heparin sulfate proteoglycans. Of the factors that have been explored, CTGF is most strongly induced by transforming growth factor-β (TGF-β).

Relation to Fibrotic Response.—Findings suggest that a CTGF response element dwells in the type 1 collagen promoter. The effect of CTGF induced by TGF-β may be a prolonged fibrotic response; only transient fibrosis occurs with either of these factors alone (Fig 2). The Smad3 protein is required for the initiation of fibrosis, and elevated phosphorylated Smad3 levels are found in the leading edge of SSc fibroblasts compared with normal fibroblasts. Therefore, an elevated Smad3 activation is linked to the initiation of the fibrotic response in SSc. Fibroblasts that are found in skin fibrotic lesions, including scleroderma, constitutively overexpress CTGF. In that CTGF promotes matrix deposition, fibroblast adhesion, and fibroblast

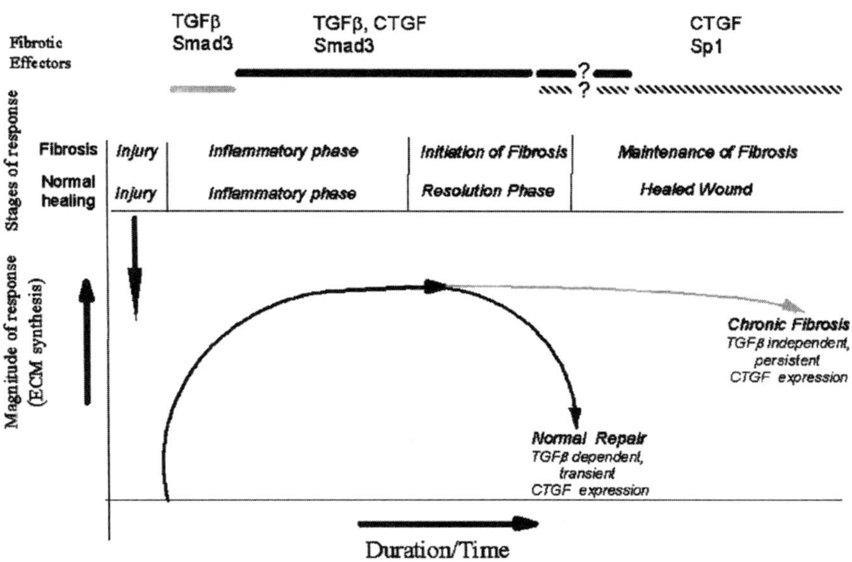

FIGURE 2.—Model of sustained, chronic fibrosis. TGF-β is necessary for initiation of normal wound healing response, including expression of extracellular matrix (*ECM*) and CTGF in dermal fibroblasts. In normal wound healing response, action of TGF-β, including induction of CTGF, is suppressed leading to proper termination of wound healing response (*solid arrow*). Conversely, in pathologic fibrosis the expression of CTGF in lesion is independent of TGF-β action. Thus, CTGF expression is not subject to controls that normally terminate wound healing response. Fibrotic response persists, leading to sustained, chronic fibrosis (*shaded arrow*). Phases of normal wound healing and fibrotic response are shown, and effectors of fibrotic response are shown at top of diagram. (Courtesy of Leask A, Denton CP, Abraham DJ: Insight into the molecular mechanism of chronic fibrosis: The role of connective tissue growth factor in scleroderma. *J Invest Dermatol* 122:1-6, 2004. Reprinted by permission of Blackwell Publishing.)

proliferation, this overexpression contributes to the phenotype of scleroderma. Elevated matrix genes in lesional SSc fibroblasts may be related to elevated Sp1 activity.

Conclusions.—The constitutive overexpression of CTGF by fibroblasts in fibrotic lesions most likely contributes directly to chronic persistent fibrosis. Thus, CTGF may be a molecular target for therapeutic interventions in persons with fibrotic disease such as SSc.

► This is a concise and timely review article of the considerable evidence that implicates CTGF in the pathogenesis of the fibrotic features of systemic sclerosis. CTGF is constitutively overexpressed in fibrotic tissue and is directly linked to both extracellular matrix production and fibroblast proliferation. There are some data that argue that TGF-β is a key initiator of the SSc fibroblast phenotype but that its effects are short lived. A more persistent effect of TGF-β is induction of CTGF and the sequence of exposures mimics the clinical, pathologic, and biochemical events of chronic fibrosis.

These issues are relevant to the clinician and clinical researcher in that "trapping" strategies, mainly monoclonal antibodies, to both CTGF and TGF-β have entered clinical trials in both scleroderma and in idiopathic pulmonary interstitial fibrosis.

While the trial data, when available, will speak for themselves, this is applied science of unusual specificity for the derangements of scleroderma. Will these agents be effective? Will one be superior to the other? Will the pleiotropic effects of TGF-β on other biologic functions, such as inflammatory response, render trapping strategies either carcinogenic or proinflammatory?

J. R. Seibold, MD

Angiotension II in the Lesional Skin of Systemic Sclerosis Patients Contributes to Tissue Fibrosis Via Angiotensin II Type 1 Receptors

Kawaguchi Y, Takagi K, Hara M, et al (Tokyo Women's Med Univ)

Arthritis Rheum 50:216-226, 2004 4–11

Introduction.—Tissue fibrosis in patients with systemic sclerosis (SSc) may be caused by excessive deposition of extracellular matrix components produced by fibroblasts in skin lesions. Angiotensin II, a vasoconstrictive peptide, is reported to have profibrotic activity consequent to induction of the extracellular matrix. The expression of angiotensin II and its type 1 (AT_2) and type 2 (AT_2) receptors in affected skin and dermal fibroblasts was evaluated in patients with SSc. The role of angiotensin II in collagen production by SSc dermal fibroblasts was also examined.

Methods.—Levels of angiotensin II in sera from patients with SSc and normal research subjects were determined by a solid-phase immobilized-epitope immunoassay. Expression of angiotensinogen in the skin was assessed by immunohistochemistry. Expression of angiotensinogen, AT_1, and AT_2 in cultured dermal fibroblasts was evaluated by reverse transcription polymerase chain reaction and immunohistochemistry. The levels of type I

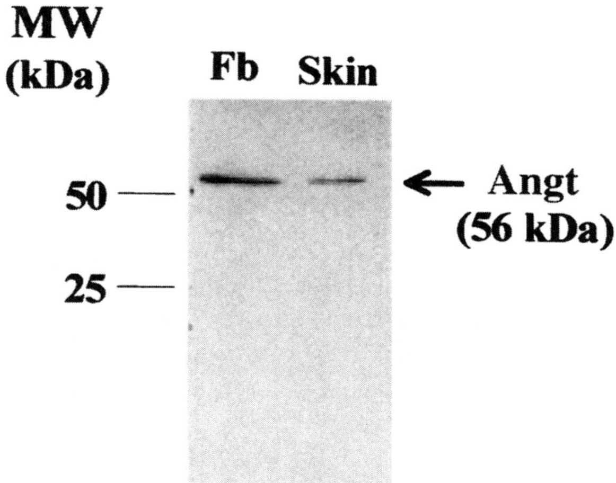

FIGURE 5.—Western blotting of angiotensins (angiotensinogen, angiotensin I, and angiotensin II) in skin and cultured dermal fibroblasts (*Fb*) from a patient with diffuse cutaneous SSc and high serum levels of angiotensin II. Proteins from lysates of skin and cultured dermal fibroblasts were subjected to electrophoresis in a sodium dodecyl sulfate-12.5% polyacrylamide gel, transferred to a polyvinylidene difluoride membrane, and the membrane was immunoblotted with antibody against human angiotensins. (Courtesy of Kawaguchi Y, Takagi K, Hara M, et al: Angiotensin II in the lesional skin of systemic sclerosis patients contributes to tissue fibrosis via angiotensin II type I receptors. *Arthritis Rheum* 50:216-226, 2004. Reprinted by permission of John Wiley & Sons, Inc.)

procollagen produced by cultured dermal fibroblasts were determined by enzyme-linked immunosorbent assay.

Results.—The serum angiotensin II levels in patients with diffuse cutaneous SSc were significantly higher than those in patients with limited cutaneous SSc and in healthy donors. Immunohistochemical and immunoblotting analyses revealed that angiotensinogen was present in the skin of patients with SSc and not in normal skin (Fig 5). Angiotensinogen mRNA was expressed in fibroblasts in patients with diffuse cutaneous SSc with high levels of serum angiotensin II and not in normal fibroblasts. AT_1 mRNA expression was observed in both SSc and normal fibroblasts. AT_2 mRNA expression was detected only in SSc fibroblasts. Exogenous angiotensin II augmented the production of both type I procollagen and transforming growth factor 1 by cultured fibroblasts through activation of AT_1 (Fig 8).

Conclusion.—Aberrant angiotensin II production might be involved in tissue fibrosis through excessive production of the extracellular matrix components in SSc dermal fibroblasts. It is likely that the use of AT_1 receptor antagonists may be a novel strategy in the treatment of tissue fibroblasts in patients with SSc.

► Angiotensin II has recognized profibrotic actions in renal and myocardial disease but has not been investigated in systemic sclerosis.

This ambitious trial demonstrated elevated levels of angiotensin II in the sera of patients with systemic sclerosis and further demonstrated high levels in involved skin in patients with diffuse scleroderma. Angiotensin mRNA was

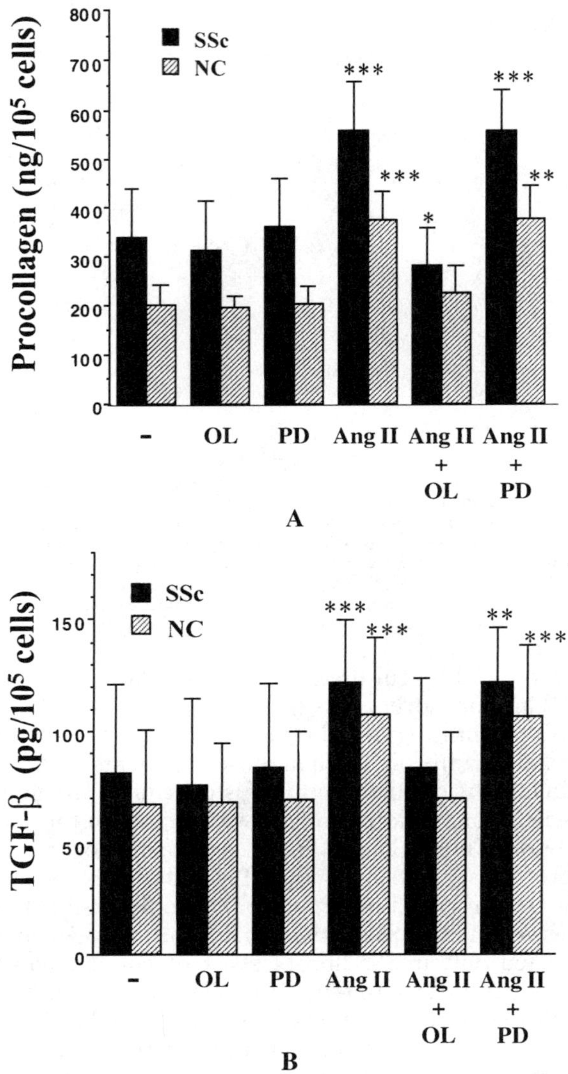

FIGURE 8.—Functional analyses of AT_1 and AT_2 receptors on cultured dermal fibroblasts from 6 patients with diffuse cutaneous systemic sclerosis and high levels of serum angiotensin II (*SSc*) and 5 normal controls (*NC*). Fibroblasts were cultured in 24-well culture plates with serum-free media containing 1 μmol/L angiotensin II, 1 μmol/L olmesartan (*OL*, an AT_1 receptor antagonist), and 10 μmol/L PD 123,319 (an AT_2 receptor antagonist). Production of procollagen (**A**) and transforming growth factor β (TGFβ) (**B**) in the supernatants was measured by enzyme-linked immunoabsorbent assays. *P = .05; **P < .01; ***P < .001 vs levels without stimuli. (Courtesy of Kawaguchi Y, Takagi K, Hara M, et al: Angiotensin II in the lesional skin of systemic sclerosis patients contributes to tissue fibrosis via angiotensin II type I receptors. *Arthritis Rheum* 50:216-226, 2004. Reprinted by permission of John Wiley & Sons, Inc.)

constitutively upregulated in diffuse scleroderma fibroblasts. Exogenous angiotensin II led to increased production of both procollagen I and TGFβ by both normal and scleroderma-derived fibroblasts.

A limited series of receptor antagonist experiments suggested that angiotensin II effects were mediated by the AT_1 receptor.

The authors remind the readership of several alternative pathways for angiotensin production that are independent of the classic renin angiotensin-converting enzyme cascade. It is known that local tissue production of angiotensin occurs and that several non–angiotensin-converting enzyme cleaving enzymes, including tissue cathepsins and chymase, can serve as alternate pathways.

This is truly novel work that deserves confirmation. Here is a system that clearly segregates between diffuse and limited scleroderma and is plausibly linked to well-described tissue and biologic events of the disease. As multiple AT_1 receptor antagonists are either available or eligible for drug development, interventional trials may actually be realized.

J. R. Seibold, MD

In Vivo Analysis of the Apoptosis-Inducing Effect of Anti–Endothelial Cell Antibodies in Systemic Sclerosis by the Chorionallantoic Membrane Assay

Worda M, Sgonc R, Dietrich H, et al (Univ of Innsbruck, Austria; Wayne State Univ, Detroit; Univ of California, Davis)

Arthritis Rheum 48:2605-2614, 2003 4–12

Background.—Systemic sclerosis is characterized by vascular lesions, immune dysregulation, and an increased deposition of extracellular matrix in the skin and internal organs. It is thought that these 3 pathogenetic processes are closely related because endothelium, mononuclear cells, and fibroblasts interact through direct contact and by cytokines, which finally result in fibrosis. The initiating event for this pathogenetic cascade has not been elucidated, and animal models are needed in the search for a cause. Vascular injury is known to occur early in the course of disease, and previous in vitro studies have suggested a primary role for antiendothelial antibodies (AECAs) in the mediation of endothelial cell apoptosis. The apoptosis-inducing effect of AECAs in vivo was analyzed.

Methods.—The University of California at Davis line 200 (UCD-200) chickens were used because these animals spontaneously develop a hereditary disease with features that closely resemble those of scleroderma in human beings. AECA-positive samples from these chickens were used for IV injection into normal CC chicken embryos on embryonic day (ED) 13 as well as for application onto chorionallantoic membranes (CAMs) of healthy control lines on ED 10. CAMs of ED 16 embryos and combs of 1-week-old CC chickens that had received the injection serum samples were analyzed for apoptotic endothelial cells by the TUNEL technique.

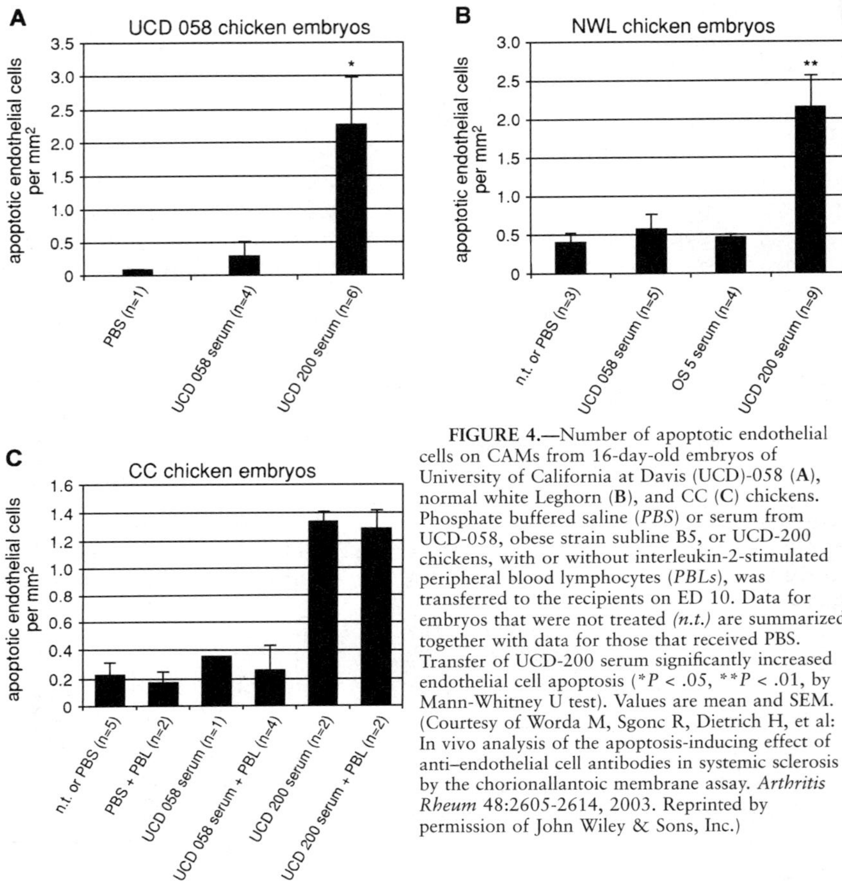

FIGURE 4.—Number of apoptotic endothelial cells on CAMs from 16-day-old embryos of University of California at Davis (UCD)-058 (**A**), normal white Leghorn (**B**), and CC (**C**) chickens. Phosphate buffered saline (*PBS*) or serum from UCD-058, obese strain subline B5, or UCD-200 chickens, with or without interleukin-2-stimulated peripheral blood lymphocytes (*PBLs*), was transferred to the recipients on ED 10. Data for embryos that were not treated *(n.t.)* are summarized together with data for those that received PBS. Transfer of UCD-200 serum significantly increased endothelial cell apoptosis ($^{*}P < .05$, $^{**}P < .01$, by Mann-Whitney U test). Values are mean and SEM. (Courtesy of Worda M, Sgonc R, Dietrich H, et al: In vivo analysis of the apoptosis-inducing effect of anti–endothelial cell antibodies in systemic sclerosis by the chorionallantoic membrane assay. *Arthritis Rheum* 48:2605-2614, 2003. Reprinted by permission of John Wiley & Sons, Inc.)

Results.—Staining from frozen CAM sections by immunofluorescence demonstrated evidence of in vivo binding of AECAs to the microvascular endothelium. Transfer of AECA-positive sera in most groups led to a significant increase in endothelial cell apoptosis as compared with control subjects (Fig 4).

Conclusions.—The first demonstration of in vivo apoptosis-inducing effects of anti-endothelial cell antibodies was provided by this study. These findings support the hypothesis of a primary pathogenetic role of AECAs in systemic sclerosis.

► Endothelial injury appears to be a fundamental initial step in the pathobiologic sequence that initiates scleroderma. The mechanism of injury remains unclear, as do the molecular events that either perpetuate injury or interfere with endothelial repair and recovery. It is intellectually defensible to consider scleroderma as primarily a vasculopathy, with extravascular fibrosis an inconsistent and sometimes short-lived event.

Several laboratories have demonstrated a high prevalence of antibody reactive with endothelium in patients with scleroderma. Remembering that antibody-mediated vasculitis is virtually never encountered in this disease, the role of these antibodies remains unclear. Do they arise as secondary to target cell injury, or do they actually participate in propagation of vascular injury?

This group has for years pursued investigations of the "scleroderma chicken"—a hereditary model with many vascular features of strong resemblance to human disease. Anti–endothelial cell antibody derived from affected adults was injected into both healthy chick embryos as well as applied onto chorioallantoic membranes of healthy control subjects. Binding to endothelium was demonstrable and associated with a marked increase in endothelial cell apoptosis by TUNEL.

These findings, if extrapolated to human disease, would offer a novel and surprising insight into potential mechanisms of tissue injury in scleroderma.

J. R. Seibold, MD

Mutant Fibrillin 1 From Tight Skin Mice Increases Extracellular Matrix Incorporation of Microfibril-Associated Glycoprotein 2 and Type I Collagen

Lemaire R, Farina G, Kissin E, et al (Boston Univ; Washington Univ, St Louis; Mount Sinai School of Medicine, New York)

Arthritis Rheum 50:915-926, 2004 4–13

Introduction.—Skin fibrosis in the tight skin (TSK) mouse, a model of skin fibrosis observed in systemic sclerosis (SSc), is caused by a large in-frame duplication in the *Fbn1* gene, *tsk-Fbn1*. An in vitro model of the TSK mouse was evaluated: (1) to determine whether *tsk-Fbn1* could cause dermal fibrosis by affecting *Fbn1* and extracellular matrices, and (2) to determine whether deposition of microfibril-associated glycoprotein 2 (MAGP-2), a protein linked with fibrillin 1 (Fbn-1), was altered in the skin of patients with SSc.

Methods.—An in vitro model of the TSK mouse was produced by conditionally expressing *tsk-Fbn1* in mouse embryonic fibroblasts (MEFs). Cell cultures were evaluated via immunofluorescence and Western and Northern blotting to ascertain the effect of *tsk-Fbn1* on the structure, expression, and deposition of Fbn-1, type I collagen, and MAGP-2. The skin of TSK mice and SSc patients was evaluated by immunohistochemistry for MAGP-2 expression.

Results.—Expression of *tsk-Fbn1* in cultured MEF cells modified the morphology of Fbn-1 fibers and increased the deposition of type I collagen into the extracellular matrix (ECM) without concomitantly altering messenger RNA expression, secretion, or processing of type I procollagen (Fig 5). The MEF cells expression *tsk-Fbn1* demonstrated increased MAGP-2 matrix, which was increased in the dermis of TSK mice. Fibrotic SSc skin also revealed higher levels of MAGP-2 in the dermis, compared with the nonfibrotic SSc skin and normal skin.

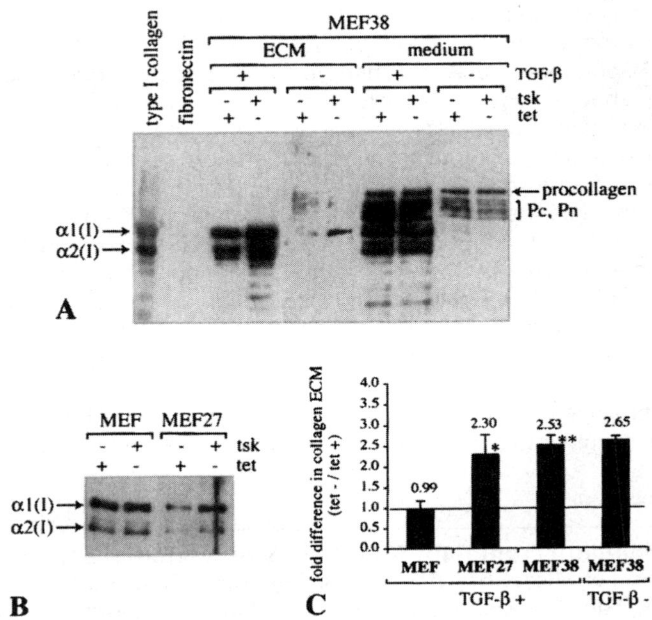

FIGURE 5.—Expression of tsk-fibrillin (tsk-Fbn-1) increases type I collagen extracellular matrix (*ECM*) deposition, but not secretion of type I procollagen. **A,** Type I collagen trichloroacetic acid precipitated from the medium or deposited into the ECM, detected by Western blot analysis of MEF38 cells cultured in the presence or absence of tetracycline, with or without transforming growth factor β (*TGFβ*) (2 ng/mL), in the presence of ascorbate. Type I collagen antibody specifically detected purified type I collagen chains while not cross-reacting with purified fibronectin. **B,** Type I collagen deposited into the FCM, detected by Western blot analysis of tsk-Fbn1–transfected cells (MEF27) and TGFβ (2 ng/mL). **C,** Graphic representation of the average tsk-Fbn1–associated change in ECM type I (α1, α2) collagen levels. Type I collagen levels were quantified by densitometry. Results are the mean and SD obtained from 3 parallel experiments for control MEF and MEF38 cells and 2 for MEF27 cells. **P* < .05 versus control MEF. ***P* < .0005 versus control MEF by Student *t* test. *Abbreviations: Pc,* Procollagen; *Pn,* partially processed collagen. (Courtesy of Lemaire R, Farina G, Kissin E, et al: Mutant fibrillin 1 from tight skin mice increases extracellular matrix incorporation of microfibril-associated glycoprotein 2 and type I collagen. *Arthritis Rheum* 50:915-926, 2004. Reprinted by permission of John Wiley & Sons, Inc.)

Conclusion.—Tsk-Fbn1 modified ECM organization and generated fibrosis by impacting the deposition of MAGP-2 or other Fbn-1-associated proteins. Alternations in microfibril structure or deposition may contribute to fibrosis in SSc.

► The TSK mouse is an excellent model for the ECM aberrations of skin involvement in human scleroderma. TSK mice have a large in-frame duplication of the *Fbn1* gene (*tsk-Fbn1*). In turn, tissue from human scleroderma, in addition to overproduction and accumulation of types I and III collagen, shows increase in a variety of ECM constituents, including alpha-smooth muscle action, glycosaminoglycan, laminin, fibronectin, and fibrillin. In addition to providing architectural framework for matrix array, fibrillin serves as a platform for the "storage" of transforming growth factor-beta.

This elegant study constructed an in vitro system that used cell cultures of embryonic murine fibroblasts. Expression of *tsk-Fbn1* in these cells increased type I collagen deposition independent of transcription. Similar effects were noted with MAGP-1. These findings offer mechanistic insight into the potential role of altered or overexpressed fibrillin and suggest that secondary ECM constituent interactions influence the matrix accumulation typical of scleroderma.

It is perhaps facile to view scleroderma as a prototypic fibrosing disease. Although accumulation of long-lived collagen is doubtless important, there are reasons to suspect that there are earlier, more fundamental and perhaps non-immune system-driven pathways to tissue fibrosis.

J. R. Seibold, MD

A Modified Model of Graft-Versus-Host–Induced Systemic Sclerosis (Scleroderma) Exhibits All Major Aspects of the Human Disease

Ruzek MC, Jha S, Ledbetter S, et al (Genzyme Corp, Framingham, Mass)

Arthritis Rheum 50:1319-1331, 2004 4–14

Introduction.—Diffuse systemic sclerosis (SSc; scleroderma) is a debilitating disease characterized by excessive dermal fibrosis and involvement of multiple physiologic systems. The disease also includes vascular or circulatory involvement and immune dysregulation manifested by inflammatory cells in affected tissues and production of autoantibodies. Many animal models resembling SSc have been evaluated, including genetic models in mice and chicken, challenge with chemicals to induce fibrosis, and models of graft-versus-host (GVH)-induced disease using certain mouse strains with differences in minor histocompatibility loci. Mice were examined to determine whether alteration of the induction of GVH-induced scleroderma could produce a model that more fully represents the human condition.

Methods.—Disease was induced via injection of spleen cells from B10.D2 mice into BALB/c mice deficient in mature T and B cells (recombination-

TABLE 1.—Comparison Between the Model of Graft-Versus-Host (GVH)–Induced Systemic Sclerosis (SSc) in Recombination-Activating Gene-2-Targeted (RAG-2KO) Mice and Human SSc

Disease Parameter	GVH SSc in RAG-2KO Mice	Human SSc
Dermal thickening in extremities	+	+
Increases in collagen expression	+	+
Vasoconstriction/vasospasm	+	+
Circulating autoantibodies	+	+
Internal organ fibrosis	+/−*	+

*Present in kidney and intestines, absent in lungs and heart, at all time points up to 9 weeks of disease.

(Courtesy of Ruzek MC, Jha S, Ledbetter S, et al: A modified model of graft-versus-host–induced systemic sclerosis (scleroderma) exhibits all major aspects of the human disease. *Arthritis Rheum* 50:1319-1331, 2004. Reprinted by permission of John Wiley & Sons, Inc.)

activating gene 2 targeted). Dermal thickening, collagen deposition, vasoconstriction, and parameters of immunity were evaluated.

Results.—Similar to the human disease, this modified GVH model of SSc showed evidence of dermal thickening, especially in the extremities, progressive fibrosis of internal organs, vasoconstriction and altered expression of vascularity markers in skin and internal organs, early immune activation, inflammation in skin and internal organs, and autoantibody generation (Table 1).

Conclusion.—This modified model of GVH-induced SSc displays all major components of human disease and may contribute to better understanding of the disease mechanism and improved treatment for patients with SSc.

► A cohesive hypothesis for the pathogenesis of SSc must account for the prominent functional and structural abnormalities of the vasculature in addition to the prominent immune derangements and accumulation of extracellular matrix constitutents, including collagen. In addition, these features are actually somewhat more consistent/characteristic of visceral features of disease rather than as directly relevant to the dermatologic features.

Animal models of scleroderma have failed to reasonably mimic human disease by either lacking visceral features or by lacking similar vascular disease. This is not the case in this creative model of GVH disease. Spleen cells from B10.D2 mice were injected into BALB/C mice deficient in mature T and B cells. Multiorgan fibrosis, vascular injury, and immune activation features were noted, although this model had little change in lung and heart.

The clinician should be reminded of the many clinical similarities between human GVH disease and SSc. These data lend credibility to the hypothesis that naturally occurring scleroderma may also be in fact a GVH mechanism, wherein the "graft" is transplacentally trafficked fetal cells.

J. R. Seibold, MD

Clinical Aspects

Genome-Wide Association Study for Regions of Systemic Sclerosis Susceptibility in a Choctaw Indian Population With High Disease Prevalence
Zhou X, Tan FK, Wang N, et al (Univ of Texas, Houston; Univ of Cincinnati, Ohio)
Arthritis Rheum 48:2585-2592, 2003 4–15

Background.—In the autoimmune connective tissue disorder systemic sclerosis (SSc), the prominent characteristics are widespread cutaneous and visceral fibrosis, obliterative small vessel vasculopathy, and autoantibodies directed against specific nuclear and nucleolar components. Clinical heterogeneity marks the extent of skin and internal organ involvement and the expression of SSc-specific autoantibodies. A complex genetic situation exists, with more than one genetic locus most likely contributing to disease susceptibility and clinical manifestations. SSc is rare and recurs infrequently in families, making conventional genetic linkage studies of multiplex families difficult. The Oklahoma Choctaw Indians have a high prevalence of SSc with a relatively homogeneous clinical expression. Previous studies found a significant relation between SSc and the fibrillin 1 gene (*FBN1*) on chromosome 15q. Additional studies have shown links with the secreted protein, acidic and rich in cysteine gene (*SPARC*), or osteonectin gene on chromosome 5q and the topoisomerase I gene (*TOPOI*) on chromosome 20q. A study was undertaken to localize chromosome regions linked with susceptibility to SSc among the Choctaw Indian group.

Methods.—Twenty Choctaw Indians with SSc and 76 ethnically matched control subjects were evaluated by a genomewide microsatellite screen at 10 cM resolution. The results of the initial screen guided the fine-scale microsatellite mapping at 1 cM or less resolution in 10 selected chromosome regions. The patients with SSc and control subjects were compared with respect to allele and marker haplotype frequencies.

Results.—Highly significant associations with SSc were found for 12 markers from the genomewide screen. Significant associations were found for 5 additional markers. The loci *D5S410, D6S422, D15S978*, and *D20S107* are near the genes *SPARC*, major histocompatibility complex (*MHC*), *FBN1*, and *TOPOI*, respectively. This confirmed the results obtained in the previous studies indicating these were potential SSc susceptibility genes in the Choctaw population. Markers that showed unique associations with SSc were *D7S510* (7p12-11), *D7S661* (7q35), *D8S514* (8q24.12), *D19S221* (19p13.2), *D19S220* (19q13.2), *D22S423* (22q13.1), *DXS1068* (Xp11.4), and *DXS8055* (Xq21-23). Assuming an inbreeding coefficient of 10%, the adjusted probability for haplotype 171, 292, 305 at the 6p22.3 region becomes 1.61×10^{-2}, indicating that shared ancestry cannot account for the significantly higher frequency of these haplotypes in individuals with SSc. This leads to the conclusion that these haplotypes are probably associated with SSc. Some markers shown to be associated with SSc are known to have linkage to systemic lupus erythematosus and occur in regions reported to be associated with lupus and other autoimmune diseases.

Conclusions.—As suspected, multiple genetic factors most likely contribute to produce SSc. In addition, SSc-specific genetic determinants are likely to combine with the genes linked to other autoimmune diseases in the pathogenesis of SSc. Candidate regions need closer examination to identify the actual predisposing genes.

► Evidence mounts that SSc has a complex genetic etiopathogenesis both for risk of disease and for subset of illness once disease is established. A carefully defined population of Choctaw native Americans living in Oklahoma has been found to have a high prevalence of disease and strikingly homogenous clinical presentation.

Previous studies of this population used "candidate" gene surveys and found strong linkage with *FBN1* as well as associations with genes for osteonectin and *TOPOI*. In this more sophisticated study, a 10-cM-density genomewide scanning technique was used. Twelve different markers of scleroderma were identified that included loci near the locations of *FBN1, osteonectin, TOPOI*, and *MHC*. Of great interest, 2 of the scleroderma markers are linked to systemic lupus erythematosus in family-based studies, whereas several others are in regions associated with both lupus and other autoimmune diseases.

This elegant study forms the basis for investigations in the non-Choctaw population. It is considered likely that a panel of markers will evolve that identifies genetic risk of disease.

J. R. Seibold, MD

Prevalence, Incidence, Survival, and Disease Characteristics of Systemic Sclerosis in a Large US Population

Mayes MD, Lacey JV Jr, Beebe-Dimmer J, et al (Univ of Texas, Houston; Natl Cancer Inst, Rockville, Md; Univ of Michigan, Ann Arbor; et al)

Arthritis Rheum 48:2246-2255, 2003 4–16

Background.—A wide variation is seen in the published estimates of the prevalence and incidence of systemic sclerosis (SSc), depending on the period of observation, methods of case identification, and geographic area of study. The survival rate of patients with SSc has improved in the past several decades, but the rate continues to be considerably diminished in comparison with that of age- and sex-matched populations. Reliable overall survival rate estimates and survival rates by disease subtypes are important factors in the determination of the effects of new treatment modalities or the documentation of the changing natural history of SSc. The prevalence, incidence, survival rate, and disease characteristics of SSc in a major urban area of the United States were assessed.

Methods.—A census of SSc cases for the years 1989 through 1991 in the Detroit area was conducted using multiple sources for case identification, including a computer search of the databases of all area hospitals, of the patient populations of hospitals and outpatient clinics affiliated with 2 university medical centers, and of data bases of patients from the practices of 70% of area rheumatologists. Diagnoses were verified by medical record reviews. Capture-recapture analysis was used to estimate the total SSc population. Cases of localized scleroderma were excluded.

Results.—On the basis of 706 verified cases of SSc, the prevalence of SSc was initially estimated to be 242 cases per million adults, with an annual incidence of 19.3 new cases per million adults per year. Capture-recapture analysis, which was based on the degree of overlap of verified cases among multiple sources, provided a revised prevalence estimate of 276 cases per million adults. Sex- and race-specific prevalence estimates were significantly higher for women than for men and for blacks than for whites. The average age at diagnosis was significantly younger for blacks than for whites. Comparison of black and white patients showed that black patients were nearly twice as likely to have diffuse disease (Fig 5). The median survival time was approximately 11 years. Factors that were found to negatively affect survival time included male sex and older age at diagnosis.

Conclusions.—Baseline estimates of SSc occurrence and characteristics were established in a large US cohort that included primarily black adults

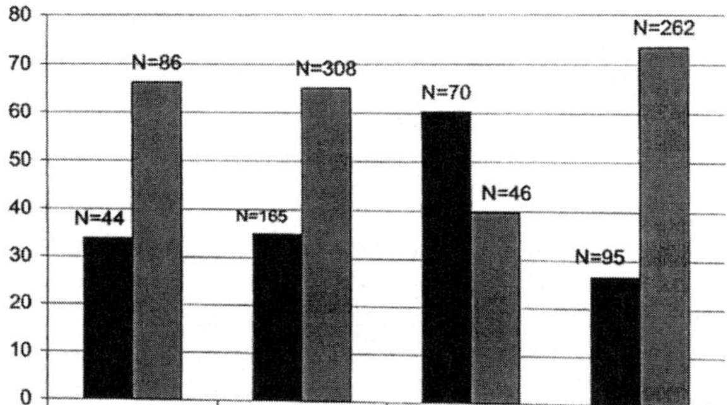

	All Incident Cases	All Prevalent Cases	Black Prevalent Cases	Non-Black Prevalent Cases
■ Diffuse %	33.8	34.9	60.3	26.6
■ Limited %	66.2	65.1	39.7	73.4

FIGURE 5.—Distribution of diffuse and limited disease in patients with systemic sclerosis. (Courtesy of Mayes MD, Lacey JV Jr, Beebe-Dimmer J, et al: Prevalence, incidence, survival, and disease characteristics of systemic sclerosis in a large US population. *Arthritis Rheum* 48:2246-2255, 2003. Reprinted by permission of John Wiley & Sons, Inc.)

and white adults. The data provided in this report should be useful in research regarding the role of geographic, ethnic, racial, and environmental factors for SSc in comparison populations.

► The relative rarity of SSc has hampered effective epidemiologic study. Many patients go undiagnosed or are misdiagnosed in community practice settings as having systemic lupus. It is nonetheless apparent that incidence of this disease is increasing, although, in part, through enhanced case recognition.

This study used multiple methods for case identification and confirmed diagnosis through a detailed review of medical records, ultimately utilizing capture-recapture analysis for refined estimates of the total patient population.

Prevalence, at least in the Detroit area, was strikingly high (estimate, 276 cases per million population). Of note, incidence was higher, and age of onset was lower in the black population who were almost twice as likely to have diffuse scleroderma.

There are no discrepant data, although few series have been as rigorously investigated. Future research in healthy services and access to both care and research participation should account for the socioeconomic and racial factors that are so key to outcomes in this disease.

J. R. Seibold, MD

Patterns of Hospital Admissions and Emergency Room Visits Among Patients With Scleroderma in South Carolina, USA

Nietert PJ, Silver RM (Med Univ of South Carolina, Charleston)
J Rheumatol 30:1238-1243, 2003 4–17

Introduction.—Data analysis from the 1995 Healthcare Cost and Utilization Project indicate that there are several types of racial disparities on a national level among hospitalized patients with systemic scleroderma (SSc). The hospitalization rate and emergency department (ED) use were examined across 3 race groups: non-Hispanic white, non-Hispanic black, and other. Predictors of referral were determined in a major referral center (Medical University of South Carolina [MUSC]) for patients with SSc.

Methods.—Data were obtained concerning all hospitalizations in South Carolina between 1996 and 2000 for patients with SSc. Hospitalizations and ED incidence rates were ascertained in conjunction with corresponding population sizes, which were obtained from the 2000 US Census. Rates were compared across race, age, and gender groups with the use of Poisson regression models. Logistic regression was used to calculate predictors of being treated at MUSC.

Results.—The incidence of hospitalization was significantly higher ($P < .05$) among black versus white patients (rate ratio [RR], 1.66; 95% CI, 1.41-1.96), as were ED incidence rate (RR, 1.78; 95% CI, 1.50-2.11) (Table 1). Even after adjusting for age, gender, median household income, primary insurance claim payor, county, and comorbidity, black patients were 60% less likely ($P < .05$) than white patients to receive inpatient treatment at MUSC. Findings were similar when comparing other nonwhite patients with white patients.

Conclusion.—The higher rate of hospitalizations and ED visits among nonwhite patients provide additional data concerning the disease burden among population groups. Despite the higher burden, nonwhite patients are less likely to be treated at a major SSc referral center.

► Scleroderma is an inherently expensive illness. Most patients have multiple simultaneous organ involvement and programs of simple organ-based management and palliation can be complex. Isolated issues, eg, pulmonary hypertension, are effectively treated with medications that start at $40,000 per year and range upwards of $250,000. The other issue is the relative rarity of the disease. Any clinician who has contacted a managed care company on behalf of a patient is aware that many can neither correctly pronounce nor appropriately code the diagnostic issues.

This study tackles the broader issues of race and economic status and their effects on patterns of health care utilization. Not surprisingly, scleroderma is quite similar to many other chronic diseases. Black patients and other "non-

TABLE 1.—Demographic and Clinical Characteristics* of Patients With SSc With a Hospitalization or Emergency Room Visit in SC from 1996 to 2000

Characteristics	All Patients, n = 785	Race Group White, n = 451	Black, n = 266	Other, n = 68	*P*
Sex, female, %	81.8	83.6	79.2	80.0	NS
Age group, yrs					
0-34	10.3	8.0	15.3	7.7	<0.0001
35-49	23.3	17.1	34.9	21.5	
50-64	31.5	30.9	30.6	38.5	
≥ 65	34.9	44.0	19.2	32.3	
Household income †, median (interquartile range), $US	37, 759 (32,090-44,822)	40, 236 (33,274-46,638)	35, 123 (30,326-41,798)	33, 675 (30,895-44,149)	<0.0001
Hospitalizations					
No. of unique patients with admission	727	427	235	65	NA
No. of admissions	2574	1441	792	341	NA
Admissions per unique patient	3.5	3.4	3.4	5.2	<0.001
Admission type, %					
Emergency	52.1	48.5	59.2	50.8	<0.05
Urgent	27.4	28.8	22.6	35.4	
Elective	20.5	22.7	18.3	13.9	
Primary payor, %					
Private	34.1	37.9	29.8	24.6	<0.0001
Public					
Medicare	49.4	54.3	38.7	55.4	
Medicaid	10.0	3.5	22.6	7.7	
Other government sponsored	0.8	0.9	0.9	0.0	
Other	5.6	3.3	8.1	12.3	
Comorbidities present, %					
Congestive heart failure	12.0	10.5	13.2	16.9	NS
Cardiac arrhythmia	10.0	12.7	6.8	4.6	<0.05
Systemic hypertension	28.3	26.2	32.3	27.7	NS
Secondary pulmonary hypertension	8.1	8.0	6.8	13.9	NS
Pulmonary fibrosis	12.0	11.5	10.6	20.0	NS
Renal failure	5.0	4.7	5.1	6.2	NS
ER visits					
No. of unique patients with ER visit	662	368	229	65	N/A
No. of ER visits	4402	2176	1531	695	N/A
ER visits per unique patient	6.6	5.9	6.7	10.7	<0.001
Primary payor (%)					
Private	33.1	37.8	29.7	18.5	<0.0001
Public					
Medicare	48.2	52.5	37.6	61.5	
Medicaid	10.1	2.5	23.6	6.2	
Other government sponsored	0.9	1.4	0.4	0.0	
Other	7.7	6.0	8.7	13.9	

*Clinical characteristics are based on patients' first hospitalization or ED visit, as appropriate.

†Median household income was derived from zip code data obtained from the 1990 US Census and inflated to 2001 dollars using an employment cost index based on estimates obtained from the US Bureau of Labor Statistics

(Courtesy of Nietert PJ, Silver RM: Patterns of hospitalization and emergency room visits among patients with scleroderma in South Carolina, USA. *J Rheumatol* 30:1238-1243, 2003.)

white" populations have significantly higher rates of both hospitalization and ED use. They appear less likely to receive care at referral centers with specific scleroderma expertise.

Black patients in particular have a higher prevalence of scleroderma, have the disease develop at an earlier age, and have more aggressive disease. Their burden of disease is magnified by societal wide problems of access to care.

J. R. Seibold, MD

Progressive Facial Hemiatrophy: Central Nervous System Involvement and Relationship With Scleroderma en Coup de Sabre

Blaszczyk M, Królicki L, Krasu M, et al (Warsaw School of Medicine, Poland)
J Rheumatol 30:1997-2004, 2003 4–18

Background.—The cause of progressive facial hemiatrophy (PFH) of Parry-Romberg is not yet known, but the disorder shows a link to epilepsy and other neurologic conditions in 10% of cases. Characteristics of PFH include self-limited hemiatrophy of the skin and subcutaneous tissues, with the underlying muscles and bones of the face affected in some cases. The clinical presentation and distribution of PFH resemble those of involutionary linear scleroderma (LS) after the regression of sclerosis. It may be difficult to differentiate PFH from LS. In addition, an ultrastructural evaluation of vessels in PFH reveals findings similar to those of scleroderma. An assessment was undertaken to identify CNS abnormalities accompanying PFH by using cerebral blood flow (CBF) revealed by single photon emission CT (SPECT), angio-MRI, and volumetric examinations.

Methods.—The 19 patients with PFH were divided into a group of 10 patients whose atrophies were preceded by cutaneous indurations and 9 patients who had no preceding indurations. Seven patients with scleroderma en coup de sabre but no PFH features were also evaluated. Among the clinical and laboratory investigations performed were indirect immunofluorescence for antinuclear antibodies. The routine neurologic examination included electroencephalography (EEG), MRI before and after contrast administration to review the integrity of the blood-brain barrier, angio-MRI to assess intracranial blood vessel anomalies, and technetium 99-HM-PAO-SPECT to determine regional CBF.

Results.—Abnormal results were obtained in the first group more often than the second group on EEG and MRI but were common in nearly all patients. SPECT revealed focal or multifocal abnormalities in 8 of the 10 patients in the first group, 5 of the 9 in the second group, and 5 of the 7 in the third group. Most changes involved the frontal and temporal areas. Blood flow was reduced but there was no direct relation to areas of involvement either cutaneously or in the brain. EEG and SPECT findings were concordant in 5 of the 10 cases in the first group, 5 of the 9 in the second group, and 2 of 6 cases in the third group. None of the groups exhibited a great number of neurologic symptoms. In the first group, 2 patients had epilepsy and 1 had transient seizures. In the second group, abnormalities such as headaches, vertigo, vision problems, and nystagmus were noted in 4 patients. In the third group, 1 patient had epilepsy. Frequent findings in both of the PFH groups were paradoxic pupillary reactivity and Horner signs. Among the patients with scleroderma en coup de sabre, MRI results were normal, but headache and dizziness plagued 4 patients and 1 had ipsilateral paresis of the facial nerve.

Conclusions.—These cases of PFH had CNS involvement whether sclerotic lesions were present or not. Scleroderma en coup de sabre with no signs of PFH also had CNS involvement. These disorders appear to be closely related as heterogeneous neurocutaneous syndromes that exist along the spectrum of scleroderma. MRI and SPECT revealed even slight CNS abnormalities, with SPECT proving most useful when there was less severe CNS involvement.

► The clinical differentiation of Parry-Romberg syndrome (PFH) and linear scleroderma of the face (coup de sabre) is frequently based on the presence of subtending abnormalities of the CNS.

This unusually large series (19 patients with PFH) was subdivided into those with and without preceding cutaneous induration and compared with a group of 7 patients with typical coup de sabre. All patients underwent detailed assessments of the CNS including MRI, SPECT, and MRI angiography.

Frequent CNS abnormalities were found in all groups and without clear association with the presence of or temporal relation of facial scleroderma. These studies argue that CNS involvement is an inherent feature of coup de sabre. The overlap of these rare syndromes indicates an extremely close relationship; in fact, so close as to represent identical syndromes. Not unexpectedly, SPECT was more sensitive than MRI in detecting abnormalities.

J. R. Seibold, MD

Age and Risk of Pulmonary Arterial Hypertension in Scleroderma

Schachna L, Wigley FM, Chang B, et al (Johns Hopkins Univ, Baltimore, Md; Univ of Maryland, Baltimore)

Chest 124:2098-2104, 2003 4–19

Introduction.—Although pulmonary arterial hypertension (PAH) is a leading cause of death in patients with scleroderma, there are few recognized predictors for this disorder. A total of 709 consecutive patients with scleroderma undergoing echocardiography were evaluated to determine whether age at disease onset is a risk factor for PAH in scleroderma.

Methods.—The risk of PAH linked with age at disease onset was modeled as both a continuous and a categoric variable. Risk estimates were adjusted for sex, race, scleroderma subtype, disease duration, smoking status, forced vital capacity, and anticentromere and antitopoisomerase I antibody status.

Results.—A total of 274 patients (38.6%) had PAH at baseline or during follow-up (272 by Doppler echocardiography; 2 by M-mode echocardiography). Of 114 patients with mild PAH (right ventricular systolic pressure [RVSP], 36-45 mm Hg), 66 had moderate PAH (RVSP, 46-55 mm Hg) and 92 had severe PAH (RVSP >56 mm Hg). A 52% increase in the risk of PAH was observed for every 10 years of age at disease onset (odds ratio [OR], 1.52; 95% confidence interval [CI], 1.31-1.76) (Table 3). Additionally, there was a 2-fold higher risk of PAH (OR, 2.30; 95% CI, 1.32-3.99) for late-onset (age ≥60 years) versus earlier-onset (<60 years) disease. These correlations remained evident and were somewhat strengthened when the analyses were limited to patients with moderate and severe PAH.

TABLE 3.—Risk of PAH Associated With Age at Disease Onset in Scleroderma

Variables	All Cases		Moderate/Severe PAH	
	Events, No.	OR (95% CI)	Events, No.	OR (95% CI)
Age modeled as a continuous variable				
Unadjusted	274	1.22 (1.10-1.36)	158	1.30 (1.13-1.51)
Adjusted for race	274	1.24 (1.11-1.39)	158	1.34 (1.15-1.55)
Adjusted for disease duration	274	1.45 (1.28-1.65)	158	1.59 (1.33-1.89)
Adjusted for FVC	254	1.21 (1.08-1.36)	147	1.33 (1.14-1.57)
Adjusted for all potential confounders*	241	1.52 (1.31-1.76)	139	1.79 (1.44-3.22)
Age modeled as a dichotomous variable				
Unadjusted	274	2.11 (1.33-3.36)	158	2.09 (1.15-3.80)
Adjusted for race	274	2.21 (1.38-3.53)	158	2.25 (1.22-4.14)
Adjusted for disease duration	274	2.60 (1.61-4.21)	158	2.55 (1.37-4.77)
Adjusted for FVC	254	1.86 (1.12-3.11)	147	1.97 (1.01-3.85)
Adjusted for all potential confounders*	241	2.30 (1.32-3.99)	139	2.53 (1.20-5.38)

*Adjusted for disease duration, sex, race, smoking status, presence or absence of American College of Rheumatology criteria, disease subtype, forced vital capacity, anticentromere antibodies, and antitopoisomerase antibody status.

(Courtesy of Schachna L, Wigley FM, Chang B, et al: Age and risk of pulmonary arterial hypertension in scleroderma. *Chest* 124:2098-2104, 2003.)

Conclusion.—Increasing age at scleroderma onset was a risk factor for PAH. Vigilance among these high-risk patients may offer an opportunity to intervene before the development of irreversible pulmonary vascular disease.

► Recognition of PAH is paramount to correct modern management of scleroderma lung disease. This series describes 709 consecutive patients in whom echocardiographic estimates of pulmonary artery pressure were available. Of the 274 (38.6%) patients with PAH at baseline or at follow-up, a 52% increase in the risk of PAH was noted for every 10 years of age at disease onset. Late age of onset (≥60 years old) patients had an OR of 2.3 compared with patients with disease onset at less than 60 years.

Patients with PAH secondary to scleroderma are generally regarded to have "blunted" responses to modern therapeutic intervention, particularly compared with primary or idiopathic PAH. No dataset has been able to assess the relative contributions of concomitant left ventricular diastolic disease, overlying interstitial lung disease, or differences in the level of irreversible vascular fibrosis. All datasets demonstrate that patients with scleroderma PAH are older and thus have comorbidities related to age and disease duration. The present data argue for a more pervasive interaction of age with risk of PAH and offer a clarion call to more vigilant monitoring in the older patient group.

The reader should note that 114 of these patients had "mild" PAH as defined by estimated RVSP of 36 to 45 mm Hg. This is the range in catheterization-based series that is associated with overestimates of pulmonary artery pressure. Also, Doppler assumes a normal wedge and by definition is inadequate to assess contributions of left ventricular diastolic dysfunction.

J. R. Seibold, MD

Prevalence and Outcome in Systemic Sclerosis Associated Pulmonary Arterial Hypertension: Application of a Registry Approach
Mukerjee D, St George D, Coleiro B, et al (Royal Free Hosp, London)
Ann Rheum Dis 62:1088-1093, 2003 4–20

Background.—Pulmonary arterial hypertension (PAH) that occurs in association with a connective tissue disease, such as scleroderma (SSc), has been regarded as a virtually untreatable condition. However, effective treatments for these patients are now becoming available. At present, little is known regarding the natural history of SSc-associated PAH (SScPAH) because no longitudinal studies have been reported involving sufficient numbers of patients during a substantial time period. Previous reports of prevalence of SScPAH have varied widely from 7% to 50%. The prevalence, outcomes, and predictive factors of mortality of SScPAH were determined in a large patient cohort.

Methods.—A prospective 4-year follow-up study was performed among 794 patients with SscPAH. All of the patients were screened for PAH with a combination of echocardiography, lung function testing, and clinical assessment. Catheterization of the right side of the heart was used to assess patients with suspected increased pulmonary artery systolic pressures of more than 35 mm Hg, carbon monoxide transfer factor (TLCO) less than 50% pre-

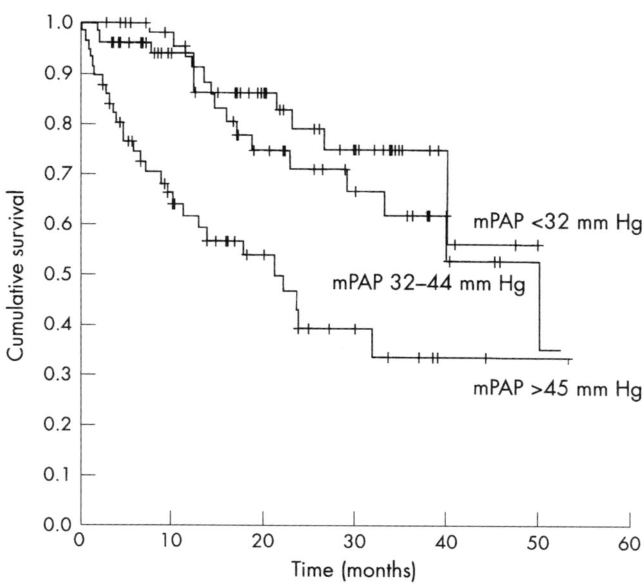

FIGURE 2.—Kaplan-Meier survival curves for 148 patients with SScPAH divided into tertiles—47 with mPAP < 32 mm Hg, 48 with mPAP = 32-44 mm Hg, and 53 with mPAP > 45 mm Hg. There was a significant difference in mortality between the three groups ($P < .01$ between each group). *Abbreviations: SScPAH,* Systemic sclerosis-associated pulmonary arterial hypertension; *mPAP,* mean pulmonary artery pressure. (Courtesy of Mukerjee D, St George D, Coleiro B, et al: Prevalence and outcome in systemic sclerosis associated pulmonary arterial hypertension: application of a registry approach. *Ann Rheum Dis* 62:1088-1093, 2003. Published courtesy of the BMJ Publishing Group.)

dicted, or a precipitous decrease in TLCO of more than 20% during 1 year with no pulmonary fibrosis. In addition, catheterization was used to assess patients with Ssc with breathlessness but with no evidence of pulmonary fibrosis. Patients with SScPAH were treated according to best practice.

Results.—Catheterization of the right side of the heart demonstrated a prevalence of PAH of 12% (89 of 722 patients). Survival rates at 1, 2, and 3 years from the diagnosis were 81%, 63%, and 56%, respectively (Fig 2). Hemodynamic indices of right ventricular failure (increased mean right atrial pressure [mRAP], increased mean pulmonary artery pressure [mPAP], and low cardiac index) were predictive of an adverse outcome. No significant difference in survival rates was observed between patients with SScPAH with pulmonary fibrosis (40 patients) and those without pulmonary fibrosis (108 patients).

Conclusions.—The prevalence of SScPAH was similar to that observed in other catheter-based studies and was less than that of previous echo-based studies. Outcomes in the SScPAH patients who were actively treated were comparable to those of the cohorts with primary PAH. The strongest hemodynamic predictor of mortality was a high mRAP. Prognosis could be improved by the implementation of future treatments at an earlier stage of disease to prevent right ventricular decompensation.

► The emergence of effective and specific therapies for PAH complicating SSc has led to radical changes in the clinical research community's approach to "scleroderma lung disease." Doppler echocardiographic estimates of pulmonary arterial systolic pressure are recommended in the assessment of all patients, most notably those with complaints of dyspnea or fatigue on exertion.

This study used a prospective registry of 794 patients and a multidisciplinary assessment that included clinical appraisals, pulmonary function testing and echocardiography. Right heart catheterization was used as the "definitive invasive test." PAH was found in 12% of patients and was associated with a notable effect on survival rate (81% at 1 year, 63% at 2 years, and 56% at 5 years) in spite of application of the best available therapies. Pulmonary fibrosis occurring as an isolated event was not found to affect survival rate.

Other point prevalence surveys have estimated the prevalence of PAH at between 28% and 40% with about half occurring as isolated vascular disease and about half as vasculopathy overlain on established interstitial disease. It is increasingly clear that outcomes of survival and late morbidity are nearly entirely due to the level of vascular involvement.

J. R. Seibold, MD

Scleroderma Patients With Combined Pulmonary Hypertension and Interstitial Lung Disease

Chang B, Wigley FM, White B, et al (Johns Hopkins Univ, Baltimore, Md)

J Rheumatol 30:2398-2405, 2003 4–21

Introduction.—Most trials differentiate scleroderma associated pulmonary hypertension and interstitial lung disease (ILD) as 2 separate pathologic entities and focus on one or the other; many patients have both conditions. The demographic, clinical features, and prognosis of persons with both vascular and ILD were reviewed.

Methods.—A retrospective, cross-sectional investigation was performed in 619 patients with scleroderma who had echocardiograph and pulmonary function testing performed within 6 months of one another. Echocardiography established the presence of pulmonary hypertension and pulmonary function testing was used to document restrictive ventilatory defect (RVD) as a marker of ILD.

TABLE 3.—Comparison of Characteristics Between Patients With No Pulmonary Disease, Isolated Pulmonary Hypertension (PHTN), Isolated Restrictive Ventilatory Defect (RVD), and Combined RVD and PHTN

	Neither, n = 249	Isolated PHTN, n = 119	Isolated RVD, n = 139	Combined RVD and PHTN, n = 112
Female, %	87.6	80.7	75.5	83.9
Age, yrs				
At diagnosis	46.3 (13.0)*	49.2 (12.5)	42.8 (13.2)*	50.2 (14.6)
At first non-Raynaud's symptom	43.2 (13.1)*	46.4 (14.1)	40.0 (12.5)*	48.0 (15.3)
At Raynaud's onset	41.4 (13.7)*	42.6 (13.9)	39.1 (13.7)*	46.4 (15.2)
Race, %				
Caucasian	85.5*	81.5*	57.6	68.8
African-American	10.4*	11.8*	32.4	28.6
Disease subtype, %				
Limited	65.9	69.7	45.3	49.1
Diffuse	34.1	30.3	54.7	50.9
ACR criteria	64.3	75.6	84.9	79.5
Serum antibodies, %				
Anticentromere	28.7*	29.2*	8.8	10.9
Antitopoisomerase	7.9*	11.5	26.3	16.3
Pulmonary function tests, (% of predicted)				
FEV1	87.3 ± 17.5*	82.6 ± 21.5*	64.7 ± 16.6	64.4 ± 15.8
FVC	89.5 ± 16.6*	82.7 ± 20.4*	62.5 ± 14.8	61.6 ± 14.2
TLC	92.3 ± 10.7*	96.0 ± 11.9*	65.6 ± 11.8	63.0 ± 11.9
VC	91.9 ± 14.7*	89.2 ± 15.4*	61.7 ± 15.2	61.3 ± 15.0
RV	102.3 ± 24.9*	109.7 ± 41.6*	75.6 ± 23.4*	67.9 ± 19.4
DLCO	62.8 ± 15.6*	47.9 ± 20.2*	41.9 ± 14.4*	37.6 ± 15.1
Echocardiography				
RVSP	28.5 ± 5*	53 ± 17	29 ± 4*	54 ± 16

*Statistically significant difference compared with patients in the combined category.

Abbreviations: FEV, Forced expiratory volume; *FVC*, forced vital capacity; *TLC*, total lung capacity; *VC*, vital capacity; *RV*, residual volume; *DLCO*, diffusing capacity of carbon monoxide.

(Courtesy of Chang B, Wigley FM, White B, et al: Scleroderma patients with combined pulmonary hypertension and interstitial lung disease. *J Rheumatol* 30:2398-2405, 2003.)

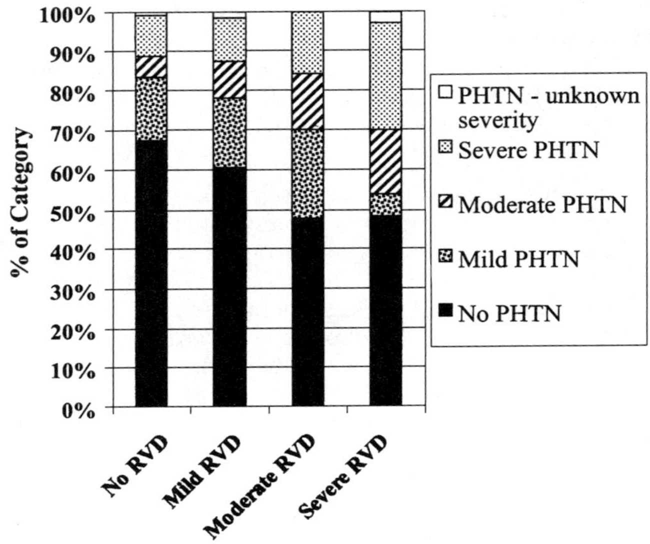

FIGURE 1.—Restriction by pulmonary function test and pulmonary hypertension (PHTN) by echocardiography in patients who had an assessment of PHTN made by the echocardiographer. Patients who did not have an RVSP estimate but a normal right heart were included among those with no PHTN. Patients with evidence of PHTN, but no RVSP estimate because of absence of tricuspid regurgitation, are categorized as PHTN - unknown severity. (Courtesy of Chang B, Wigley FM, White B, et al: Scleroderma patients with combined pulmonary hypertension and interstitial lung disease. *J Rheumatol* 30:2398-2405, 2003.)

Results.—Of 619 patients with scleroderma, 139 (22.5%) had isolated RVD, 119 (19.2%) had isolated pulmonary hypertension, and 112 (18.1%) had combined RVD and pulmonary hypertension. Persons with combined RVD and pulmonary hypertension resembled those with isolated RVD in that they had a high degree of diffuse skin involvement and antitopoisomerase positivity; yet, they were older at diagnosis and at disease onset ($P < .01$) (Table 3). In persons with mild RVD, 39.2% had pulmonary hypertension versus those with severe RVD, in whom 51.4% had pulmonary hypertension (Fig 1). Compared with individuals without pulmonary disease, the mortality risk ratio for patients with isolated pulmonary hypertension, combined RVD, and pulmonary hypertension, and RVD was 2.9, 2.4, and 1.61, respectively.

Conclusion.—Patients with features of combined schleroderma lung disease are more likely to have diffuse disease, represent an older group of patients, and have a prognosis similar to individuals with isolated pulmonary hypertension. These patients may represent a distinct subpopulation of those diagnosed with schleroderma.

► Pulmonary hypertension is increasingly recognized as the leading cause of death in scleroderma. The availability of highly specific and fully licensed therapies has radically changed the approach to assessment and management. One issue that is not widely appreciated by the community physician is the systematic exclusion from clinical trials of patients with pulmonary hypertension in the setting of concomitant interstitial lung disease. A "cookie cutter" template for Food and Drug Administration approval of pulmonary hypertensive therapies has emerged in which short-term studies (16-18 weeks) that use a surrogate marker (6-minute walk test) are the standard. Individuals with forced vital capacity under 80% are typically excluded.

This large (619 patient) single-center survey gathered Doppler echocardiographic and pulmonary function results and stratified patients into no lung disease, isolated pulmonary vascular syndromes, isolated restrictive lung disease, and overlapping RVD. Among the study group, isolated RVD (22.5%), isolated pulmonary hypertension (19.2%), and combined restrictive disease/ pulmonary hypertension (18.1%) were surprisingly equally distributed. The relative risks of mortality compared with subjects without lung involvement was 2.9 for isolated pulmonary hypertension; 2.4 for combined restrictive disease/pulmonary hypertensive, but only 1.6 for isolated restrictive disease.

This large high-quality data set shows (1) pulmonary hypertensive has a prevalence of around 40% in scleroderma, (2) vascular injury occurs independent of the degree of interstitial disease, and (3) in both circumstances has a major impact on survival. Pulmonary hypertension should be suspected in all subjects with dyspnea in the setting of scleroderma.

J. R. Seibold, MD

N-Terminal Pro–Brain Natriuretic Peptide as a Diagnostic Marker of Early Pulmonary Artery Hypertension in Patients With Systemic Sclerosis and Effects of Calcium-Channel Blockers

Allanore Y, Borderie D, Meune C, et al (Paris V Univ)

Arthritis Rheum 48:3503-3508, 2003 4–22

Background.—The generalized disturbance of the microcirculation that characterizes systemic sclerosis (SSc) may lead to pulmonary artery hypertension (PAH). As a result of improved treatment of renal crises in SSc, most deaths from SSc are attributable to cardiopulmonary involvement. PAH is widely recognized as a major complication of both limited and diffuse SSc. Established, severe PAH is difficult to treat, and the prognosis is poor. Cardiac evaluation in patients with PAH has been improved by the systemic measurement of ventricular (left and right) hormone secretion. The brain natriuretic peptide (BNP) gene encodes a prohormone (proBNP) that is cleaved on secretion to generate BNP and N-terminal proBNP (NT-proBNP). NT-proBNP was evaluated as a marker of early PAH and to study changes in the levels of this marker after treatment with dihydropyridine-type calcium-channel blocker (DTCCB) in patients with SSc.

Methods.—A group of 40 consecutive patients with SSc who had been hospitalized for follow-up care were studied. The patients had a (mean ± SD) age of 56 ± 11 years and a mean duration of cutaneous disease of 9 ± 9 years. There were 27 patients with limited cutaneous disease and 13 with diffuse cutaneous disease and with no clinical symptoms of heart failure and had a normal left ventricular ejection fraction. At baseline, 10 patients had PAH,

TABLE 3.—Long-term Effects of DTCCB on Plasma Concentrations of NT-proBNP and Proportion of SSc Patients With High Concentrations of NT-proBNP at Baseline, Assessment 1, and Assessment 2

	Baseline (n = 20)	Assessment 1 (n = 20)	*P* vs. Baseline	Assessment 2 (n = 20)	*P* vs. Baseline
SSc patients without PAH (n = 10)					
NT-proBNP concentration, pg/ml					
Mean ± SD	144 ± 125	78 ± 51	0.04	72 ± 50	0.02
Proportion with high values	0	0	ND	0	ND
SSc patients with PAH (n = 10)					
NT-proBNP concentration, pg/ml					
Mean ± SD	267 ± 125	118 ± 90	0.005	178 ± 92	0.06
Proportion with high values	9/10	2/10	0.02	4/10	0.06

To study long-term effects of DTCCB treatment in patients with SSc with and without PAH, levels NT-proBNP were determined at baseline (after discontinuation of DTCCB treatment for 72 hours), after taking 3 doses of DTCCB after treatment reinitiation (assessment 1), and after 6 to 9 months of continuous DTCCB treatment (assessment 2).

Abbreviation: ND, Not determined.

(Courtesy of Allanore Y, Borderie D, Meune C, et al: N-terminal pro–brain natriuretic peptide as a diagnostic marker of early pulmonary artery hypertension in patients with systemic sclerosis and effects of calcium channel blockers. *Arthritis Rheum* 48:3503-3508, 2003. Reprinted by permission of John Wiley & Sons, Inc.)

defined as a systolic pulmonary artery pressure greater than 40 mm Hg as measured by echocardiography. Levels of NT-proBNP were determined at baseline (after discontinuation of DTCCB treatment for 72 hours), after taking 3 doses of DTCCB after treatment reinitiation (assessment 1), and after 6 to 9 months of continuous DTCCB treatment (assessment 2) in the 20 patients who attended regular appointments (including the 10 patients with PAH at baseline (Table 3).

Results.—At baseline, 13 patients had high NT-proBNP values for their ages. High NT-proBNP levels identified patients with PAH with a sensitivity of 90%, a specificity of 90.3%, a positive predictive value of 69.2%, and a negative predictive value of 96%. At the first assessment the number of patients with PAH and high levels of NT-proBNP had decreased from 9 of 10 to 2 of 10. This decrease was sustained in 4 of 10 patients at the second assessment.

Conclusions.—NT-proBNP was shown to be a useful biologic marker that can be used in the diagnosis of early PAH in patients with SSc without clinical heart failure. The measurement of NT-proBNP may be a valuable diagnostic tool for the evaluation of treatment with DTCCB and vasodilators in patients with PAH.

► PAH is the leading cause of death in SSc. A high index of clinical suspicion coupled with appropriate use of Doppler echocardiography, pulmonary function testing, and right heart catheterization leads to early recognition. A variety of effective and highly specific therapies are available.

The issue in the community is that the work-up requires an interested cardiopulmonary specialist, and too frequently the clinical rheumatologist is left in the situation of having to guide the work-up. It is nothing less than "the ignorant leading the disinterested," although referral to a pulmonary hypertension or scleroderma clinical center would represent the most obvious solution.

The availability of a screening blood test would advance this field considerably. NT-proBNP is emerging as a candidate marker. While traditionally viewed as a marker of left ventricular failure, several studies, including this one, have suggested excellent specificity and sensitivity for recognition of PAH.

This editor would discount the use of calcium channel blockers of any sort as inappropriate in the modern era of PDE-5 inhibitors, endothelin antagonists, and prostacyclins, but the sensitivity to change of BNP in this experiment suggests utility as a measure of clinical efficacy.

J. R. Seibold, MD

Analysis of Systemic Sclerosis in Twins Reveals Low Concordance for Disease and High Concordance for the Presence of Antinuclear Antibodies

Feghali-Bostwick C, Medsger TA Jr, Wright TM (Univ of Pittsburgh, Pa)
Arthritis Rheum 48:1956-1963, 2003 4–23

Background.—Systemic sclerosis (SSc) is an autoimmune condition that has an incidence of 10 to 19 new cases per million per year. The cause of SSc has not been determined, but some case studies have implicated some environmental factors. The findings in studies investigating the relative contribution of genetic factors and/or environmental factors to the pathogenesis of SSc have been inconclusive. The study of twins is the classic approach to the assessment of the role of genetic versus environmental factors in disease pathogenesis. The concordance of SSc in monozygotic (MZ) and dizygotic (DZ) twins was investigated.

Methods.—MZ and DZ twins were recruited nationwide. Zygosity was confirmed by DNA fingerprint analysis. The presence of antinuclear antibodies (ANAs) was determined by means of indirect immunofluorescence with HEp-2 cells as substrate. Serum autoantibodies associated with SSc were identified by immunoprecipitation and double immunodiffusion. Major histocompatibility complex class II alleles were identified by polymerase chain reaction-restriction fragment length polymorphism analysis.

Results.—The concordance for SSc was similar in both the MZ and DZ twins; the overall concordance for SSc was low (4.7%). The concordance for the presence of ANAs was significantly higher in the MZ twins than in the DZ twins. SSc-associated serum autoantibodies were found only in patients with SSc. The distribution of SSc-associated serum autoantibodies was found to be similar to that observed in a large database of SSc patients (Fig 2). DZ twins were found to have increased HLA allele sharing independent of disease concordance.

Conclusions.—The development of SSc cannot be explained solely by inherited genetic factors. The suggestion from these data is that inheritance may be a factor in the development of serum autoantibodies in the "healthy" twin sibling of a patient with SSc.

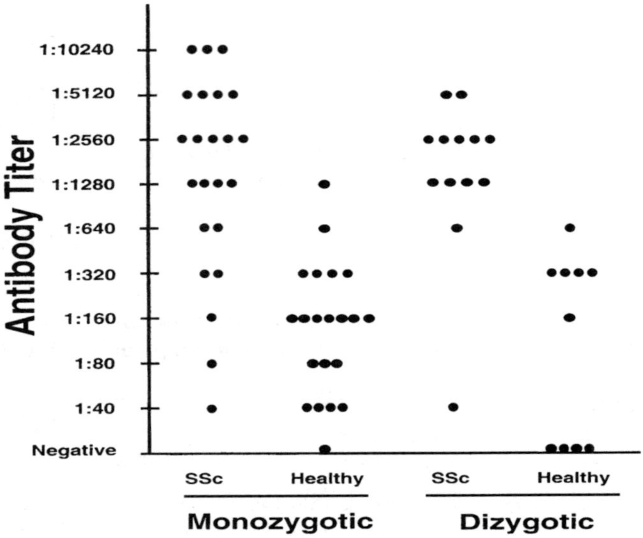

FIGURE 2.—Titers of antinuclear antibodies in the era of systemic sclerosis (SSc) patients and their healthy twin controls. Significant differences were found using the Wilcoxon signed rank test. (Courtesy of Feghali-Bostwick C, Medsger TA Jr, Wright TM: Analysis of systemic sclerosis in twins reveals low concordance for disease and high concordance for the presence of antinuclear antibodies. *Arthritis Rheum* 48:1956-1963, 2003. Reprinted by permission of John Wiley & Sons, Inc.)

► Using an extensive and prolonged national recruitment effort, this team was able to identify 42 twin pairs in which 1 of the 2 had confirmed SSc. This has been a most basic approach in seeking evidence of genetic contribution to the development of disease. In contrast to illnesslike lupus and rheumatoid arthritis, concordance for SSc was surprisingly low (4.7% or 2 of 42 twin pairs). While this far exceeds the general population prevalence of SSc (estimated at 240-300 per million population), it is, nonetheless, compelling evidence against both a dominant proscleroderma genotype and indirect evidence against shared environmental exposures as etiologic factors.

Monozygosity was confirmed in 41 of the twin pairs. Nonspecific low-titer ANA was found in unaffected twins, confirming older reports, but serologic findings, specific for SSc, including antitopisomerase-I, anti-U3 RNP and anticentromere antibodies, were restricted to those individuals with diagnosable SSc.

Data derived from larger family studies have suggested a risk of SSc in 0.4% of siblings of patients. These data would infer that genetic monozygosity increases the risk of scleroderma, perhaps, 10-fold. This sort of labor-intensive, high-risk research deserves our attention and appreciation. If there's indeed a genetic basis for scleroderma, it would increasingly appear that it has a complex multigene basis and that exogenous triggers must also occur in a genetically susceptible environment.

J. R. Seibold, MD

Significance of Plasma N-terminal Pro-brain Natriuretic Peptide in Patients With Systemic Sclerosis-related Pulmonary Arterial Hypertension

Mukerjee D, Yap LB, Holmes AM, et al (Royal Free Hosp, London)
Respir Med 97:1230-1236, 2003 4–24

Introduction.—The role of brain natriuretic peptide in patients with systemic scleroderma (SSc) has never been examined. Brain natriuretic peptide is an independent predictor of mortality in patients with primary arterial hypertension (PAH). This peptide is found in the circulation in 2 forms: a 76 amino acid peptide N-terminal probrain natriuretic peptide (N-T proBNP) molecule and a 32 amino acid physiologically active BNP peptide. A single center pilot investigation was conducted (1) to determine whether circulating N-T proBNP levels could discriminate between patients with and without pulmonary arterial hypertension (PAH) in the setting of SSc, and (2) to ascertain whether absolute N-T proBNP levels in patients with SSC and PAH correlated with hemodynamic and functional indices of disease severity.

Methods.—Of 49 patients with SSc, 23 and 26 did not have PAH. Right ventricular hemodynamic variables, 6-minute walk test, and plasma N-T proBNP levels were documented in patients who were catheterized for suspected PAH (23 with PAH and 11/26 without PAH).

Results.—The mean value of N-T proBNP for patients with SSC and PAH was 3365 pg/mL versus 347 pg/mL for patients without PAH. There was a statistically significant association ($P < .05$) between N-T proBNP values and mean pulmonary artery pressure ($r = 0.53$) (Fig 2), right ventricular end diastolic pressure ($r = 0.59$), and pulmonary vascular resistance ($r = 0.49$).

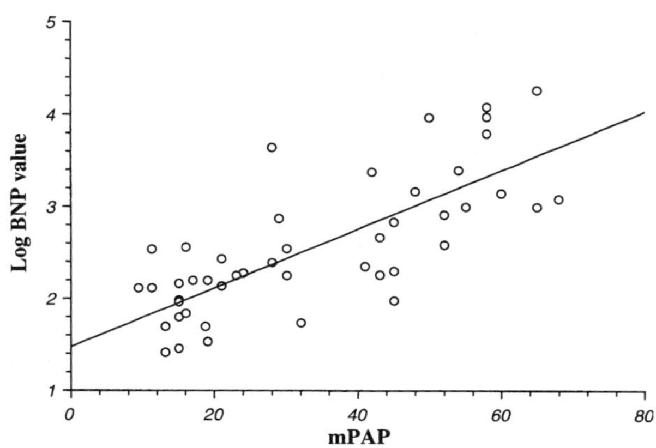

FIGURE 2.—Correlation between N-T proBNP values (pg/mL) and mean PAP (mm Hg) on cardiac catheter. Correlation coefficient $r = 0.53$ ($r^2 = 0.28$; $P < .05$), SE = 26.8. NOTE: BNP log scale used due to wide variation in values. *Abbreviation: PAP*, Pulmonary artery pressure. (Reprinted from Mukerjee D, Yap LB, Holmes AM, et al: Significance of plasma N-terminal pro-brain natriuretic peptide in patients with systemic sclerosis-related pulmonary arterial hypertension. *Respir Med* 97:1230-1236, 2003, by permission of the publisher, WB Saunders Company Limited London.)

Receiver operator characteristic curve analysis revealed that a cutoff value of 395.34 pg/mL had a sensitivity of 0.69 and a specificity of 1.0.

Conclusion.—The N-T proBNP estimation in SSc-associated PAH is a potentially beneficial diagnostic tool with high specificity and negative predictive value. It has the potential to have an important role in both risk stratification and monitoring of therapy.

► The prevalence of pulmonary hypertension in scleroderma appears to be in the 30% to 40% range, with about half having isolated pulmonary vascular disease and the remainder pulmonary vascular disease in the setting of interstitial lung disease. The high impact of this complication coupled with this range of prevalence inevitably draws focus to cost-effectiveness, sensitivity and accuracy, and accessibility of screening tests. The classic paradigm is to consider pulmonary hypertension in all patients who are dyspneic or in whom there is isolated or disproportionate reduction in pulmonary diffusing capacity. Doppler estimate of pulmonary artery systolic pressure (PASP) by echocardiographic study is the standard noninvasive test. In some settings, Doppler is more expensive than right-heart catheterization. It is increasingly recognized that the accuracy of Doppler in early, mild disease (PASP 31-45 mm Hg) is unacceptably low (50%-60%).

A biologic marker of pulmonary hypertension would thus be of great use in clinical settings. BNP derives from ventricular myocardium and is elevated in a variety of left ventricular disorders. More recently, BNP levels have been found to correlate with right ventricular function in patients with primary pulmonary hypertension.

This single center study of 49 patients with scleroderma found that plasma BNP levels were around 9-fold that in patients with catheterization documented pulmonary hypertension in comparison with patients who have normal pulmonary hemodynamics. Levels correlated with PAP and right ventricular pressure, as well as pulmonary vascular resistance. Sensitivity was 0.69 and specificity 1.0.

Application of these findings to a broader population and one with earlier stage disease is needed as are serial assays to assess the usefulness of BNP as a noninvasive monitoring test of therapeutic efficacy.

J. R. Seibold, MD

Erectile Dysfunction Associated With Scleroderma: A Case-Control Study of Men With Scleroderma and Rheumatoid Arthritis

Hong P, Pope JE, Ouimet JM, et al (Univ of Ottawa, Ontario, Canada; Univ of Western Ontario, London, Canada; Univ of Medicine and Dentistry of New Jersey, New Brunswick)

J Rheumatol 31:508-513, 2004 4–25

Background.—In the chronic autoimmune disease scleroderma (SSc), there are abnormalities in the blood vessels and fibrosis with vasculopathy in multiple organs. Men often have erectile dysfunction (ED), but a direct link

TABLE 2.—Raynaud's Phenomenon (RP), Erectile Dysfunction (ED), and Associated Variables for Research Subjects with Scleroderma (SSc) and RA (Control Subjects)

ED Related Factors	SSc	RA (Controls)	*P*	RR	95% CI for RR
n	43	23	—	—	—
Erectile dysfunction, %	81	48	0.005	4.77	(1.55, 14.66)
Noticed a change in sexual function, %	84	59	0.03	3.56	(1.10, 11.52)
Change in sexual function was rapid (vs gradual), %	22	46	0.10	0.33	(0.90, 1.28)
ED began after disease diagnosis, %	77	82	0.74	0.75	(0.13, 4.20)
Time from disease onset until impotence, yrs, mean ± SEM (min, max)	2.7 ± 1.2 (−12, 24)	3.3 ± 2.2 (−9, 21)	0.82	—	—
RP*, %	86	19	0.0001	27.0	(6.75, 107.96)
Men with both ED and RP, %	71	14	0.0001	15.83	(3.94, 63.54)
ED among patients with RP, %	81	75	0.80	1.38	(0.12, 15.36)
Time from disease onset until RP, yrs, mean ± SEM (min, max)	−0.9 ± 0.7 (−19, 7)	−1.0 ± 2.5 (−3, 0)	0.97	—	—

Note: Relative risk (RR) was calculated for men with SSc relative to men with RA.
*Values were significantly different between American and Canadian men with SSc.
(Courtesy of Hong P, Pope JE, Ouimet JM, et al: Erectile dysfunction associated with scleroderma: A case-control study of men with scleroderma and rheumatoid arthritis. *J Rheumatol* 31:508-513, 2004.)

between SSc and ED has not been elucidated. The prevalence of ED in a sample of men with SSc was compared with its prevalence in men with RA. Associations between ED and other comorbidities or other factors were sought, as was any temporal relationship between the diagnosis and/or symptom onset of SSc and ED in comparison to RA.

Methods.—Questionnaires were mailed to 89 men with SSc and to 42 with RA; approximately 50% of each group responded. The items provided an assessment of ED and related factors, as well as gathering information on the individual's overall health and rheumatic disease status.

Results.—Eighty-one percent of the men with SSc and 48% of the men with RA had ED (Table 2). A change in sexual functioning was reported by 84% of the men with SSc and by 59% of those with RA. ED was noted fairly soon after the men's disease onset (mean lag, 2.7 years for SSc and 3.3 years for RA). ED began at the time of diagnosis in most cases. Eighty percent of men who had Raynaud's phenomenon (RP) also had ED; 50% of men who did not have RP had ED. Eighty-six percent of men who had SSc had RP; 71% of men with SSc had both RP and ED. Only 14% of men with RA had both RP and ED. The SSc group had higher Health Assessment Questionnaire scores than did the RA group, but the difference did not reach statistical significance. ED was found more often among men who had diabetes and who had nerve damage than among men not having these confounding factors. Testing for hormone levels revealed that problems with testosterone or prolactin levels were uncommon among men with SSc and could not be used to explain the presence of ED.

Conclusions.—The prevalence of ED among men with SSc was approximately 80%; men having SSc were about 5 times more likely to have ED than were men with RA. ED was a very early manifestation of SSc but occurred after disease onset and diagnosis. This clinical finding may be further confirmation of the presence of SSc but is not diagnostic. RP was not found to be an independent risk factor for the development of ED.

► Scattered reportage of individual cases and case series has suggested that ED is common in men with SSc. The literature has further suggested that this is an early disease feature and is, thus, a clinical presentation related to the underlying vasculopathy.

This case–control study demonstrated that ED had an 81% prevalence in a population of men with SSC and that the onset was 2.7 ± 1.2 years after the diagnosis of SSc. RP was associated with ED in both SSc and RA.

State-of-the-art management of SSc is supportive and involves attention to details, particularly in those areas that affect quality of life. Predominantly a disease of women, SSc presents unique clinical issues for men, which this study emphasizes. The total literature suggests a disorder of penile blood flow and, thus, a syndrome that may be amenable to phosphodiesterase-5 inhibitors or local prostacyclins.

J. R. Seibold, MD

Frequency and Analysis of Factors Closely Associated With the Development of Depressive Symptoms in Patients With Scleroderma

Matsuura E, Ohta A, Kanegae F, et al (Saga Med School, Japan; Eguchi Hosp, Saga, Japan)

J Rheumatol 30:1782-1787, 2003 4–26

Background.—The pathogenesis of systemic sclerosis (SSc) is unknown, and few truly effective therapies have been identified. Thus, the disease may often cause decreased physical functioning and various psychosocial problems, and quality of life may decline gradually during a long disease course. Depression or a depressive state is increasingly recognized as a significant problem in systemic rheumatic diseases because the depressive state is an important factor causing decreased quality of life. The frequency of depressive symptoms and factors closely associated with their development were investigated in patients with SSc.

Methods.—Fifty patients with SSc were evaluated for factors associated with depressive symptoms by using a variety of established scales, including the Beck Depression Inventory; the Rheumatology Attitude Index for measuring helplessness; the Sense of Coherence scale (a measure of an individual's resilience when experiencing stress and the capacity to cope with it); the modified Health Assessment Questionnaire for physical disability, working, and social function; support domains of Arthritis Impact Measurement Scales version 2; and a visual analog pain scale. Disease severity of SSc, including skin thickness and internal organ involvement, was also evaluated. Factors that correlated with depressive symptoms were determined by multiple regression analysis.

Results.—Depressive symptoms ranging from mild to severe were observed in 46% of patients. Total Beck Depression Inventory scores were significantly correlated with low working ability, low social activity, low sense

TABLE 4.—Comparison of SSc Severity Scores Between Patients With High Beck Depression Inventory (BDI) Scores and Those With Low BDI Scores

	Mean SSc Severity Score (Range)		
	BDI < 17 (n = 40)	BDI ≥ 17 (n = 10)	*P*
General	0.38 (0-3)	0.2 (0-1)	NS
Peripheral vascular	1.73 (0-4)	1.8 (0-3)	NS
Skin	1.23 (0-2)	1.5 (0-3)	NS
Joint/tendon	0.35 (0-4)	0.3 (0-2)	NS
Muscle	0.28 (0-2)	0.5 (0-1)	NS
Gastrointestinal tract	0.5 (0-2)	0.7 (0-1)	NS
Lung	0.7 (0-4)	1 (0-2)	NS
Heart	0.4 (0-2)	0.3 (0-1)	NS
Kidney	0.03 (0-1)	0.1 (0-1)	NS

Differences in severity scores between high BDI group and low BDI group were statistically evaluated by Fisher exact probability method.

(Courtesy of Matsuura E, Ohta A, Kanegae F, et al: Frequency and analysis of factors closely associated with the development of depressive symptoms in patients with scleroderma. *J Rheumatol* 30:1782-1787, 2003.)

of coherence, pain, and helplessness and were not associated with disease severity variables, including skin score and internal organ involvement (Table 4). Multiple regression analysis showed that a high level of helplessness and a low level of SOC may occur in association with depressive symptoms in patients with SSc.

Conclusions.—It would appear from these findings that depressive symptoms are a frequent occurrence in patients with SSc. It is recommended that medical staffs be attentive to the possible risk factors for depressive symptoms in these patients, such as helplessness and low level of sense of coherence.

▶ The burden of disease faced by the patient with SSc is considerable. The cause is unknown and effective disease-modifying therapies are lacking. Modern medicine is increasingly able to assist patients through the hectic first several years of disease activity, but the issue in scleroderma is that more activity usually leads to even more damage. The burden of disease, including day-to-day symptoms and interference with quality of life in general, increases with disease duration.

It should come as no surprise that these patients suffer many of the common secondary characteristics of both chronic disease and chronic pain syndromes. Notable among these would be reactive depression. It is surprising how little organized research has been performed in this area.

This excellent survey from Japan is a notable contribution. Fifty patients underwent a standard battery of depression assessment modalities. Depressive symptoms were found in 46%. Measures of helplessness and lowered sense of coherence were closely associated with depression. These areas are clearly amenable to intervention.

Comprehensive management, including patient education, self-help, attention to social support systems, and mood elevating medication, are linchpins in modern care of scleroderma.

J. R. Seibold, MD

Delayed Gastric Emptying in Patients With Diffuse Versus Limited Systemic Sclerosis, Unrelated to Gastrointestinal Symptoms and Myoelectric Gastric Activity

Franck-Larsson K, Hendenström H, Dahl R, et al (Univ Hosp, Uppsala, Sweden)
Scand J Rheumatol 32:348-355, 2003 4–27

Background.—The gastrointestinal (GI) tract is frequently involved in systemic sclerosis (SSc). All areas of the GI tract can be involved, with the possible exception of the gallbladder. Included in gastric involvement in SSc are gastric ulcer, vascular ectasia (sometimes accompanied by bleeding), and impaired motility. Gastric function has been studied primarily in symptomatic patients only or without regard to symptoms. The different subtypes of SSc have seldom been evaluated in terms of gastric involvement. Gastric emptying and myoelectric activity in patients with SSc were investigated in relation to type of disease; the relations between symptoms and gastric function were also studied.

Methods.—Scintigraphic gastric emptying and recording of the myoelectric signals of the stomach were evaluated in 15 patients with diffuse SSc (dSSc), in 13 patients with limited SSc (lSSc), and in 15 healthy control subjects. The frequency of upper GI symptoms was determined by questionnaire.

Results.—Patients with dSSc had slower gastric emptying than control subjects and patients with lSSc (scintigraphic gastric half-emptying time: median, 103 minutes vs 70 minutes vs 76 minutes) (Fig 3). There was no difference among the groups in electrographic recordings. Symptoms tended to be more abundant in dSSc patients than in lSSc patients, although patients with a high frequency of symptoms did not differ from those with a low fre-

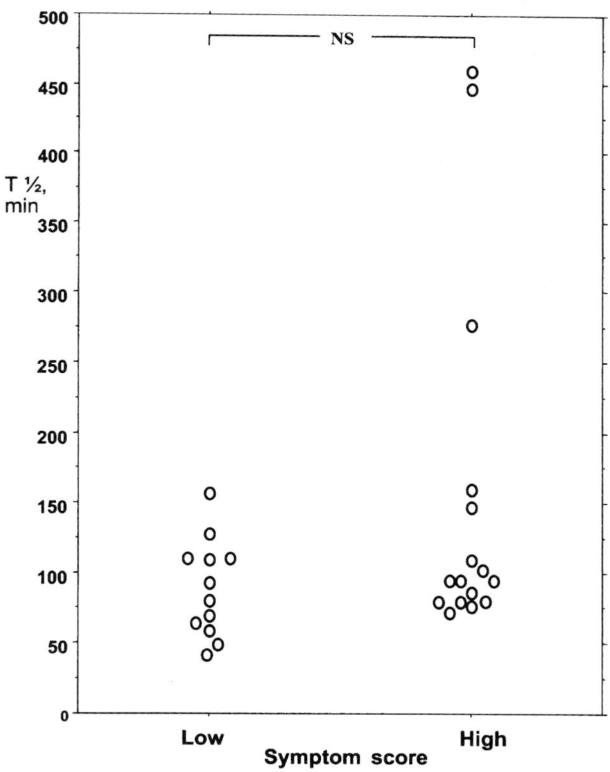

FIGURE 3.—Gastric emptying in SSc patients with low and high degree of symptoms. Low symptom score: no more dyspeptic symptoms than control subjects, such as bloating up to several times a week and epigastric pains occasionally, but no nausea, emesis, or early satiety. High symptom score: more frequent dyspeptic symptoms than control subjects for at least 1 of the symptoms, that is, daily bloating, epigastric pain more than once a week, presence of nausea, emesis, and/or early satiety. (Courtesy of Franck-Larsson K, Hedenström H, Dahl R, et al: Delayed gastric emptying in patients with diffuse versus limited systemic sclerosis, unrelated to gastrointestinal symptoms and myoelectric gastric activity. *Scand J Rheumatol* 32:348-355, 2003. Published by Taylor & Francis, Ltd. at http://www.tandf.cc.uk/journals.jsp.htm.)

quency of symptoms in gastric function as determined by scintigraphic gastric emptying or electrogastrography. Delayed gastric emptying could not be predicted by EGG or a thorough review of upper GI symptoms.

Conclusions.—The higher prevalence of delayed gastric emptying in patients with SSc indicates a more severe involvement of the GI tract in dSSc than in lSSc. The importance of differentiating between the subtypes of SSc patients is underscored by these findings. The lack of correlation between electrogastrography dysrhythmia and gastric emptying suggests that factors other than defective myoelectric signals may have a role in disturbed gastric function in patients with diffuse and limited SSc.

► After skin involvement and Raynaud's phenomenon, the GI tract is the most frequently involved organ system in SSc. Involvement is so frequent that prevention of involvement as a clinical trial outcome measure seems impractical. Level of damage is also somewhat difficult to assess given the expensive and invasive nature of most available testing modalities.

This interesting study examined electrogastrographic recordings of myoelectric activity and scintigraphic studies of gastric emptying time in patients with well-defined diffuse and limited scleroderma. Electrogastrographic results were not found to differ between subgroups, whereas gastric emptying was more impaired in diffuse versus limited disease. This objective evidence of more extensive GI damage and dysfunction was not necessarily clinically apparent, although all patients with low body mass index had evidence of impaired emptying.

While many clinicians feel that GI issues seem more prevalent in longstanding limited disease, this study confirms past reports of more extensive and clinically important levels of damage in diffuse disease. Agents of reasonable effectiveness for enhancing motility are desperately needed in this clinical population. There is good reason to challenge "therapeutic nihilism" in GI involvement since the level of damage seems so fundamental to basic issues of patient outcome.

J. R. Seibold, MD

Aberrant Serum Hyaluronan and Hyaluronidase Levels in Scleroderma

Neudecker BA, Stern R, Connolly MK (Univ of California, San Francisco)

Br J Dermatol 150:469-476, 2004 4–28

Background.—Systemic sclerosis (scleroderma) is characterized by aberrations of extracellular matrix deposition. These aberrations occur in parallel with the early stages of wound healing when increased deposition of hyaluronan (HA) and collagen occur. The result of both of these processes is the formation of fibrotic scar tissue. Activities of the enzymes HA synthase and hyaluronidase, which synthesize and degrade HA, are critical in the turnover of HA. Levels of both enzymes are increased in the setting of matrix deposition. The deposition of HA is an early event in the wound healing process, and increases in HA deposition have been reported in the circulation of scleroderma patients. It has been proposed that an increase in both HA and hyaluronidase may be indicators of early-stage disease in scleroderma, in parallel with early changes observed in wound healing. Topical and IV hyaluronidase administrations have been used in the past as treatment modalities to reduce HA accumulation and the associated fibrosis in scleroderma tissues. It has been suggested that hyaluronidase enzyme activity is a component of the disease process, and it has now been recognized that the hyaluronidases are an enzyme family. The somatic hyaluronidase Hyal-1 is the only activity present in human serum. The levels of HA and Hyal-1 in the sera of scleroderma patients at various disease stages were determined.

Methods.—The study included 25 patients with scleroderma whose levels of HA and Hyal-1 activity were determined and a control group of 25 age- and sex-matched subjects (Fig 1). The patients were separated into 2 groups: those in the early stage of disease, with duration of 2 years or less; and those in the late stages, with disease duration of more than 2 years.

Results.—In the patients with early-stage scleroderma, levels of HA were significantly increased (as predicted) in comparison with those of late-stage scleroderma patients and control subjects. Levels of HA in the late stage of the disease were comparable to levels found in the sera from control subjects. In contrast, levels of Hyal-1 activity were normal in early-stage patients, similar to those in control subjects, but were decreased in late-stage patients, even to a point less than that found in control subjects (Fig 2).

Conclusions.—These findings provide confirmation that circulating levels of HA are increased in scleroderma, but also provide the first evidence that

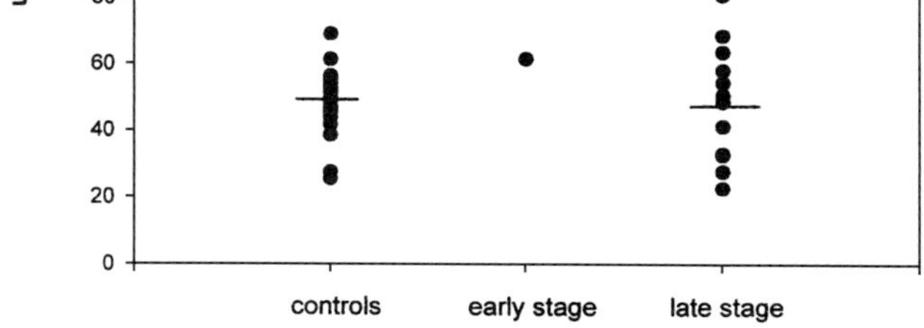

FIGURE 1.—Hyaluronan (HA) levels were determined in serum samples from 25 scleroderma patients, and from a group of 25 age- and sex-matched controls. The patients were separated into two groups, patients with early-stage disease, of duration of 2 years or less (n = 13), and late-stage patients, with disease of more than 2 years' duration (n = 12). The HA was determined in serum using a microtitre assay, based on a biotinylated HA-binding peptide, coupled to an avidin-biotin reaction. Assays were performed in triplicate. The HA levels were significantly higher in early-stage patients, in comparison with late-stage patients and the control group ($P < .0001$). (Courtesy of Neudecker BA, Stern R, Connolly MK: Aberrant serum hyaluronan and hyaluronidase levels in scleroderma. *Br J Dermatol* 150:469-476, 2004. Reprinted by permission from Blackwell Publishing.)

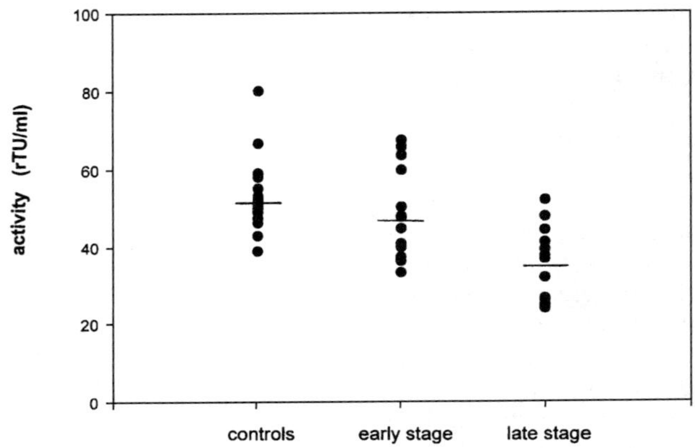

FIGURE 2.—Hyaluronidase Hyal-1 levels in serum samples from 25 scleroderma patients and from a group of age- and sex-matched controls. The patients were divided into two groups, patients with early-stage disease, duration of 2 years or less (n = 13), and late-stage scleroderma patients, with disease of more than 2 years' duration (n = 12). Activity was measured in serum in triplicate, using a microtitre-based assay. Values are shown in relative turbidity-reducing units (rTU), using a known standard (Wydase; Wyeth-Ayerst). The rTU unit has been defined previously. (Courtesy of Neudecker BA, Stern R, Connolly MK: Aberrant serum hyaluronan and hyaluronidase levels in scleroderma. *Br J Dermatol* 150:469-476, 2004. Reprinted by permission from Blackwell Publishing.)

these increases occur predominantly in early-stage disease. Serum Hyal-1 activity is decreased in patients with late-stage disease, which may be a reflection of decreased levels of HA turnover. These findings also provide the first determination of hyaluronidase activity levels in patients with scleroderma.

► HA levels were found to be significantly elevated in patients with scleroderma of less than 2 years' duration, whereas in later-stage patients, levels approached that of normal controls. These findings mimic those of wound healing wherein collagen and HA occur in concert in early stages of fibrosis. These findings also serve to remind the reader that scleroderma is not simply a disorder of aberrant expression of collagen but is better thought of as an "across the board" stimulation of multiple components of extracellular matrix, including collagens, laminin, fibronectin, fibrillin, and α-smooth muscle actin. It is unlikely that an intervention directed solely at collagen biology would significantly affect later fibroproliferative features of disease.

In the case of scleroderma, hyaluronidase levels do not increase commensurate with hyaluronan, although later-stage patients actually have depressed levels of this principal enzyme governing HA degradation.

J. R. Seibold, MD

Digital Necrosis Related to Carboplatin and Gemcitabine Therapy in Systemic Sclerosis

Clowse MEB, Wigley FM (Johns Hopkins Univ, Baltimore, Md)

J Rheumatol 30:1341-1343, 2003 4–29

Background.—In systemic sclerosis (SSc), patients have Raynaud's phenomenon and an increased risk for painful digital ulcers and catastrophic loss of their digits. Therapies promote vasoconstriction or thrombosis but also increase the risk for ischemia. A patient with SSc who received carboplatin and gemcitabine before incurring multiple severe digital infarcts illustrates the risks of chemotherapeutic agents for these patients.

Case Report.—A 50-year-old woman was diagnosed with SSc in 1996, with symptoms including digital ulcers and sclerodactyly. Carpal tunnel syndrome, Raynaud's phenomenon, sicca syndrome, and mild dysphagia were also present. No symptomatic pulmonary complaints were present, but pulmonary function tests revealed restrictive lung disease with a vital capacity of 69% of predicted value and a diffusion capacity of 80% of predicted. Hilar adenopathy and bilateral pulmonary nodules were found in 2000, and further tests led to a diagnosis of poorly differentiated carcinoma. Before beginning chemotherapy, the patient had a small ulcer develop on her first finger without evidence of cyanosis or critical ischemia. The chemotherapy regimen consisted of a 21-day cycle of carboplatin on day 1 and gemcitabine on days 1 and 8. She had some swelling of the right hand and left foot after 1 cycle, but these spontaneously resolved. A blue hue and pain developed on her finger on the first day of her second cycle; a calcium channel blocker, prednisone, cephalexin, gabapentin, and 2 stellate ganglion blocks were used without significant effect. After 4 months she had SSc skin changes and telangiectasia of the hands, forearms, face, and both upper and lower legs as well as critical ischemia with advanced gangrenous changes in multiple fingers (Fig 1). Several fingers required amputation. Her laboratory results were normal. The lymph nodes and pulmonary nodules were notably smaller at this time. The digital ischemia prompted discontinuance of gemcitabine and carboplatin. The patient was lost to follow-up.

Conclusions.—This case illustrates the possibility that chemotherapy and SSc vascular disease interacted and led to digital ischemia that required amputation. It is possible that this patient's ischemic digits resulted purely from the SSc, but the corresponding development of ischemia and use of chemotherapy suggests the drugs were a contributing factor. Thus, the combination of carboplatin and gemcitabine should be avoided in patients with SSc.

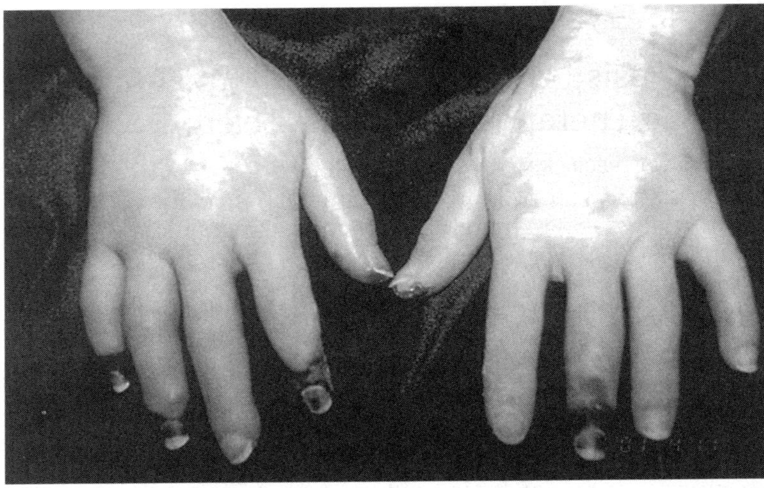

FIGURE 1.—Dry gangrene on multiple digits before amputation. (Courtesy of Clowse MEB, Wigley FM: Digital necrosis related to carboplatin and gemcitabine therapy in systemic sclerosis. *J Rheumatol* 30:1341-1343, 2003.)

► Gemcitabine is widely used in the treatment of lung, pancreatic, and certain testicular cancers. Adverse events of both venous and arterial thrombotic events are well described.

This case report describes the rapid development of critical ischemia of multiple digits in a patient with SSc receiving gemcitabine and carboplatin for poorly differentiated lung carcinoma. The implication is that patients with the vasculopathy of scleroderma are uniquely susceptible to the important vasculopathic complications of these therapies.

The editor has seen a similar case in which mild Raynaud's became gangrenous change of all 10 digits after 2 cycles of gemcitabine for pancreatic carcinoma and is aware of similar cases through discussions with colleagues.

Lung cancer is increased in patients with scleroderma. It is generally accepted that lung irradiation is contraindicated secondary to an enhanced risk of radiation pneumonitis. This case and the discussion it has stimulated would argue that gemcitabine therapy should be avoided in patients with SSc.

J. R. Seibold, MD

Therapy

Minocycline Is Not Effective in Systemic Sclerosis: Results of an Open-Label Multicenter Trial

Mayes MD, O'Donnell D, Rothfield NF, et al (Univ of Texas-Houston; Wayne State Univ, Detroit; Univ of Connecticut, Farmington; et al)
Arthritis Rheum 50:553-557, 2004 4–30

Introduction.—Minocycline has been reported to be effective treatment for systemic sclerosis (SSc) in an open-label trial of 9 patients. A treatment

TABLE 2.—Change in Modified Rodnan Skin Thickness Score for Minocycline Study Patients Including Intent-to-Treat Patients, Minocycline Noncompleters, and Minocycline Completers Compared With D-Penicillamine Completers in the Second Year of the D-Penicillamine Study

Feature	All Minocycline (ITT) Patients (n = 31)	Minocycline Noncompleters (n = 14)	Minocycline Completers (n = 17)	D-Pen Completers (n = 68)
MRSS at study entry, mean ± SD (range)	22.7 ± 7.7 (12-43)	23.7 ± 8.1 (12-43)	21.9 ± 7.5 (12-37)	17.0 ± 9.8 (2-44)*
MRSS at final visit, mean ± SD (range)	18.6 ± 9.3 (2-48)	23.5 ± 9.9 (8-48)	14.6 ± 6.7 (2-26)	14.3 ± 5.0 (0-44)†
Unit change in MRSS, mean ± SD (95% CI)‡	−4.1 ± 7.19 (1.46, 6.73)	−0.2 ± 8.39 (−4.63, 5.06)	−7.3 ± 3.96 (5.26, 9.33)	−2.8 ± 13.7 (−0.58, 6.08)

*At month 12.
†At month 24.
‡None of the differences between groups were statistically significant.
Abbreviations: ITT, Intent to treat; *MRSS*, modified Rodnan skin thickness score; *CI*, confidence interval; *D-Pen*, D-penicillamine; *SD*, standard deviation.
(Courtesy of Mayes MD, O'Donnell D, Rothfield NF, et al: Minocycline is not effective in systemic sclerosis: Results of an open-label multicenter trial. *Arthritis Rheum* 50:553-557, 2004. Reprinted by permission of John Wiley & Sons, Inc.)

effect of 30% improvement in the modified Rodnan skin thickness score (MRSS) was selected as likely to represent a clinically significant change that could not be attributed to the natural history of the disease.

Methods.—The 30% or higher level is a level of improvement not likely to occur in the natural history of SSc, as determined by recent controlled trials. Patients with SSc of 5 or more years duration were treated with oral minocycline for 1 year. The major outcome measure was the MRSS. Data from the D-penicillamine (D-PEN) trial was used to estimate expected skin score change in a comparator group of 68 participants.

Results.—Thirty-one of 36 patients returned for at least 1 follow-up visit and were included in a modified intent-to-treat analysis. The mean age of 23 women and 8 men was 51.7 years (range, 26-82 years). The mean disease duration was 23.5 months (range, 6-60 months). The mean MRSS at entry was 22.7 (range, 12-43); at final visit, it was 18.6 (range, 2-48). No statistically significant difference was observed in the change in skin scores between the minocycline-treated participants and participants previously reported in the D-PEN trial.

Additionally, when adjusted for disease duration, a comparison of MRSS in the minocycline trial participants (including all persons active at each time point) and the previously reported D-PEN trial participants demonstrated no difference and no treatment effect. Fourteen participants did not complete all 12 months of treatment; 10 withdrew due to disease progression. Noncompleters had a significantly shorter disease duration, compared to completers ($P < .03$) (Table 2).

Conclusion.—The extent of change in the MRSS was similar to that expected in the natural course of this disease. Minocycline is not effective therapy for patients with SSc.

► The lesson here, I think, is an obvious one, that trials must be controlled. I can no longer count the number of "open," uncontrolled observations "hyped" for treating rheumatic diseases, particularly SSc, that have proven valueless. I like minocycline; I use it occasionally for RA and am intrigued about some of the animal data for osteoarthritis (though the human data are far less impressive) but found it hard to imagine how a metalloproteinase inhibitor would be useful for SSc. Guess it wasn't.

R. S. Panush, MD

► A description of scleroderma therapeutics attributed to the late Sir Eric Bywaters is "No drug has been proven totally ineffective until it's been tried in scleroderma." Well-designed randomized controlled trials are now the rule in scleroderma and it seems the better the trial is designed, the more likely the results will be negative. In 2004, there are NO therapies that have been demonstrated effective for the overall treatment of the disease and there are no therapies that have been confidently demonstrated to effect even protean basic features such as skin thickening. To the contrary, placebo response is the rule in studies of skin involvement. Some of this represents spontaneous arrest and reversal of skin thickening after the first year or so of diffuse scleroderma whereas in other instances, evolution to skin atrophy is mistaken as a measure of improvement.

Against this background of improved rigor in scleroderma clinical research, the bizarre and unseemly observations still pop up from time to time. In 1998, low dose minocycline was reported to be an effective therapy for scleroderma on the basis of an open label trial involving but 9 subjects. This flimsy observation was embraced with enthusiasm by the patient community and was further nurtured by self-promotion and the news media. Lacking legitimate pilot data or even a reasonable underlying scientific hypothesis, minocycline advocacy approached that of D-penicillamine, DMSO and Potaba. The core research community made several attempts to obtain funding for a placebo controlled randomized clinical trial but this proved unsuccessful.

This study can be viewed as a public service. With minimal funding and a strong commitment to the patient with scleroderma, three U.S. centers conducted an open label study of 36 appropriate patients. Briefly, many patients worsened and dropped out of the trial. Those whose clinical course was more stable to improved remained on therapy but had clinical responses comparable to that expected with placebo. Even viewed liberally as a pilot trial by veteran observers, there was no evidence in support of the use of or further investigation of this therapy.

J.R. Seibold, MD

Scleredema Adultorum of Buschke Treated With Radiation

Bowen AR, Smith L, Zone JJ (Univ of Utah, Salt Lake City)

Arch Dermatol 139:780-784, 2003 4–31

Background.—Three variants of scleredema adultorum of Buschke have been recognized. The first variant is accompanied by an acute febrile illness and resolves over several months; the second variant follows a slow, progressive course with no apparent underlying disease. The third variant is associated with diabetes mellitus. Therapeutic options are limited, and no treatment has been shown to be consistently effective in treating large numbers of patients. Radiation therapy has been reported to be successful in the treatment of scleredema in a patient with associated monoclonal hypergammaglobulinemia and in some patients with diabetes-associated scleredema. Three patients with severe restrictive scleredema associated with type 2 diabetes mellitus who responded to radiation treatment after other treatment had failed were described.

Methods.—Angle of shoulder abduction was used to obtain an objective measurement of improvement in these patients, each of which had a 2- to 30-year history of type 2 diabetes mellitus and a 2- to 15-year history of slowly progressive neck thickening and, in 1 patient, restrictive lung disease. All 3 patients were treated with either electron beam or a combination of electron-beam and photon irradiation.

Results.—All 3 patients had improvement that lasted from 1 to 1.5 years. Objective improvements tended to plateau over time, but improvements remained well above baseline in all 3 patients. The duration of subjective improvement was variable, lasting from a few months to the end of the observation time of 2.5 years.

Conclusions.—Although the effects of radiation therapy in the treatment of scleredema adultorum of Buschke were not consistently durable, radiation therapy is a viable treatment option in extreme cases.

► Adult scleredema involves the face, cape, and mantle and can be both chronic and debilitating. It is seen as a dermatologic feature of plasma cell dyscrasia and appears to improve with treatment of the underlying disease. However, the most common form is seen as a complication of diabetes mellitus. The treatment literature is nearly entirely anecdotal and has included reports of efficacy of psoralen ultraviolet A-range, cyclosporine, extracorporeal photopheresis, methotrexate, and others.

This case series utilized irradiation therapy in 3 cases of high clinical severity associated with impaired shoulder girdle function. Electron beam to 200 total rad was well tolerated. Shoulder abduction improved, as did a number of patient subjective symptoms. Duration of effect ranged from several months to as long as 2.5 years.

Small case series such as this offer more questions than answers but patient selection and mode of assessment were reasonably robust. Responses are clearly beyond that expected from placebo effect. Larger controlled trials across a broader spectrum of disease, including earlier patients, are clearly indicated.

J. R. Seibold, MD

Raynaud's Phenomenon

Raynaud's Phenomenon in Children: A Retrospective Review of 123 Patients

Nigrovic PA, Fuhlbrigge RC, Sundel RP (Harvard Med School, Boston)

Pediatrics 111:715-721, 2003 4–32

Background.—Few data are available on Raynaud's phenomenon (RP) in children. The clinical presentation and disease associations of RP in children and adolescents were reported.

Methods and Findings.—One hundred thirty-two patients younger than 19 years were included in the systematic chart review. Approximately 70% of these patients did not have a recognized underlying connective tissue disorder. Approximately 80% of patients with primary or secondary RP were female. The mean age of onset was similar in the primary and secondary RP groups. Biphasic or triphasic color changes were not as common as monophasic changes and were equally common in the primary and secondary RP groups. Only the presence of antinuclear antibodies and abnormal nailfold capillaries predicted secondary RP. At some time, at least 21% of patients with primary or secondary RP had antiphospholipid antibodies.

Conclusions.—As in adulthood, RP in childhood and adolescence mainly affects girls. It is often unassociated with connective tissue disease. In this series, antiphospholipid antibodies were surprisingly common, the implications of which are not clear.

► This article deals with a fascinating phenomenon, RP in children. This reviewer had no idea that RP was such a significant problem in children, who are individuals less than 19 years old. The curious thing was that 70% of the 123 cases described here from a large hospital database had no underlining connecting tissue disease and also that 80% of the patients, as in the adult populations, were female. The amazing finding in this article is that 36% of the children with primary RP and 30% with secondary RP had at least 1 abnormal titer of antiphospholipid antibody. The significance of this is really unclear, since there may be some stimulus which is really unknown and which the authors discuss that may be responsible for these antibodies; but the true reasons for these antibodies in these children are not clear, particularly, since in the normal population of children, the control subjects, these antibodies are not observed at all. One last note is that nail capillary examination and other antinuclear antibodies are the most useful discriminating tests for primary versus secondary RP for patients who have other conditions—for adults as well as for the pediatric age group.

R. G. Lahita, MD, PhD

Severe Raynaud's Phenomenon With Yohimbine Therapy for Erectile Dysfuntion

Johnson S, Iazzetta J, Dewar C (Univ of Toronto; Sunnybrook and Women's College Health Sciences Centre, Toronto; Lions Gate Hosp, North Vancouver, BC, Canada)

J Rheumatol 30:2503-2505, 2003 4–33

Background.—The selective α-2 adrenoreceptor antagonist yohimbine is extracted from the bark of the African *Pausinystalia yohimbe* tree. It increases the release of noradrenaline and the firing rate of central noradrenergic cells. This produces increased sympathetic tone and decreased blood outflow from the corporeal bodies of the penis, which facilitates erection. Raynaud's phenomenon (RP) can develop in any acral area of the body and results from various causes, including drugs. A Raynaud's-like phenomenon developed in association with yohimbine use.

Case Report.—Man, 65, had a history of 3 years of RP related to calcinosis, esophageal dysfunction, sclerodactyly, and telangiectasia (CREST syndrome). All of his toes and fingers were affected, as was his penis. The episodes lasted 10 to 15 minutes, with painful symptoms in the penis. He had been taking yohimbine for 3 months to treat erectile dysfunction (ED), which was determined to be nonpsychogenic. He was also taking felodipine. The patient noted increased frequency and severity of the digital RP while he was taking yohimbine, with episodes lasting over 60 minutes and occurring many times daily; these were unrelieved by heat, which had been successful earlier. The patient kept a detailed daily record of his RP while continuing to take yohimbine for 4 weeks.

His RP improved significantly within 48 hours of discontinuing yohimbine, with shorter episodes, less pain, improved sensation, and the ability to return to his work on the computer. More severe RP developed within 48 hours of rechallenge with yohimbine. The patient's ED did not improve once yohimbine was discontinued and only felodipine was being used. An application of 1 inch of nitroglycerin (NTG) ointment to his penis produced a dramatic improvement in ED. His digital RP also improved. He was prescribed sildenafil, which was successful in treating the ED, but chose to use topical NTG and felodipine to control both RP and ED, avoiding the risk of severe hypotension that accompanies the use of topical NTG with sildenafil.

Conclusion.—The patient experienced an acute exacerbation of RP when he was using yohimbine for ED. This is the first report linking an aggravation of RP with the use of yohimbine and showing the improvement in RP and ED resulting from treatment with felodipine and topical NTG.

▶ I couldn't resist this selection. Obviously, this patient didn't see any of the Super Bowl ads.

R. S. Panush, MD

Effects of Cilostazol in Patients With Raynaud's Syndrome

Rajagopalan S, Pfenninger D, Somers E, et al (Univ of Michigan, Ann Arbor)

Am J Cardiol 92:1310-1315, 2003 4–34

Background.—Cyclic adenosine monophosphate concentrations can be increased by cilostazol, which produces vasodilation. Other effects of cilostazol include increasing the sensitivity to endogenous vasodilators, decreasing platelet aggregation in response to agonists, increasing nitric oxide production, and, theoretically, ameliorating endothelial functioning through favorable effects on lipids. Conditions with reduced vasodilator reserve and abnormalities in endothelial functioning can be improved by cilostazol. Short-term treatment with cilostazol was postulated to have a positive effect on conduit and resistance vessel responsiveness in Raynaud's syndrome (RS).

Methods.—Forty subjects with RS, 19 of whom had primary RS and 21 of whom had secondary RS, were randomly assigned to receive placebo or 100 mg cilostazol twice daily for 6 weeks. At the beginning of the study and at its completion, research subjects had tests of brachial artery vasoreactivity, laser Doppler fluxmetry, and cold pressor testing.

Results.—The mean brachial artery diameter after 6 weeks was significantly increased in patients taking cilostazol but not in those receiving placebo. No statistically significant difference was found between the groups in terms of the flow-mediated dilation (FMD) in either primary or secondary RS. When adjustment was made for the change in baseline brachial diameter obtained with cilostazol, FMD showed a net improvement in both primary and secondary RS groups. The slope of brachial responsiveness to cold was positively influenced by cilostazol. With respect to microvascular responses to provocative reactive hyperemia stimulus, the attack rate for the cilostazol group was 2.3 times greater among patients with primary RS than in the placebo group (Table 3). No association was noted between treatment and attack rates in patients with secondary RS. Side effects reported by patients included headaches, found in 35% of patients receiving cilostazol and in none of the placebo patients, and palpitations, which affected 2 patients taking cilostazol. Ten percent of patients experienced gastrointestinal side effects, regardless of the treatment received.

Conclusions.—Vessel diameter was increased in patients with primary as well as secondary RS when cilostazol was taken. FMD was also improved in both patient groups. Baseline perfusion and cutaneous resistance vessel responses to reactive hyperemia did not change. The response to cold was posi-

TABLE 3.—Comparison of Attack Frequency and Severity Between Treatment Groups, Stratified According to Primary and Secondary Raynaud's Syndrome (RS)

	Primary			Secondary		
	Placebo	Cilostazol	*P* Value	Placebo	Cilostazol	*P* Value
Attacks	17 (14)	36 ± 21.5*	0.028	45 (27)	46 (51)	0.96
Attack incidence/d	0.4 (0.3)	0.9 ± 0.6*	0.022	1 (0.7)	1 (1)	0.99
Severity score	2.5 (2)	3.0 (2)	0.536	2.6 (1)	3.0 (2.5)	0.64
Composite frequency and severity score†	84 (68)	116 (71)	0.330	100 (53)	116 (101)	0.68

*Results reported as mean ± SD.
†Composite score based on area under the curve approach.
(Reprinted by permission of the publisher from Rajagopalan S, Pfenninger D, Somers E, et al: Effects of cilostazol in patients with Raynaud's syndrome. *Am J Cardiol* 92:1310-1315, Copyright 2003 with permission from Excerpta Medica, Inc.)

tively influenced by cilostazol in patients with primary RS, but this was not found in those with secondary RS.

► Cilostazol is a type III phosphodiesterase inhibitor that results in increased vascular smooth muscle cyclic adenosine monophosphate concentrations. This effect as well as secondary actions of increasing endothelial nitric oxide production and decreasing platelet agonist response would suggest effectiveness in a variety of structural vasculopathies. Because cilostazol is licensed for intermittent claudication, one might expect a beneficial perfusion effect in individuals with RS.

This is an extremely well done trial in which well-described populations of patients with primary and secondary RS were treated in a double-blind crossover fashion for 6 weeks with 100 mg twice a day. The study accommodated for winter temperatures and used a variety of vascular laboratory techniques to assess physiologic responses. The brachial artery diameter improved in both primary and secondary RS groups. Neither population had a clinical benefit, and the adverse effect of a headache was common (35%). No changes occurred in FMD, nitroglycerin-mediated dilatation, or microvascular flow by laser Doppler.

RS remains a therapeutic challenge. Patients with primary RS are thought to have structurally normal vessels and are theoretically amenable to antivasospastic interventions. Individuals with secondary RS, particularly those with scleroderma or lupus, have sufficient evidence of irreversible structural injury to the distal circulation coupled with chronic dysfunction in endothelial-related vasodilatation.

J. R. Seibold, MD

5 Osteoarthritis and Osteoporosis

Introduction

Osteoarthritis and osteoporosis are the two most common chronic musculoskeletal conditions among persons aged 65 and older. Both are associated with significant morbidity, measured by functional limitation and reduced quality of life, and high levels of health care utilization and costs. This chapter includes new information on the epidemiology and pathophysiology of both osteoarthritis and osteoporosis, clinical evaluation of patients with osteoarthritis, as well as treatment of both osteoarthritis and osteoporosis. In addition, there is a separate section devoted to glucocorticoid-induced osteoporosis, a common complication of glucocorticoid therapy.

I have chosen two lead articles, one for the section on osteoarthritis and one for the section on osteoporosis. The former presents data from a 2-year longitudinal cohort study of patients with osteoarthritis of the knee followed with magnetic resonance imaging. These are some of the first longitudinal data using this technology and provide further evidence for the validity of this technique in the measurement of outcomes in patients with osteoarthritis. The latter article reports results from the pivotal phase III trial of strontium renalate in women with postmenopausal osteoporosis. This agent is unique in having both antiresorptive as well as anabolic effects. Despite these positive data, it has not been submitted for consideration for approval in the United States.

Marc C. Hochberg, MD

Osteoarthritis

Lead Article

Quantitative Magnetic Resonance Imaging Evaluation of Knee Osteoarthritis Progression Over Two Years and Correlation With Clinical Symptoms and Radiologic Changes

Raynauld J-P, Martel-Pelletier J, Berthiaume M-J, et al (Université de Montréal; ArthroVision, Montreal; Université de Québec à Montréal; et al)

Arthritis Rheum 50:476-487, 2004 5–1

Background.—Recent technologic advances in MRI have facilitated significant improvements in spatial resolution and contrast, which has made it possible for researchers to evaluate anatomic damage of joint structures in the axial, coronal, and sagittal planes. More recently several investigators have developed a system for quantifying cartilage volume in osteoarthritis (OA) by using MRI acquisitions combined with sophisticated software. The change in OA knee cartilage volume over a 2-year period was assessed by MRI and correlated with radiologic changes.

Methods.—MRI of the knee was performed at baseline and at 6, 12, 18, and 24 months in 32 patients with symptomatic knee OA. Loss of cartilage volumes were computed and contrasted with changes in clinical variables

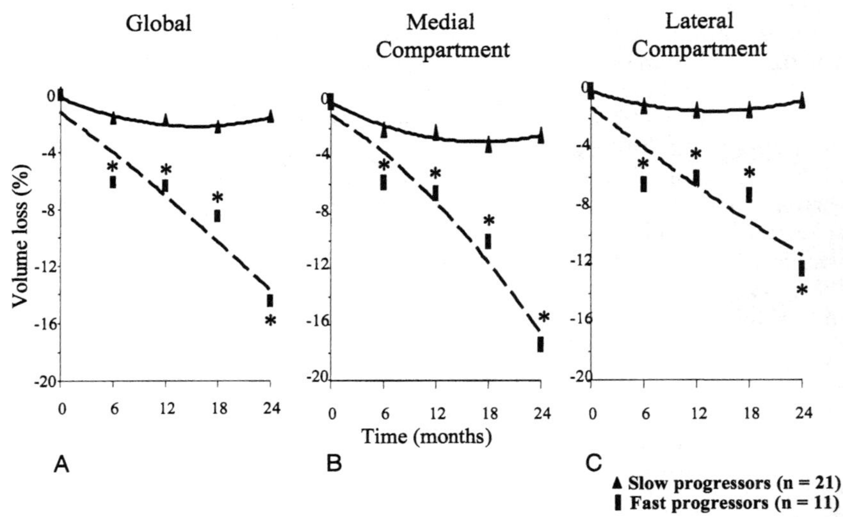

FIGURE 1.—Changes in cartilage volume in slow versus fast progressors at different time points over 2-year follow-up period. A, Global knee cartilage. B, Medial compartment cartilage. C, Lateral compartment cartilage. Values are mean loss of cartilage volume (%). In fast progressors, loss of cartilage volume at all time points vs baseline was statistically significantly different (*$P < .0001$ by t test) regardless of area evaluated. (Courtesy of Raynauld J-P, Martel-Pelletier J, Berthiaume M-J, et al: Quantitative magnetic resonance imaging evaluation of knee osteoarthritis progression over two years and correlation with clinical symptoms and radiologic changes *Arthritis Rheum* 50:476-487, 2004. Reprinted by permission of John Wiley & Sons, Inc.)

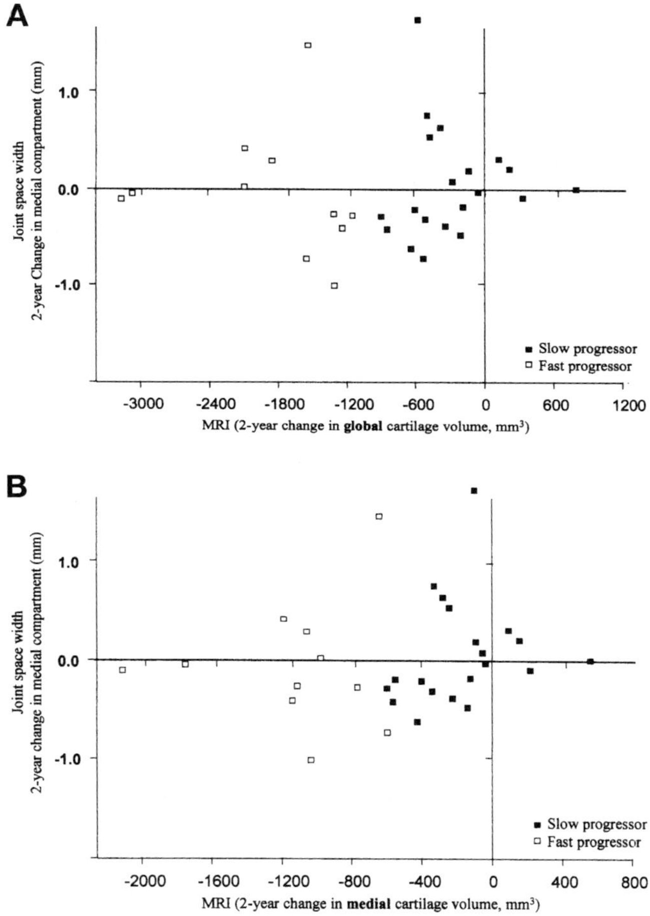

FIGURE 4.—Scatterplots contrasting changes in global cartilage volume (**A**) and medial cartilage volume (**B**), as measured by MRI, vs changes in joint space width, as measured by standardized radiography of medial compartment, over 2-year period in 31 patients with knee OA. No correlation between changes in cartilage volumes and changes in joint space width was found. (Courtesy of Raynauld J-P, Martel-Pelletier J, Berthiaume M-J, et al: Quantitative magnetic resonance imaging evaluation of knee osteoarthritis progression over two years and correlation with clinical symptoms and radiologic changes *Arthritis Rheum* 50:476-487, 2004. Reprinted by permission of John Wiley & Sons, Inc.)

for OA and with standardized semiflexed knee radiographs at baseline and at 1 and 2 years.

Results.—There was a statistically significant progression of cartilage loss at all follow-up points. The mean (±SD) global cartilage loss was 3.8% ± 5.1% at 6 months, 3.6% ± 5.1% at 12 months, and 6.1% ± 7.2% at 24 months. Medial compartment loss was 4.3% ± 6.5% at 6 months, 4.2% ± 7.5% at 12 months, and 7.6% ± 8.6% at 24 months. Two groups of patients were identified on discriminant function analysis: those who progressed slowly (<2% of global cartilage loss; 21 patients) and those who progressed rapidly (>15% of global cartilage loss; 11 patients) over a 2-year period (Fig 1). At baseline there was a greater proportion of women, a lower range of motion, a greater circumference and higher level of pain and stiffness in the study knee, and a higher body mass index in the fast progressor group compared with the slow progressor group (Fig 4). No statistical correlation was evident between cartilage volume loss and radiographic changes.

Conclusions.—These findings demonstrated that quantitative MRI can provide precise measurement of the progression of knee OA and can aid in the identification of patients with rapidly progressing disease. It appears that MRI could be helpful in the assessment of the effects of treatment with structure-modifying agents in OA.

► MRI has been shown to be more sensitive than standard radiography for identifying osteophytes, cartilage lesions, synovial thickening, and joint effusions in patients with knee OA. Furthermore, articular cartilage volume can be quantified by MRI.[1] These authors studied a volunteer sample of 40 patients with symptomatic radiographic knee OA to determine whether changes in cartilage volume correlate with changes in joint space width on radiographs and clinical features. Only one third of patients had a decline in cartilage volume over a 2-year period. The authors were unable to demonstrate significant correlations between change in cartilage volume and clinical parameters or joint space width over time. These findings increase the level of confusion about the role of cartilage volume on MRI and joint space width on radiographs as surrogate end points for clinical trials of disease-modifying agents in OA.[2]

M. C. Hochberg, MD

References

1. Raynauld J-P, Kauffmann C, Beaudoin G, et al: Reliability of a quantification imaging system using magnetic resonance images to measure cartilage thickness and volume in human normal and osteoarthritis knees. *Osteoarthritis Cart* 11:351-360, 2003.
2. Altman RD, Brandt KD, Hochberg MC, et al: Design and conduct of clinical trials in patients with osteoarthritis: Recommendations from a task force of the Osteoarthritis Research Society. *Osteoarthritis Cart* 4:217-243, 1996.

Epidemiology/Clinical

Association of Radiographic Hand Osteoarthritis With Radiographic Knee Osteoarthritis After Meniscectomy

Englund M, Paradowski PT, Lohmander LS (Lund Univ, Sweden; Med Univ Hosp, Lodz, Poland)

Arthritis Rheum 50:469-475, 2004 5–2

Background.—Meniscectomy of the knee is associated with a high risk of knee osteoarthritis (OA) and knee disability at long-term follow-up. It has been suggested that the OA disease process that usually follows such injury depends on local biomechanical factors associated with the acute trauma and chronic overload on the joint cartilage that are produced by the loss of

TABLE 3.—The Association Between Radiographic Hand OA and Radiographic Knee OA 20 Years After Meniscectomy

	Index (Operated) Knee (n = 170)			Contralateral (Nonoperated) Knee (n = 130)		
Radiographic Hand OA	Knee OA, No. (%)	OR	95% CI	Knee OA, No. (%)	OR	95% CI
Absent	53/113 (47)	1.0	Reference	9/86 (10)	1.0	Reference
Present						
Crude estimate	41/57 (72)	2.9	1.5-5.8	17/44 (39)	5.4	2.1-13.5
Adjusted for age, sex, and BMI		2.9	1.3-6.4		2.6	0.9-7.5
Adjusted for all variables*		3.0	1.2-7.5		3.5	1.0-12.2

Abbreviations: OR, Odds ratio; *CI,* confidence interval; *BMI,* body mass index.

*Age, sex, BMI, occupational workload, spare-time physical activity level, meniscectomy compartment, and type of meniscal tear.

(Courtesy of Englund M, Paradowski PT, Lohmander LS: Association of radiographic hand osteoarthritis with radiographic knee osteoarthritis after meniscectomy. *Arthritis Rheum* 50:469-475, 2004. Reprinted by permission of John Wiley & Sons, Inc.)

meniscal tissue. This process may be further exacerbated by other risk factors, such as obesity. However, there is recent evidence that the risk of developing symptomatic or radiographic OA after a meniscal tear is high even after limited meniscal resection. These findings have led to speculation that, in addition to knee trauma and loss of meniscal function, an endogenous susceptibility to OA may contribute to the risk of meniscal tears and OA. Such a relation would provide an example of the interaction between heredity and environment for a common and genetically complex disease. The association between radiographic hand OA, a disease with a significant hereditary component, and radiographic knee OA was evaluated in patients treated with meniscectomy.

Methods.—A retrospective review was used to identify 170 patients (mean age, 54 years; range, 33 to 87 years) who had undergone isolated meniscectomy an average of 20 years earlier (range, 17 to 22 years). Patients with cruciate ligament injury were excluded. All the study subjects were examined by standardized knee and hand radiography. The association between radiographic hand OA and radiographic knee OA was evaluated by using logistic regression.

Results.—Radiographic hand OA was present in 57 patients (34%), and radiographic knee OA was identified in 105 patients (62%) within 94 index knees (55%) and 47 contralateral knees (28%). Multivariate analysis showed that radiographic hand OA was associated with an increased likelihood of radiographic OA in the index knee (Table 3).

Conclusions.—Radiographic hand OA was found to be associated with an increased frequency of radiographic knee OA after meniscectomy, which provides confirmation of the findings of an earlier study that reported an interaction between hereditary and environmental risk factors for OA. It is recommended that the development of OA after a meniscal tear and the resulting meniscal surgery not be considered of secondary origin only.

► Radiographic hand OA is associated with radiographic knee OA,[1] and part of this association can be explained by the hereditary predisposition to hand OA.[2]

This study, conducted in a cohort of 170 patients who had undergone meniscectomy in either 1973 or 1978, confirmed this association, not only in the index (operated) knee but also in the contralateral (nonoperated) knee. The authors interpret their findings as providing evidence of a genetic-environmental interaction in the development of knee OA; specifically, that the genetic predisposition to hand OA influences the risk of developing knee OA after meniscectomy. The absence of a control group without prior meniscectomy but with otherwise similar risk of developing knee OA limits their conclusions.

M. C. Hochberg, MD

References

1. Hirsch R, Lethbridge-Cejku M, Scott WW Jr, et al: Association of hand and knee osteoarthritis: Evidence for a polyarticular disease subset. *Ann Rheum Dis* 55:25-29, 1996.
2. Jonsson H, Manolescu I, Stefansson SE, et al: The inheritance of hand osteoarthritis in Iceland. *Arthritis Rheum* 48:391-395, 2003.

Is Osteoarthritis a Systemic Disorder of Bone?

Rogers J, Shepstone L, Dieppe P (Univ of East Anglia, Norwich, England; Univ of Bristol, England)

Arthritis Rheum 50:452-457, 2004 5–3

Background.—Radiography is the standard for the diagnosis of osteoarthritis (OA), even though it can provide only a unidimensional representation and radiographic findings in the joints relate poorly to pain and disability. Because OA was first differentiated from other forms of joint disease on the basis of the hypertrophic changes seen in bone, osteology is the proper area in which to look for further insights into the disease. The osteologic findings associated with OA in a variety of joints were described.

Methods.—Visual examinations were performed on 563 skeletons in which 80% or more of the skeleton was available. The skeletons were obtained from an archeologic site in England. The surfaces and margins of several different joints (shoulders, elbows, wrists, hips, hands, knees, and ankles) were studied for evidence of eburnation and osteophytes, respectively. The entire skeleton was examined for evidence of generalized enthesophyte formation. The main outcome measures were associations between changes in different joint sites and between enthesophyte formation and evidence of OA.

Results.—There were strong associations evident between eburnation and osteophyte formation at the hand, hip, and knee and eburnation and osteophytes at other joint sites not commonly thought to be prone to OA, including the wrist and elbow. Only the ankle was rarely involved. A strong relation was also found between both bone eburnation and osteophytes and generalized enthesophyte formation. The statistical significance of these findings persisted after adjustment for the age, sex, and historic period of the skeletons.

Conclusions.—It appears that skeletal OA is more widespread in the body than is apparent from clinical studies. The findings of this study are consistent with other data that have suggested that OA is a disease that depends primarily on systemic predisposition to a particular type of bone response to mechanical stress.

► OA is a disease characterized by morphologic changes in both the articular cartilage and subchondral bone. This study of 563 adult skeletons excavated from a single site in Northeastern England found an association between osteophytes and eburnation of subchondral bone, not only in individual joints commonly affected by OA (eg, hips, knees, hand), but also in joints not typically affected by OA (eg, elbow, wrist). Furthermore, there was a significant relation to "bone former" status, defined by the presence of enthesophytes at ligament and tendon attachments.[1] The authors interpret their findings as consistent with the hypothesis that OA is a disorder characterized by "a systemic predisposition to a certain type of bone response to mechanical stress." Perhaps alteration in this bone response by pharmacologic intervention might affect the development or progression of OA? So far, evidence in human beings does not exist to support this, although preclinical data in animal models of OA treated with nitrogen-containing bisphosphonates suggest that this approach might be effective.

M. C. Hochberg, MD

Reference

1. Rogers J, Shepstone L, Dieppe P: Bone formers: Osteophyte and enthesophyte formation are positively associated. *Ann Rheum Dis* 56:85-90, 1997.

Collagen Type I α1 Sp1 Polymorphism, Osteoporosis, and Intervertebral Disc Degeneration in Older Men and Women

Pluijm SMF, van Essen HW, Bravenboer N, et al (VU Univ, Amsterdam)
Ann Rheum Dis 63:71-77, 2004 5–4

Background.—Osteoporosis and osteoarthritis (OA) are common skeletal disorders that cause pain, physical limitations, and disability in later life. Studies have shown that osteoporosis is inversely related to spinal degeneration diseases or intervertebral disc degeneration. There has been no clear explanation for this inverse relation, but it has been suggested that it may be attributed to a shared set of genetic factors that underlie both disorders. A likely candidate gene is the collagen type I α 1 gene (*COLIA1*), which encodes a part of type I collagen, the major protein in bone. Whether *COLIA1* Sp1 polymorphism is associated with osteoporosis or intervertebral disc degeneration in older people was determined.

Methods.—*COLIA1* genotype was determined in 966 men and women (≥65 years) of the Longitudinal Aging Study Amsterdam. The guanine (G) to thymidine (T) polymorphism in the first intron of the *COLIA1* gene was detected by polymerase chain reaction and Mscl digestion. Quantitative US measurements, serum osteocalcin, and urine deoxypyridinoline were assessed. Fractures were followed up every 3 months. In a subsample, total body bone mineral content (485 patients) and bond mineral density of the hip and lumbar spine (512 patients) were measured by dual energy x-ray absorptiometry. Prevalent vertebral deformities and intervertebral disc degeneration were identified on radiographs (517 patients).

Results.—Persons with the TT genotype had a higher risk of disc degeneration than persons with the GG and GT genotypes. Among men, higher levels of osteocalcin were found in persons with the T allele than in those without it. *COLIA1* polymorphism was not significantly associated with other measures of osteoporosis in either men or women.

Conclusions.—*COLIA1* Sp1 polymorphism may be a genetic risk factor related to intervertebral disc degeneration in older people. However, the results of this study did not provide confirmation of previously reported associations between the *COLIA1* Sp1 genotype and lower bone mineral density or quantitative ultrasound values, higher levels of urine deoxypyridinoline, and an increased fracture risk in either men or women.

► Genetic factors have been shown to be associated with intervertebral disc degeneration.[1,2] These authors studied the association of genotypes of the Sp1 binding site of *COLIA1* and intervertebral disc degeneration in 517 older adults participating in the Longitudinal Aging Study Amsterdam. Homozygosity for the T/T genotype was significantly associated with severe disc degeneration, characterized by large osteophytes and severe disc space narrowing, even after adjustment for potential confounders. The association was no longer significant when case status was defined by moderate or severe disc degeneration; unfortunately, data were not presented on the genotype frequency by severity of disc degeneration. Further studies are needed to confirm this association and, if confirmed, evaluate the biologic mechanisms underlying the association.

M. C. Hochberg, MD

References

1. Sambrook PN, MacGregor AJ, Spector TD: Genetic influences of cervical and lumbar disc degeneration: A magnetic resonance imaging study in twins. *Arthritis Rheum* 42:366-372, 1999.
2. Bijkark C, Houwing-Duistermaat JJ, Valkenburg HA, et al: Heritabilities of radiologic osteoarthritis in peripheral joints and of disc degeneration of the spine. *Arthritis Rheum* 42:1729-1735, 1999.

PATHOPHYSIOLOGY

Increased Apoptosis in Human Osteoarthritic Cartilage Corresponds to Reduced Cell Density and Expression of Caspase-3

Sharif M, Whitehouse A, Sharman P, et al (Univ of Bristol, England)
Arthritis Rheum 50:507-515, 2004 5–5

Background.—Apoptosis of chondrocytes has been described in both human and experimentally induced osteoarthritis (OA), but the importance of chondrocyte apoptosis in the etiopathogenesis of OA is unclear. The rate of chondrocyte apoptosis was determined by different methods and the relation between chondrocyte apoptosis and cartilage cellularity, expression of proapoptotic molecules, and expression of antiapoptotic molecules was investigated in articular cartilage obtained from patients with OA and from nonarthritic control subjects.

Methods.—The extent of apoptosis was examined in OA cartilage from the knee (10 specimens) and hip (9 specimens) and nonarthritic control cartilage (7 specimens) by using expression of caspase-3, an enzyme that mediates the final stage of cell death by apoptosis, and by the TUNEL method. Immunohistochemistry was used to analyze the expression of a panel of proapoptotic and antiapoptotic molecules that regulate apoptosis in articular cartilage in an effort to determine whether the rate of apoptosis is associated with the expression of these molecules.

Results.—The median percentage of TUNEL-positive chondrocytes in knee OA cartilage was 3.11 (range, 1.67 to 3.67) in the knee cartilage, 1.86 (range, 1.22 to 2.89) in the hip cartilage, and 0.39 (range, 0.00 to 1.78) in the control cartilage (Fig 2). Pooling of all cartilage samples demonstrated a strong inverse correlation with cellularity. The percentage of cells expressing caspase-3 in the 3 groups was 15.70 (range, 7.40 to 20.50) for the knee,

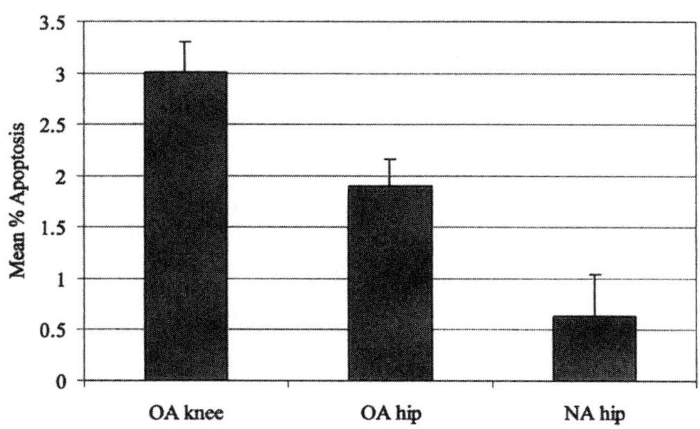

FIGURE 2.—Mean and SEM percentage in apoptosis in cartilage obtained from 10 patients with knee OA, 9 patients with hip OA, and 7 nonarthritic (*NA*) control subjects. (Courtesy of Sharif M, Whitehouse A, Sharman P, et al: Increased apoptosis in human osteoarthritic cartilage corresponds to reduced cell density and expression of caspase-3. *Arthritis Rheum* 50:507-515, 2004. Reprinted by permission of John Wiley & Sons, Inc.)

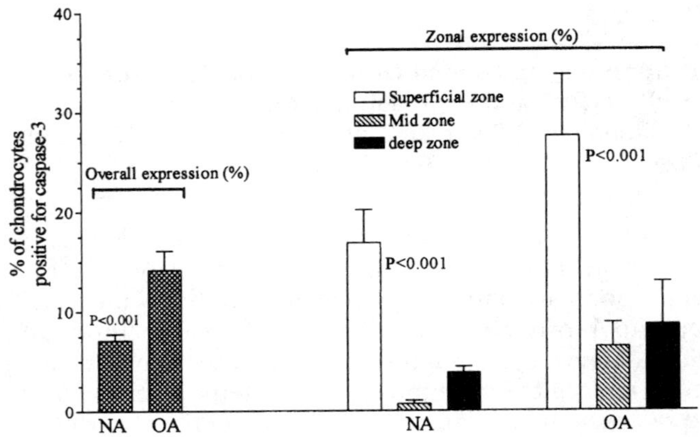

FIGURE 5.—Percentage of chondrocytes expressing caspase-3 in nonarthritic (*NA*) and OA cartilage. *Bars* show mean and SEM. (Courtesy of Sharif M, Whitehouse A, Sharman P, et al: Increased apoptosis in human osteoarthritic cartilage corresponds to reduced cell density and expression of caspase-3. *Arthritis Rheum* 50:507-515, 2004. Reprinted by permission of John Wiley & Sons, Inc.)

15.77 (range, 7.42 to 20.5) in the hip, and 7.40 (range, 5.90 to 8.00) for the control cartilage specimens. One-way analysis of variance showed that the difference between groups of both TUNEL-positive cells and expression of caspase-3 were statistically significant (Fig 5). There was also a significant positive correlation between TUNEL-positive cells and the expression of caspase-3.

Conclusions.—It would appear from these findings that there is an increase in apoptosis of 2- to 4-fold (on average) in osteoarthritic cartilage. Because OA is a slowly progressing disease, such an increase in the rate of apoptosis in the articular cartilage could be an important component in the disease process.

▶ Chondrocyte apoptosis has been related to decreased cartilage anabolism in patients with osteoarthritis.[1] This report confirmed that chondrocyte apoptosis was more frequent in cartilage from hips and knees from patients who underwent total joint arthroplasty for OA than in nonarthritic control cartilage. Apoptotic chondrocytes, defined by expression of caspase-3 on immunostaining, were more commonly observed in the superficial than in the mid and deep zones of cartilage. These results support a role for apoptosis in explaining the reduced cellularity of osteoarthritic articular cartilage and resultant decreased anabolism of the cartilage matrix. Furthermore, apoptotic bodies may contribute to increased catabolism of cartilage matrix by increasing production of autocrine cytokines and proinflammatory molecules. Agents that prevent apoptosis may be of benefit in the prevention and treatment of OA.

M. C. Hochberg, MD

Reference

1. Hashimoto S, Ochs RL, Komiya S, et al: Linkage of chondrocyte apoptosis and cartilage degradation in human osteoarthritis. *Arthritis Rheum* 41:1632-1638, 1998.

TRAIL Induces Apoptosis of Chondrocytes and Influences the Pathogenesis of Experimentally Induced Rat Osteoarthritis

Lee SW, Lee HJ, Chung WT, et al (Dong-A Univ, Busan, South Korea)

Arthritis Rheum 50:534-542, 2004 5–6

Background.—It has long been postulated that reduced cartilage cellularity has a role in the pathogenesis of osteoarthritis (OA). In recent studies it was shown that, in OA, articular chondrocytes appeared to be eliminated by apoptosis. Apoptosis of chondrocytes was initially reported in relation to development and growth, such as in the differentiation of hypertrophic chondrocytes and the ossification of the growth plate. It has also been reported that several stimuli, such as nitric oxide, prostaglandin E_2, Fas ligand (FasL), and tumor necrosis factor α (TNFα), induced apoptosis in chondrocytes, indicating that those molecules may have a role in the pathogenesis of OA. TRAIL is a type II transmembrane protein of the TNF superfamily. Recent studies have shown that TRAIL induced apoptosis in untransformed normal cells. Whether TRAIL influences the pathogenesis of OA was investigated.

Methods.—A recombinant adenoviral vector system (Ad-TRAIL) was used in this experiment. The expression of TRAIL in a rat chondrocyte cell line (RCJ3.1C.18) and alterations in the expression of death and decoy receptors after Ad-TRAIL infection were measured by Western blot assay. Western blot assay, mitochondrial membrane potential ($\delta\psi m$) measurement, Hoechst staining, and DNA electrophoresis were conducted. The expression of TRAIL and death and decoy receptors was examined by immunochemistry in primary cultured chondrocytes and on cartilage obtained from rats with experimentally induced OA.

Results.—Ad-TRAIL infection induced expression of TRAIL in RCJ3.1C.18 cells, increased expression of death receptor 4 (DR4), and decreased expression of DR5 and decoy receptor 1 (DcR1). Ad-TRAIL, at doses of 10 and 100 multiplicities of infection, decreased the viability of chondrocytes 4 days after infection. Reduction of $\delta\psi m$, cytochrome c release, nuclear condensation, activation of caspase 3 and poly(adenosine diphosphate ribose) polymerase, and DNA fragmentation proved the induction of apoptosis. Activation of caspase 8 was also observed. Ad-TRAIL also induced apoptosis in primary cultured chondrocytes, in which alterations in expression of TRAIL and death receptors were similar to those observed in RCJ3.1C.18 cells. Cartilage obtained from rats in which OA was experimentally induced showed increased expression of TRAIL and DR4 and decreased expression of DR5 and DcR1 compared with control cartilage.

Conclusions.—TRAIL was found to induce chondrocyte apoptosis in a rat model. It would appear from these findings that there may be a role for TRAIL-induced chondrocyte apoptosis in the pathogenesis of OA.

► Chondrocyte apoptosis has been related to decreased cartilage anabolism in patients with osteoarthritis.[1] Several stimuli have been reported to induce chondrocyte apoptosis, including nitric oxide, prostaglandin E_2, Fas ligand, and

TNFα. This report demonstrates that chondrocyte apoptosis is mediated in part by TRAIL, a transmembrane protein of the TNF superfamily that functions with 3 related proteins: TNFα, CD95 (Fas ligand), and TWEAK/APO-3L. Agents that modulate TRAIL expression and prevent apoptosis may be of benefit in the prevention and treatment of OA.

M. C. Hochberg, MD

Reference

1. Hashimoto S, Ochs RL, Komiya S, et al: Linkage of chondrocyte apoptosis and cartilage degradation in human osteoarthritis. *Arthritis Rheum* 41:1632-1638, 1998.

Inhibition of Endogenous TGF-β During Experimental Osteoarthritis Prevents Osteophyte Formation and Impairs Cartilage Repair

Scharstuhl A, Glansbeek HL, van Beuningen HM, et al (Univ Med Ctr, Nijmegen, The Netherlands)

J Immunol 169:507-514, 2002 5–7

Background.—Transforming growth factor-β (TGF-β) has been suggested as an important factor in the pathogenesis of osteoarthritis (OA), in part because of the significant levels of active TGF-β in the synovial fluid of patients with OA. Although it has been implicated in the pathologic process, TGF-β has also been suggested as a beneficial factor in cartilage repair. Thus, TGF-β appears to have a dual role in OA, providing protection against cartilage damage but inducing the formation of osteocytes. The role of endogenous TGF-β during experimental OA was determined.

Methods.—To determine the role of endogenous TGF-β on osteophyte formation and articular cartilage, TGF-β activity was blocked in a murine model by a scavenging soluble TGF-β-RII.

Results.—Enhanced expression of TGF-β1 and -β3 was expressed in developing osteophytes and articular cartilage in murine experimental osteoarthritis. Inhibition of endogenous TGF-β almost completely prevented the formation of osteophytes. In contrast, treatment with recombinant soluble TGF-β-RII resulted in significant enhancement of articular cartilage proteoglycan loss and reduction in the thickness of articular cartilage.

Conclusions.—These findings are the first demonstration that endogenous TGF-β is a crucial factor in the process of osteocyte formation and performs an important role in protection against cartilage loss.

► Previous studies demonstrated a role for TGF-β in OA through the formation of osteophytes by the process of endochondral ossification as well as maintenance of cartilage proteoglycan levels by inhibition of interleukin-1 (IL-1) induced matrix catabolism by matrix metalloproteinases (MMPs). These authors selectively blocked endogenous TGF-β by systemic administration of a recombinant soluble TGF-β receptor in a murine model of papain-induced OA. Inhibition of TGF-β resulted in decreased cartilage proteoglycan content and decreased cartilage thickness mediated by lack of inhibition of IL-1–induced MMP-3 and MMP-13 expression as well as smaller osteophyte size. These data suggest that locally administered TGF-β may have a potential role for disease modification in patients with OA in preventing cartilage loss; this potential benefit would need to be balanced by the possible growth in osteophyte size.

M. C. Hochberg, MD

Evaluation

Reliability of the Knee Examination in Osteoarthritis: Effect of Standardization

Cibere J, Bellamy N, Thorne A, et al (Arthritis Research Centre of Canada, Vancouver, BC; Univ of Queensland, Brisbane, Australia; Univ of British Columbia, Canada; et al)

Arthritis Rheum 50:458-468, 2004 5–8

Background.—Knee examination is a key component in the assessment of patients with osteoarthritis (OA). Many different signs and techniques are included in the recommendations for the physical examination of the OA knee. The clinical diagnostic criteria for knee OA according to the American College of Rheumatology (ACR) include assessments for crepitus, bony swelling, bony tenderness, and warmth. However, the reliability of these and other signs by physical examination has not been evaluated comprehensively. The reliability of physical examination of the OA knee by rheumatologists was examined, and the benefits of standardization of knee examination techniques were evaluated.

Methods.—An evaluation of 42 physical signs and techniques for examination of the knee was conducted with a 6 × 6 Latin square design. Patients with mild to sever knee OA on the basis of physical and radiographic signs were examined in random order before and after standardization of techniques. For signs with dichotomous scales, agreement among the rheumatologists was calculated as the prevalence-adjusted, bias-adjusted kappa. For the signs with continuous and ordinal scales, a reliability coefficient was calculated by analysis of variance. A prevalence-adjusted, bias-adjusted kappa of more than 0.60 and a reliability coefficient of more than 0.80 were considered indicative of adequate reliability.

Results.—Adequate poststandardization reliability was attained for 30 (71%) of 42 physical signs/techniques. The most reliable signs identified by physical examination of the OA knee were alignment by goniometer, bony swelling, general passive crepitus, gait by inspection, effusion bulge sign, quadriceps atrophy, medial tibiofemoral tenderness, patellofemoral tenderness on grind test, and flexion contracture. Standardization of the knee examination provided substantial improvements in reliability for evaluation of several physical signs, although little or no effect of standardization was noted for some signs. After standardization, warmth, medial instability at 30° flexion, and lateral instability at 30° flexion were the only 3 signs that were highly unreliable.

Conclusions.—It appears that, except for physical examinations for instability, a comprehensive knee examination can be performed with adequate reliability. Standardization of the knee examination provides further improvement in the reliability of some physical signs and findings. Use of these findings in regard to standardization in future OA studies will help to improve the assessment of outcomes in patients with OA.

► This study shows that the examination of the knee can be standardized and that all the usual maneuvers, except for the evaluation for instability and warmth, can be conducted with very good to excellent reliability (substantial or almost perfect agreement). All rheumatologists involved in teaching physical examination techniques to medical students, residents, and postdoctoral fellows should read this article and implement these techniques with their colleagues before conducting teaching sessions.

M. C. Hochberg, MD

Validation and Reproducibility of Ultrasonography in the Detection of Synovitis in the Knee: A Comparison With Arthroscopy and Clinical Examination

Karim Z, Wakefield RJ, Quinn M, et al (Univ of Leeds, England)

Arthritis Rheum 50:387-394, 2004 5–9

Background.—The most frequent presenting sign of inflammatory arthritis is synovitis, which has a central role in the progression of joint damage in rheumatoid arthritis. Synovitis is also seen frequently in osteoarthritis, particularly with advanced structural damage, and has recently been associated with the degree of pain and the predicted progression of cartilage loss in the knee. Clinical assessment of the knee for synovitis has poor sensitivity and reproducibility, and there is a need for a more reliable method for detecting and quantifying synovitis. The validity and reproducibility of US in the detection of synovitis of the knee was evaluated by comparing US findings with those of arthroscopy and clinical examination.

Methods.—Clinical examination and US were performed immediately before knee arthroscopy on 60 consecutive patients with knee pain resulting from various arthritides. All 3 assessments were performed by different clinicians who were blinded to the results obtained with the other modalities. US and clinical examination were compared with arthroscopically detected synovitis as the gold standard. Data from a subset of patients were used to calculate the interreader and intrareader reproducibility of US results by using a standard dichotomous (absence/presence of synovitis) as well as a graded (absence/grade of synovitis) scoring system.

Results.—Measured against the use of arthroscopy as the gold standard, US was found to have a higher sensitivity (98% vs 85%), specificity (88% vs 25%), accuracy (97% vs 77%), positive predictive value (98% vs 88%), and negative predictive value (88% vs 20%) compared with clinical examination. The Cohen kappa values for interreader and intrareader reproducibil-

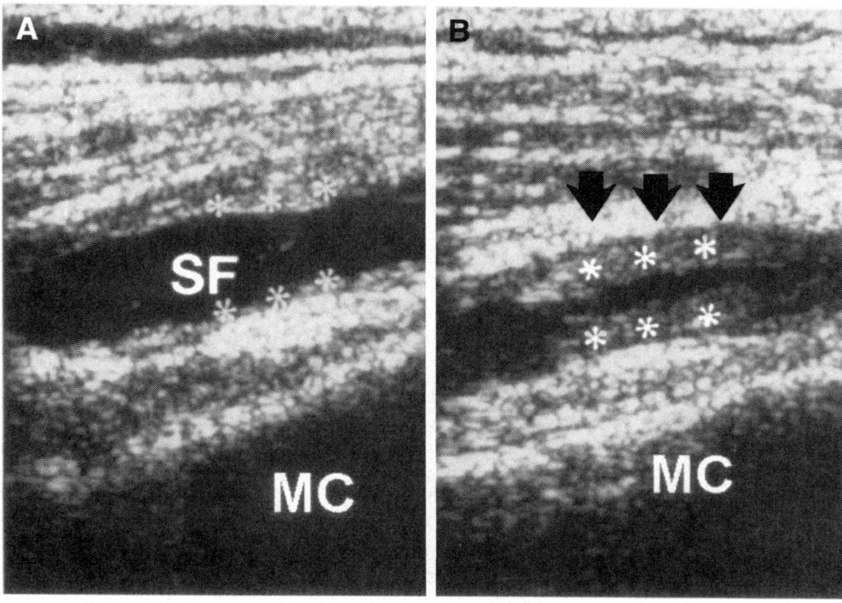

FIGURE 2.—US, with effusion demonstrated by transducer ballottement: longitudinal view of suprapatellar pouch with knee flexed. **A**, Image obtained under normal transducer pressure. **B**, Increased transducer pressure or ballottement. *Arrows* indicate apposition of synovial membrane (*) under pressure from transducer. *Abbreviations: SF*, Synovial fluid; *MC*, medial condyle. (Courtesy of Karim Z, Wakefield RJ, Quinn M, et al: Validation and reproducibility of ultrasonography in the detection of synovitis in the knee: A comparison with arthroscopy and clinical examination. *Arthritis Rheum* 50:387-394, 2004. Reprinted by permission of John Wiley & Sons, Inc.)

ity of US for distinguishing between presence and absence of synovitis were 0.71 and 0.85, respectively (Fig 2). The weighted kappa values for distinguishing grade of synovitis were 0.65 for interreader and 0.74 for intrareader reproducibility. The kappa value for intrareader reproducibility of arthroscopy results was 0.88.

Conclusions.—These findings demonstrated that US is a valid, reproducible technique for the detection of synovitis in the knee, with greater accuracy than is obtained with clinical examination. US may be valuable as a tool in studies that investigate pain, diagnosis, and treatment response in knee arthritis.

► Synovitis is associated with pain[1] and has been recognized to be a predictor of progression in patients with osteoarthritis of the knee. Assessment of synovitis on clinical examination is imprecise, and noninvasive methods of detecting the presence of synovitis are needed. This study found that US, performed by a single experienced physician, had a sensitivity and specificity of 98% and 88%, respectively, compared with arthroscopy for detecting synovitis in a sample of 60 patients, 19 with osteoarthritis. Unfortunately, the authors failed to analyze their data by underlying diagnosis; hence, we don't know if US is as valid in patients with osteoarthritis as in those with rheumatoid arthritis or other inflammatory arthropathies. Nonetheless, this technique holds promise for clinical practice, assuming that training and costs are not prohibitive and that insurance companies will reimburse rheumatologists for its use in routine office practice.

M. C. Hochberg, MD

Reference

1. Hill CL, Gale DG, Chaisson CE, et al: Knee effusions, popliteal cysts, and synovial thickening: Association with knee pain in osteoarthritis. *J Rheumatol* 28:1330-1337, 2001.

How Does Tibial Cartilage Volume Relate to Symptoms in Subject With Knee Osteoarthritis?

Wluka AE, Wolfe R, Stuckey S, et al (Monah Univ, Prahan, Victoria, Australia)
Ann Rheum Dis 63:264-268, 2004 5–10

Background.—The relation between the clinical symptoms of knee osteoarthritis (OA), such as pain and function, and the structural changes of OA measured radiographically is unclear. It has been well established that the prevalence of knee pain increases with increasing radiographic severity of knee osteoarthritis. However, the severity of pain is not related to the degree of radiographic OA, and radiographic change has been consistently linked with symptoms of disease. Determined were the relationship between symptoms of knee OA and tibial cartilage volume, whether pain is predictive of loss of cartilage in knee OA, and whether change in cartilage volume of time is related to change in symptoms over the same period.

Methods.—A total of 132 subjects with symptomatic early (mild to moderate) knee OA were studied. MRI scans were performed and the patients completed questionnaires at baseline and again 2 years later to quantify symptoms of knee OA (knee-specific WOMAC: pain, stiffness, function) and general physical and mental health (SF-36). Tibial cartilage volume was determined for the MRI images.

TABLE 5.—Correlation Between the Change in Symptoms of Knee OA With the Loss of Cartilage Volume

	Correlation Coefficient*	*P* Value
Increased pain score†	−0.28	0.002
Increased stiffness score†	−0.17	0.07
Increased function score†	−0.21	0.02
Decreased physical function score‡	0.11	0.26
Decreased mental function score‡	−0.08	0.39

*Spearman's correlation coefficient.

†WOMAC pain, stiffness, and function subscales (higher score indicates worse symptoms).

‡results of SF-36 standardized to Australian normal values (lower score indicates worse function).

(Courtesy of Wluka AE, Wolfe R, Stuckey S, et al: How does tibial cartilage volume relate to symptoms in subjects with knee osteoarthritis? *Ann Rheum Dis* 63:264-268, 2004, copyright BMJ Publishing Group.)

Results.—Complete data were available for 117 (89%) subjects. A weak association was evident between tibial cartilage volume and symptoms at baseline. The severity of symptoms of knee OA at baseline was not predictive of subsequent tibial cartilage loss. However, weak associations were noted between worsening of symptoms of OA and increased cartilage loss (Table 5).

Conclusions.—It appears that there is a weak association between tibial cartilage volume and symptoms in knee osteoarthritis. A weak association was observed between loss of tibial cartilage and worsening of symptoms, which suggests that although cartilage does relate to the symptoms of OA, it is not a major determinant of symptoms.

► MRI has been shown to be more sensitive than standard radiography for identifying osteophytes, cartilage lesions, synovial thickening, and joint effusions in patients with knee OA. Furthermore, articular cartilage volume can be quantified by MRI.[1] These authors studied a volunteer sample of 132 patients with symptomatic radiographic knee OA to determine whether changes in cartilage volume correlate with changes in clinical features. Over a 2-year period pain, stiffness, and function significantly improved overall, while cartilage volume declined by a mean of approximately 10%. The authors found a significant but weak correlation between change in cartilage volume and clinical parameters over time. These findings differ from those reported by Raynauld et al[1]; potential explanations include differences in sample size/power, characteristics and treatment of the patients, and acquisition and analysis of the MRI scans, among others. Clearly, further longitudinal studies are needed before cartilage volume can be used as a surrogate end point for outcome studies in knee OA.

M. C. Hochberg, MD

Reference

1. Raynauld J-P, Kauffmann C, Beaudoin G, et al: Reliability of a quantification imaging system using magnetic resonance images to measure cartilage thickness and volume in human normal and osteoarthritis knees. *Osteoarthritis Cart* 11:351-360, 2003.

Therapies

Efficacy of Knee Tape in the Management of Osteoarthritis of the Knee: Blinded Randomised Controlled Trial

Hinman RS, Crossley KM, McConnell J, et al (Univ of Melbourne, Australia)
BMJ 327:135-140, 2003 5–11

Introduction.—Limited progress has been made toward curing osteoarthritis (OA), so symptom management is the mainstay of treatment. Simple, inexpensive treatments that increase the range of options for patients with OA are warranted. Knee taping relieves pain in patients with OA of the knee, probably by improving alignment of the patellofemoral joint or unloading inflamed soft tissues. The effect of therapeutic knee taping on pain and disability in patients with symptoms of knee OA was evaluated, along with any benefits maintained after cessation of treatment.

Methods.—Eighty-seven patients with symptoms of knee OA, as defined by the American College of Rheumatology, participated in a randomized, single-blind, controlled trial with 3 intervention arms (therapeutic tape, control tape, and no tape) of 3 weeks' duration and 3 weeks of follow-up (Fig 1). Outcome evaluations were performed in a university-based laboratory. Taping interventions were performed by 4 physiotherapists at a university and 8 in private practice. Therapeutic taping provided medial glide, medial tilt, and anteroposterior tilt to the patella (Fig 2). The primary outcome measure was pain as measured by visual analogue scale and participant-perceived rating of change. The secondary measures of pain and disability included the Western Ontario and MacMaster universities OA index, the knee pain scale, and the Short Form-36.

Results.—Participants in the therapeutic tape group reported a greater decrease in pain on all primary outcomes compared with the other 2 groups. A significant correlation was evident between intervention and change in pain at 3 weeks ($P = .000$), with 73% (21/29) of the therapeutic group reporting improvement, compared to 49% (14/29) of the control tape group and 10% (3/29) of the no tape group. Significantly greater improvements in pain and disability were seen in most secondary outcomes in the therapeutic group

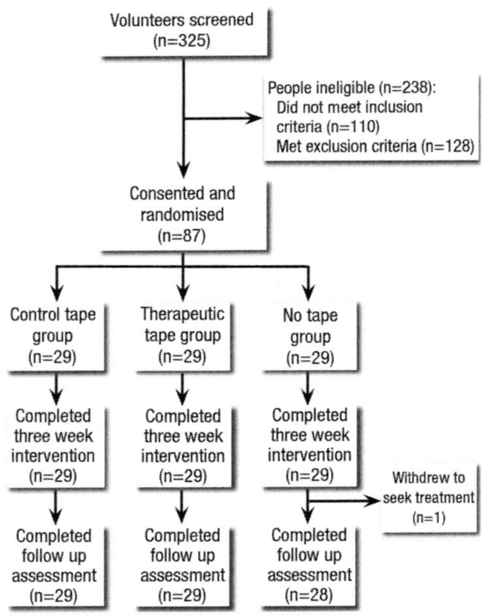

FIGURE 1.—Trial profile. (Courtesy of Hinman RS, Crossley KM, McConnell J, et al: Efficacy of knee tape in the management of osteoarthritis of the knee: Blinded randomised controlled trial. *BMJ* 327:135-140, 2003. With permission from the BMJ Publishing Group.)

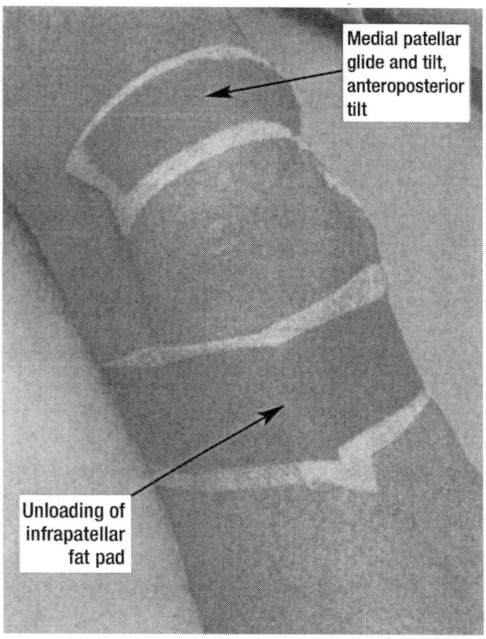

FIGURE 2.—Positioning of therapeutic knee tape (Courtesy of Hinman RS, Crossley KM, McConnell J, et al: Efficacy of knee tape in the management of osteoarthritis of the knee: Blinded randomised controlled trial. *BMJ* 327:135-140, 2003. With permission from the BMJ Publishing Group.)

versus the no tape group. The benefits of therapeutic tape were maintained 3 weeks after treatment cessation.

Conclusion.—Therapeutic knee taping is an efficacious treatment for management of pain and disability in patients with knee OA.

► It seems our British colleagues emphasize simple, easy approaches like this more than we do. I will try to incorporate this into my practice.

R. S. Panush, MD

Efficacy and Safety of 5% Ibuprofen Cream Treatment in Knee Osteoarthritis: Results of a Randomized, Double-Blind, Placebo-Controlled Study

Trnavský K, Fischer M, Vögtle-Junkert U, et al (Postgraduate Med School, Prague, Czech Republic; ClinResearch GmbH, Cologne, Germany; Dolorgiet Pharmaceuticals, St Augustin/Bonn, Germany)

J Rheumatol 31:565-572, 2004 5–12

Background.—Oral nonsteroidal anti-inflammatory drugs (NSAIDs) such as ibuprofen are standard therapy for rheumatic diseases, but topical preparations of these agents are less well appreciated. A cream containing

5% ibuprofen has been used safely for 20 years with good success, but randomized controlled trials have been lacking. The guidelines of the European Committee for Proprietary Medicinal Products and the International Conference on Harmonisation were used in a randomized controlled trial investigating the efficacy and safety of a 5% ibuprofen cream (Dolgit).

Methods.—Both male and female patients 40 to 75 years of age took part. All had score for pain on motion of at least 40 mm on a visual analog scale, a Lequesne index score between 5 and 13, and a Kellgren-Lawrence radiographic score between grades II and III. Patients were randomly assigned to receive the study medication or placebo. The study medication was applied in a 10-cm strip containing approximately 200 mg ibuprofen 3 times a day for 7 days on the knee with the most pain. The reduction of pain on motion was evaluated by the patient using a 100-mm visual analog scale. A response was defined as a reduction of pain on motion of at least 18 mm or 23% in comparison to baseline values. Other measures included the mean changes in pain with motion, pain at rest, and overall pain between the beginning and end of the study; improvement in algofunctional disability; patient and investigator assessments of efficacy; documentation of adverse events; and patient and investigator assessments of safety.

Results.—After 8 days, all 12 patients who received ibuprofen and 2 of 13 who received placebo responded to the intervention. At the second analysis, 21 of the 25 patients receiving ibuprofen and 10 of the 25 receiving placebo responded. The difference between the response rates of 84% and 40% was highly significant. Ibuprofen consistently relieved pain, and the most pronounced reduction was seen by the fourth day after the intervention began.

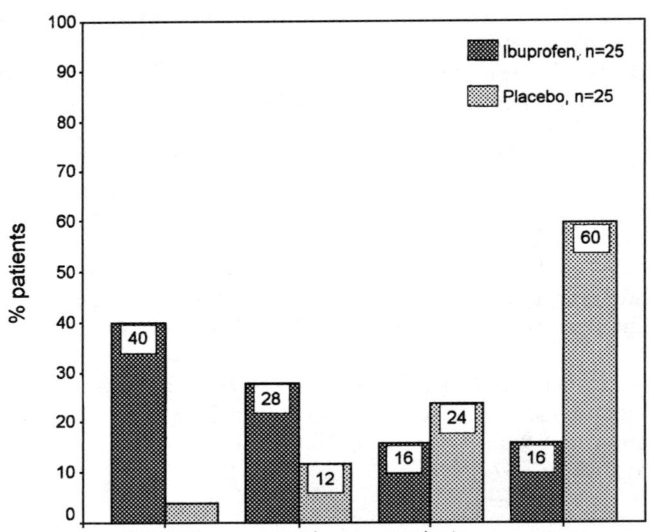

FIGURE 3.—Overall assessment of efficacy. (Courtesy of Trnavský K, Fischer M, Vögtle-Junkert U, et al: Efficacy and safety of 5% ibuprofen cream treatment in knee osteoarthritis: Results of a randomized, double-blind, placebo-controlled study. *J Rheumatol* 31:565-572, 2004.)

The reduction of pain with placebo was slight and held nearly constant over the study period. Lequesne index values decreased 27.5% for the ibuprofen group and 10.7% for the placebo group. No adverse events occurred during the study. The efficacy of ibuprofen cream was rated very good by 40% of the research subjects, good by 28%, moderate by 16%, and poor by 16%. In comparison, the efficacy of placebo was rated very good in 4%, good in 12%, moderate in 24%, and poor in 60% (Fig 3).

Conclusions.—Patients receiving topical ibuprofen cream had an 84% response rate; those receiving placebo had only a 40% response rate. The ibuprofen cream worked quickly to reduce pain, and most responses occurred before 4 days of therapy. No adverse events developed. Thus, ibuprofen cream is both efficacious and safe for use in treating knee osteoarthritis.

► Topical NSAIDs may turn out to be one of those adjunctive therapies that may help certain patients with localized or regional musculoskeletal disorders. I occasionally prescribe topical capsaicin and would like to have a broader menu of possibilities to consider. I'd want to be sure topical NSAIDs were not appreciably absorbed and did not sensitize, and I'd like to see comparisons with other agents, including other topical agents.

R. S. Panush, MD

Aspirin, Ibruprofen, and Mortality After Myocardial Infarction: Retrospective Cohort Study

Curtis JP, Wang Y, Portnay EL, et al (Yale Univ, New Haven, Conn; Denver Health Med Ctr, Colo)

BMJ 327:1322-1323, 2003 5–13

Introduction.—Observational trials and in vivo experiments have raised concern that the cardioprotective effects of aspirin therapy are blocked by the nonsteroidal anti-inflammatory drug (NSAID), ibuprofen, by competitively inhibiting aspirin's binding site on platelets. A retrospective search was performed to ascertain whether prescribing aspirin and ibuprofen after myocardial infarction (MI) was linked with increased risk of death.

Methods.—A database compiled by the Cooperative Cardiovascular Project was composed of 234,769 Medicare patients in the United States who were hospitalized with MI between 1994 and 1996. Patients with MI who were aged 65 years or older and who were prescribed aspirin on hospital discharge were included. The outcome measure was time to death within 1 year of discharge, which was determined by the Medicare enrollment database.

Baseline characteristics were compared in patients prescribed only aspirin, prescribed aspirin and ibuprofen, and prescribed aspirin and other NSAIDs. Survival was analyzed. A Cox proportional hazards mortality model was developed, including demographics, medical history, admission presentation, hospital course, and discharge care.

Results.—Aspirin was prescribed for a total of 70,316 patients at hospital discharge; 66,739 were prescribed aspirin alone, 844 aspirin and ibuprofen, and 2733 aspirin and other NSAIDs. Patients in the aspirin only group had more co-morbidity and experienced more complications in the hospital. A total of 11,546 (17.5%) patients in the aspirin only group, 118 (14.0%) in the aspirin and ibuprofen group, and 432 (15.8%) in the aspirin and other NSAIDs group died within 1 year after discharge ($P = .004$). The multivariate model revealed that patients prescribed aspirin and ibuprofen on discharge had a risk of death similar to that of patients prescribed aspirin alone (hazard ratio, 0.84; 95% confidence interval, 0.70-1.01) or those prescribed aspirin and another NSAID (hazard ratio, 0.96; 95% confidence interval, 0.86-1.06).

Conclusion.—Aspirin and ibuprofen did not adversely interact in this series of patients aged 65 years or older who were discharged after MI. It is likely that the pharmacodynamic interaction of aspirin and ibuprofen may not have a significant impact on patient outcomes.

► I commented at length on the confounding issues of aspirin, NSAIDs, and cardioprotection in the 2003 YEAR BOOK.[1] If the ability of ibuprofen to block binding of aspirin to cyclooxygenase (and mitigate cardioprotection) translated to clinical significance, then patients taking both agents should have a higher incidence of MI. In the 2004 YEAR BOOK,[2] I included an article suggesting exactly that. This selection contains contradictory observations. I conclude (for now) that we don't know, but if there is a clinical effect, it would seem to be small. We'll see.

R. S. Panush, MD

Reference

1. 2003 YEAR BOOK OF RHEUMATOLOGY, ARTHRITIS, AND MUSCULOSKELETAL DISEASE, pp 1-16.
2. 2004 YEAR BOOK OF RHEUMATOLOGY, ARTHRITIS, AND MUSCULOSKELETAL DISEASE, pp 19-21.

Methodological Differences in Clinical Trials Evaluating Nonpharmacological and Pharmacological Treatments of Hip and Knee Osteoarthritis

Boutron I, Tubach F, Giraudeau B, et al (Université Paris VII; INSERM CIC 202, Tours, France)

JAMA 290:1062-1070, 2003 5–14

Introduction.—Randomized controlled trials are widely accepted as the most dependable means for ascertaining the effectiveness of specific therapies. The quality of articles addressing pharmacologic and nonpharmacologic treatments of hip and knee osteoarthritis (OA) were compared to identify specific methodological issues associated with the evaluation of nonpharmacologic treatments.

Methods.—MEDLINE and the Cochrane Central Register of Controlled Trials were searched for articles of randomized controlled trials published between January 1, 1992 and February 28, 2002 in 28 general medical and specialty journals with high impact factors and assessment of pharmacologic and nonpharmacologic treatment of patients with hip or knee OA. The quality of the methods in the articles was examined by 2 independent investigators who used the Jadad scale, the Delphi list, and guidelines from the *Users' Guides to the Medical Literature*. The investigators used a checklist of items to analyze trial characteristics.

Results.—One hundred and ten articles were analyzed: 50 (45.5%) examined nonpharmacologic treatments and 60 (54.5%) evaluated pharmacologic treatments. Articles reporting nonpharmacologic treatments had a lower global quality score than did articles reporting pharmacologic treatments, as determined by the Jadad scale (mean [SD] score, 1.4 [1.3] vs 4.0 [1.3]) and the Delphi list (mean [SD] score, 5.2 [1.5] vs 7.5 [1.1]). Lack of reporting sufficient random sequence generation and intention-to-treat analyses were identified in articles reporting nonpharmacologic or pharmacologic treatments. Nonpharmacologic treatments were less often compared with a placebo than were pharmacologic treatments (28.0% vs 71.7%). Compared with articles reporting pharmacologic treatments, articles reporting nonpharmacologic treatments less often described blinding of patients (26.0% vs 96.7%), care providers (6.0% vs 81.7%), and outcome assessors (68.0% vs 98.3%). Care providers' skill levels could have affected the treatment effect in 84.0% of nonpharmacologic articles versus in 23.3% of pharmacologic articles.

Conclusion.—Nonpharmacologic articles scored lower in quality than did pharmacologic articles of patients with hip and knee OA. Investigations of nonpharmacologic treatments need to consider additional methodological issues.

► Of course. As long as the pharmaceutical has no immediate telling properties (eg, peculiar taste or odor), there is no excuse for a flawed trial design. I believe strongly that the same assertion pertains to elective surgical interventions. There is no excuse for designs that avoid sham surgery to establish effectiveness and randomization to various interventions to establish relative effectiveness.

However, most other nonpharmacologic interventions are not simply "modalities," they are treatment acts in which the therapist is as critical as the modality that is purveyed. In that sense, modalities such as acupuncture, manipulation, and education become difficult, if not impossible, to control adequately. The operator would have to be trained to feign the same sort of indifference or enthusiasm whether applying a sham or the study modality. There will always be uncertainty and debate regarding the effectiveness of treatment acts.

N. M. Hadler, MD

Gastrointestinal Health Care Resource Utilization With Chronic Use of COX-2–Specific Inhibitors Versus Traditional NSAIDs

Laine L, Wogen J, Yu H (Univ of Southern California, Los Angeles; Inst for Effectiveness Research, Bridgewater, NJ)
Gastroenterology 125:389-395, 2003 5–15

Introduction.—The use of nonsteroidal anti-inflammatory drugs (NSAIDs) is associated with increased risk of ulcers and gastrointestinal (GI) clinical events, including bleeding and dyspepsia. In controlled trials, cyclo-oxygenase 2 (COX-2)–specific inhibitors (coxibs) reduce the development of ulcers, GI clinical events, and GI health resource utilization compared with traditional nonselective NSAIDs. It is not known whether these findings are observed in clinical practice. An integrated administrative database of medical and pharmaceutical claims of more than 8 million lives was examined to evaluate GI-associated resource use in patients switching from long-term NSAID therapy to long-term coxib therapy in a longitudinal, retrospective cohort investigation. The use of resources was compared in patients beginning long-term NSAID therapy with that of patients starting long-term coxib therapy.

Methods.—A total of 2246 patients who switched from NSAID to coxib therapy were evaluated during the 12-month periods before and after the initial prescription. The proportions of patients with GI resource use (odds ratio [OR] adjusted for relevant covariates) and costs were compared for traditional NSAIDs versus long-term coxib.

Results.—The adjusted OR for any GI resource use (coxib vs NSAID period) was 0.86 (95% CI, 0.74-0.99) for patients switching therapies. The reduction was due to less GI cotherapy (OR, 0.82; 95% CI, 0.69-0.97). The costs did not decrease significantly after switching to coxibs (mean difference, –$19; 95% CI, –$139 to $55). After adding NSAID/coxib costs, the total cost in the coxib period was significantly greater (mean increase, $377; 95% CI, $271-$488). The adjusted OR for GI resource use for patients new

TABLE 3.—Crude Proportions of Patients With GI Healthcare Resource Utilization and Adjusted Odds Ratios in Patients Initiating Chronic NSAID Versus Chronic Coxib Therapy

GI Resource Use	New-to-Therapy NSAID (n = 25,989)	New-to-Therapy Coxib (n =2125)	Adjusted OR (95% CI) Coxib vs. NSAID
Any GI resource*	32.6%	51.0%	1.04 (0.92-1.16)
GI prescription	21.9%	41.5%	1.13 (1.0-1.29)
GI outpatient/ED visit	19.8%	27.3%	0.98 (0.88-1.10)
GI hospitalization	1.6%	2.5%	.90 (0.66-1.23)

*Adjusted for patient age; sex; prior GI diagnoses; number of prior GI prescriptions; number of GI-related outpatient, inpatient, or ED visits; chronic disease score; timing of initiation of NSAID/coxib therapy; and number of NSAID/coxib prescriptions.

Abbreviations: GI, Gastrointestinal; *NSAID*, nonsteroidal anti-inflammatory drug; *Coxib*, cyclo-oxygenase 2–specific inhibitor; *ED*, emergency department.

(Courtesy of Laine L, Wogen J, Yu H: Gastrointestinal health care resource utilization with chronic use of COX-2-specific inhibitors versus traditional NSAIDs. *Gastroenterology* 125:389-395, 2003.)

to coxib therapy versus patients new to NSAID therapy was 1.04 (95% CI, 0.92-1.16) (Table 3); the GI costs were significantly lower in the new-NSAID group.

Conclusion.—In the group of patients who switched from long-term NSAID therapy to long-term coxib therapy, a slight reduction was seen in the proportion using GI-associated resources, but a reduction was not seen in GI-related costs. When NSAID/coxib drug costs were included, costs were slightly less for NSAIDs than for coxibs. The potential GI-associated cost savings indicated in coxib clinical trials may not be fully realized in the clinical setting.

The Cost-Effectiveness of Cyclooxygenase-2 Selective Inhibitors in the Management of Chronic Arthritis

Spiegel BMR, Targownik L, Dulai GS, et al (Univ of California, Los Angeles)

Ann Intern Med 138:795-806, 2003 5–16

Background.—Nonsteroidal anti-inflammatory drugs (NSAIDs) are widely used for the treatment of chronic arthritis pain and account for 3% of the US prescription market. Despite the association of NSAIDs with clinically significant peptic ulcer complications, these drugs are a mainstay of treatment. Cyclo-oxygenase-2 selective inhibitors, including rofecoxib and celecoxib (coxibs), have been developed as safer alternatives to nonselective NSAIDs. Rofecoxib and celecoxib have been found to effectively treat chronic arthritis pain and to reduce ulcer complications by 50% compared with NSAIDs. However, the absolute risk reduction of the coxibs is small, and the cost-effectiveness of treatment has not been established. Whether the degree of risk reduction of gastrointestinal complications by coxibs offsets their increased cost compared with a generic nonselective NSAID was determined.

Methods.—A systematic review of MEDLINE and published abstracts that included patients with osteoarthritis or rheumatoid arthritis who were not taking aspirin and who required long-term NSAID therapy for moderate to severe arthritis pain was used for this cost-utility analysis. Naproxen, 500 mg twice daily, and coxib, once daily, were administered. Patients' therapy was switched to a coxib if they could not tolerate naproxen. The main outcome measure was the incremental cost per quality-adjusted life-year (QALY) gained. Base-case and sensitivity analyses were performed.

Results.—The base-case analysis showed that the use of a coxib instead of a nonselective NSAID in average-risk patients cost an incremental $275,809 per year to gain 1 additional QALY. The sensitivity analysis showed that the incremental cost per QALY gained decreased to $55,803 when the analysis was limited to the subset of patients with a history of bleeding ulcers. The coxib strategy was dominant when the cost of coxibs was reduced by 90% of the current average wholesale price. A probabilistic sensitivity analysis showed that if a third-party payer was willing to pay $150,000 per QALY gained, then 4.3% of average-risk patients would fall within the budget.

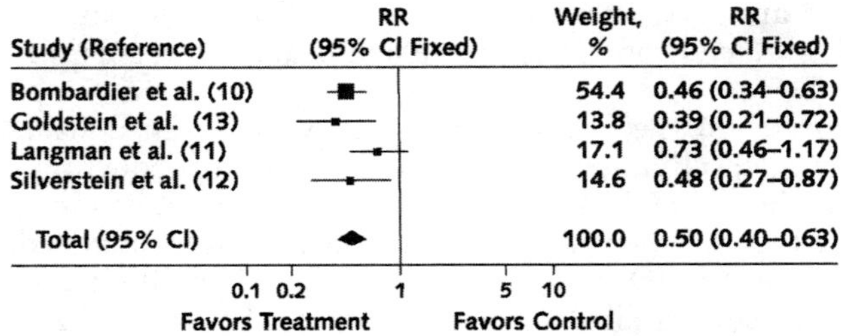

FIGURE 3.—Meta-analysis with the use of the fixed-effects model of randomized controlled trials that report clinically significant ulcer complications (symptomatic ulcer, ulcer hemorrhage, or ulcer perforation) in patients receiving a cyclo-oxygenase-2–selective inhibitor versus a nonselective nonsteroidal anti-inflammatory drug. The summary estimate is the relative risk (RR). (Courtesy of Spiegel BMR, Targownik L, Dulai GS, et al: The cost-effectiveness of cyclooxygenase-2 selective inhibitors in the management of chronic arthritis. *Ann Intern Med* 138:795-806, 2003.)

Conclusions.—The risk reduction (Fig 3) obtained with coxibs does not offset their increased cost compared with nonselective NSAIDs in the treatment of average-risk patients with chronic arthritis. However, the incremental cost-effectiveness ratio of coxibs may be acceptable when they are used in the subgroup of patients with a history of bleeding ulcers.

► I have never prescribed a coxib.

I find the behavior of "Big Pharma" in marketing these agents to be egregious and the behavior of the medical community in being seduced, if not co-conspiratorial, to be unconscionable.

I have said so before and written so in more than one publication. I did not need these 2 papers to bear me out: the data that underpin my reproach are available for all to see. However, I will not pass up the opportunity to make the point and raise the ethical issues yet again, to wit,

1. There is not a hint in the literature that coxibs are more effective than aspirin in any clinical setting.
2. Long-term toxicity is still to be defined.
3. Therefore, the only justification for prescribing the agents relates to short-term safety, as they are no more convenient than NSAIDs available over the counter, and the only short-term safety issue for which there are data relates to GI toxicity.
4. The article by Laine et al (see Abstract 5–15) should debunk all claims of safety in general use. In fact, Table 3 suggests that traditional NSAIDs have the edge in all ways!
5. The myth of safety grew out of the trials that Spiegel et al (see Abstract 5–16) rely on for their econometric analysis. Of these the CLASS trial[1] (denoted as *Silverstein et al* in Fig 3) and the VIGOR trial (denoted as *Bombardier et al*) were considered in detail by the US Food and Drug Administration (FDA) when the manufacturers petitioned for labeling as "safe." It is the CLASS trial that is given most weight by Spiegel et al (Fig 3). That's disconcerting. The FDA reviewers were not convinced that there was any safety margin afforded by celecoxib over the course of 6 months studied in the CLASS trial. Furthermore, Pharmacia and their investigators had much to

explain; they were aware of the results after 12 months at the time of the *New England Journal of Medicine* publication. At 12 months, there was not even a hint of safety. Shame.

Come the revolution . . .

N. M. Hadler, MD

References

1. Silverstein FE, Faich G, Goldstein JL, et al: Gastrointestinal toxicity with celecoxib vs nonsteroidal anti-inflammatory drugs for osteoarthritis and rheumatoid arthritis: The CLASS study: A randomized controlled trial. Celecoxib Long-term Arthritis Safety Study. *JAMA* 284:1247-1255, 2000.
2. Bombardier C, Laine L, Reicin A, et al: Comparison of upper gastrointestinal toxicity of rofecoxib and naproxen in patients with rheumatoid arthritis. VIGOR Study Group. *N Engl J Med* 343:1520-1528, 2000.

Nonsteroidal Antiinflammatory Drugs or Acetaminophen for Osteoarthritis of the Hip or Knee? A Systematic Review of Evidence and Guidelines

Wegman A, van der Windt D, van Tulder M, et al (VU Univ Med Ctr, Amsterdam)

J Rheumatol 31:344-354, 2004 5–17

Introduction.—Primary care physicians treat most patients who have symptoms of osteoarthritis (OA). Nonpharmacologic interventions, including patient education, exercise, and occupational therapy, are mainstays of treatment. Oral medication is frequently an important component of therapy. Because prolonged pharmacotherapy is often associated with side effects and costs, it is important to carefully consider evidence and recommendations concerning pharmacology. A systematic review of randomized, controlled trials (RCT) was performed to gather data regarding the quality and content of clinical guidelines for pharmacologic treatment of OA.

Methods.—Published reports of RCT and clinical guidelines were identified via a systematic search of bibliographic databases and relevant Web sites. The quality of RCT was examined by 2 independent reviewers who used a standardized checklist. Data from the RCT were used to ascertain pooled differences between groups for pain and disability. The methodology of identified guidelines was assessed using the Appraisal of Guidelines for Research and Evaluation (AGREE) instrument.

Results.—Five RCT met all inclusion criteria. Statistical pooling of data from 3 trials with adequate methodology and data presentation yielded a pooled standardized mean difference for general pain of 0.33 (95% CI), suggesting a small effect in favor of nonsteroidal anti-inflammatory drugs (NSAID). The pooled estimates for other outcome measures were insignificant. Three of 9 identified guidelines satisfied more AGREE criteria, compared with others, especially concerning rigor of development. Stakeholder involvement, applicability, and editorial independence were not well described in most guidelines. The content of recommendations concerning the use of NSAID versus acetaminophen was somewhat consistent.

Conclusion.—Acetaminophen is frequently effective in OA and is linked with fewer adverse reactions, compared with NSAID. Available evidence supports recommendations of recent guidelines concerning the use of acetaminophen as the initial therapy for OA in addition to nonpharmacologic interventions.

► There is so much at stake in the on-going press to capture the pharmaceutical market for the treatment of OA. Of course, the vaunted treatment has little to do with OA and much with joint pain. And regional musculoskeletal pain is an intermittent and remittent fact of life. The marketing involves turning such a life predicament into a disease, ie, medicalizing regional pain and labeling it "OA." That's what is happening with the direct-to-consumer schemes, such as showing a famous ice skating champion whose looks belie her middle age, and who claims to be able to skate thanks to her pills. We visited this marketing scene elsewhere in this volume (Abstracts 5–15 and 5–16). This article is a refreshing breath of objectivity unfettered by overt conflicts of interest. It offers several important messages:

Before marauding marketing, rheumatologists would consider the pharmaceutical options and concluded that there was no compelling reason to treat "OA" with an NSAID, given that acetaminophen seemed to have a more favorable benefit/risk ratio.

After marauding marketing, "thought leaders" among the rheumatologists thought better of the NSAIDs, particularly the newer prescription NSAIDs. These "thought leaders" have peppered the literature with their convictions.

There is very little science to stem this dialectic. The authors of this article could only find 5 randomized trials contrasting acetaminophen with an NSAID for this indication.

However, there are 5 trials, and not too terribly flawed trials at that. Several recruited about 200 patients. On the basis of this science, the early advice of the rheumatologists who were unfettered by the marauding marketing proves prescient.

N. M. Hadler, MD

Heterotopic Ossification Prophylaxis With Indomethacin Increases the Risk of Long-Bone Nonunion

Burd TA, Hughes MS, Anglen JO (Univ of Missouri, Columbia)

J Bone Joint Surg Br 85-B:700-705, 2003 5–18

Introduction.—Indomethacin is often administered for prophylaxis of heterotopic ossification (HO) after surgical treatment of acetabular fractures. Nonsteroidal anti-inflammatory drugs (NSAIDs), including indomethacin, have been linked with delayed healing of fractures and mechanically weaker callus. The risk of nonunion in patients with associated fractures of the long bone was examined in patients who received indomethacin for prophylaxis against HO.

Methods.—Between July 1992 and January 2001, 282 patients who underwent open reduction and internal fixation of an acetabular fracture were evaluated. Patients at risk of HO were randomly assigned to treatment with either radiation therapy (XRT) or indomethacin.

Results.—Of 282 patients evaluated, 112 had at least 1 concomitant fracture of a long bone, 36 did not need prophylaxis, 38 underwent focal irradiation, and 38 received indomethacin. Fifteen patients had 16 nonunion fractures. A significant difference was found in the rate of nonunion fractures in patients who received indomethacin compared with those who did not (26% vs 7%; $P = .004$).

Conclusion.—Patients with concurrent fractures of the acetabulum and long bone who receive indomethacin are at significantly increased risk of nonunion fractures of the long bone compared with patients who receive XRT or no prophylaxis.

► This is a secondary analysis of data generated in a prospective randomized controlled trial (RCT) comparing oral indomethacin with external XRT as prophylaxis for HO complicating repair of acetabular fractures. Analysis of the primary data discerned no difference between the treatments in a trial that was adequate in design to be reassuring. Indomethacin and several other NSAIDs, but particularly indomethacin, has accumulated a lot of baggage since it was introduced as a unique, potent anti-inflammatory in 1963. Indomethacin is an indole derivative that was destined to supplant phenylbutazone, the last of the aminopyrenes to find a home in the formulary. No newer NSAID has been shown to be more powerful than indomethacin (or aspirin, for that matter). The NSAID wars have been fought for 50 years over claims of tolerability and safety. Indomethacin has more CNS side effects, manifesting as headaches and confusion in the elderly and dyspepsia in younger patients. Nonetheless, it is not a bad drug. In fact, there is the impression that it is peculiarly effective for gouty attacks and hip pain, and systematic studies have documented its effectiveness in reactive arthritis, particularly Reiter's syndrome and psoriatic arthritis.

Indomethacin's baggage is more alive in the orthopedic literature. Indomethacin, perhaps more than other NSAIDs, can interfere with bone healing in murine fracture models. However, murine models are hardly perfect models for human musculoskeletal diseases. For example, indomethacin will cure many murine models of erosive arthritis, whereas in man, there is no such suggestion. The primary analysis of this RCT is more reassuring than this secondary analysis is off-putting.

N. M. Hadler, MD

Gastrointestinal Tolerability and Effectiveness of Rofecoxib Versus Naproxen in the Treatment of Osteoarthritis: A Randomized, Controlled Trial

Lisse JR, for the ADVANTAGE Study Group (Univ of Arizona, Tucson; et al)
Ann Intern Med 139:539-546, 2003 5–19

Background.—Nonsteroidal anti-inflammatory drugs (NSAIDs) are often used to treat symptoms of osteoarthritis. Gastrointestinal (GI) toxicity is a common side effect of dual cyclooxygenase (COX)-1– and COX-2–inhibiting NSAIDs. GI toxicity in older patients is increased by concomitant aspirin use, previous GI intolerability, and other comorbid conditions. In these patients, intolerable GI symptoms may necessitate the discontinuation

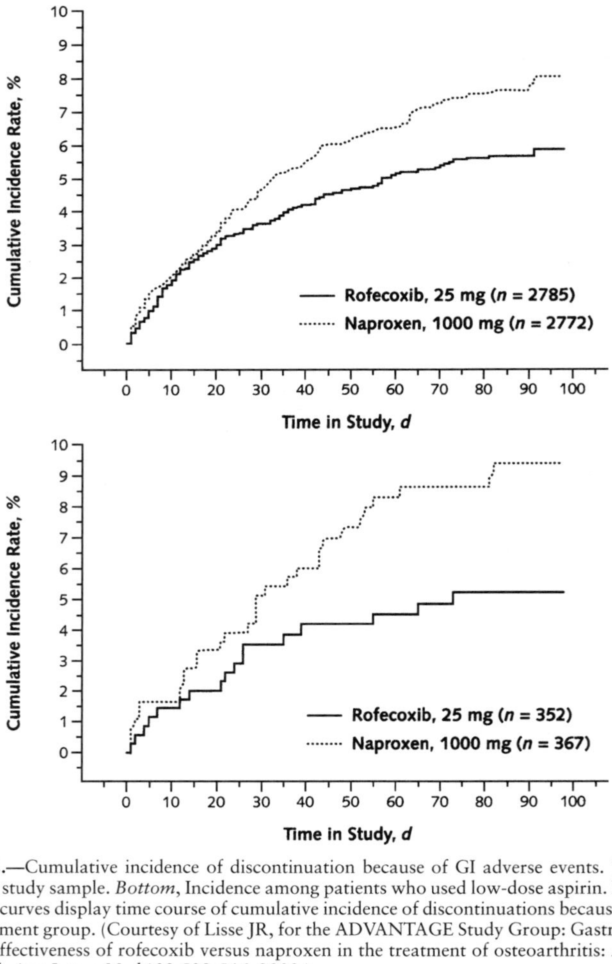

FIGURE 2.—Cumulative incidence of discontinuation because of GI adverse events. *Top*, Incidence among overall study sample. *Bottom*, Incidence among patients who used low-dose aspirin. For both parts, Kaplan-Meier curves display time course of cumulative incidence of discontinuations because of GI adverse events by treatment group. (Courtesy of Lisse JR, for the ADVANTAGE Study Group: Gastrointestinal tolerability and effectiveness of rofecoxib versus naproxen in the treatment of osteoarthritis: A randomized, controlled trial. *Ann Intern Med* 139:539-546, 2003.)

of therapy. Unlike NSAIDs, rofecoxib targets only the COX-2 isoform. The tolerability of rofecoxib was compared with naproxen for the treatment of osteoarthritis.

Methods.—This randomized, controlled trial was conducted in 600 office and clinical research sites and included 5557 patients (mean age, 63 years) with a baseline diagnosis of osteoarthritis of the knee, hip, hand, or spine. Patients received either rofecoxib 25 mg/day or naproxen 500 mg twice daily. The patients were allowed to use routine medications, including aspirin. The main outcome measure was the discontinuation of therapy because of GI adverse events. The secondary outcome measure was the use of concomitant medication to treat GI symptoms. Efficacy was determined by patient-reported global assessment of disease status and the Australian/Canadian Osteoarthritis Hand Index and discontinuations resulting from a lack of efficacy. Patients were evaluated at baseline and at weeks 6 and 12.

Results.—The rates of cumulative discontinuation for GI adverse events were statistically significantly lower in the rofecoxib group than in the naproxen group (5.9% vs 8.1%), as were the rates of cumulative use of medication to treat GI symptoms (9.1% vs 11.2%) (Fig 2). Subgroup analysis of patients who used low-dose aspirin (13%) and those who previously discontinued arthritis medication because of GI symptoms (15%) demonstrated a relative risk similar to the overall sample for discontinuation resulting from GI adverse events. There was no statistically significant difference noted between the 2 treatments for efficacy in the treatment of osteoarthritis or for occurrence of other adverse events.

Conclusions.—This study in patients treated for 12 weeks for osteoarthritis found that rofecoxib 25 mg was as effective as naproxen 500 mg twice daily, but rofecoxib had statistically significantly superior GI tolerability and therefore less use of concomitant GI medications. The benefits of rofecoxib in subgroup analysis of these findings were consistent with the findings in the overall sample.

▶ This 12-week randomized controlled trial in more than 5500 patients with osteoarthritis demonstrated that participants who received rofecoxib at a dose of 25 mg once daily had a lower rate of discontinuation for GI adverse events in both the overall study cohort and in the subgroup of patients taking concomitant low-dose aspirin than those participants who received naproxen 500 mg twice daily. Results for outcomes of GI perforations, symptomatic ulcers, and bleeding episodes and for myocardial infarctions were consistent with findings from the VIGOR trial; there were fewer GI perforations, symptomatic ulcers, and bleeding episodes and more myocardial infarctions in patients randomly assigned to rofecoxib than in those assigned to naproxen.[1,2] No differences in efficacy were noted between treatment groups. Rofecoxib should be considered for treatment of symptomatic OA in patients who are at increased risk of serious upper GI side effects from nonselective nonsteroidal anti-inflammatory drugs.

M. C. Hochberg, MD

References

1. Bombardier C, Laine L, Reicin A, et al: Comparison of upper gastrointestinal toxicity of rofecoxib and naproxen in patients with rheumatoid arthritis. VIGOR Study Group. *N Engl J Med* 343:1520-1528, 2000.
2. Konstam MA, Weir MR, Reicin A, et al: Cardiovascular thrombotic events in controlled, clinical trials of rofecoxib. *Circulation* 104:R15-R23, 2001.

Cardiovascular Thrombotic Events in Arthritis Trials of the Cyclooxygenase-2 Inhibitor Celecoxib

White WB, Faich G, Borer JS, et al (Univ of Connecticut, Farmington; Pharmaceutical Safety Assessments, Inc, Narberth, Pa; Cornell Univ, New York)
Am J Cardiol 92:411-418, 2003 5–20

Background.—Studies have provided substantial evidence in support of the decreased gastrointestinal toxicity of cyclooxygenase-2 (COX-2) specific inhibitors compared with nonsteroidal anti-inflammatory drugs (NSAIDs). However, it has also been hypothesized that COX-2 inhibitors may increase cardiovascular thrombotic risk because COX-2 inhibition, unlike simultaneous inhibition of both COX-1 and COX-2 by NSAIDs, does not inhibit platelet thromboxane synthesis and so does not result in inhibition of platelet aggregation. Whether celecoxib, a COX-2 inhibitor, affects cardiovascular thrombotic risk was determined.

Methods.—The incidence of cardiovascular events was analyzed for celecoxib, placebo, and NSAIDs in the entire controlled, arthritis clinical trial database for celecoxib. End points for this study were those used in the Antiplatelet Trialists' Collaboration, including cardiovascular, hemorrhagic, and unknown deaths; nonfatal myocardial infarction; and nonfatal stroke. Other secondary thrombotic events were also examined. Separate analyses were performed for all patients and for those not taking aspirin. The analyses included data from all controlled, completed arthritis trials of 4 or more weeks' duration, including new drug application studies and 2 large postmarketing trials (CLASS and SUCCESS). The entire 15-trial database was searched for possible serious thrombotic events and to identify all deaths. Patients were randomly assigned to celecoxib at doses from 100 to 400 mg twice daily, diclofenac 50 to 75 mg twice daily, ibuprofen 800 mg 3 times daily, naproxen 500 mg twice daily, or placebo.

Results.—The incidences of primary and secondary end points were not significantly different between the celecoxib and placebo groups or between the celecoxib group and the NSAIDs group, regardless of aspirin use and type of NSAID (Fig 1).

Conclusions.—In these comparative analyses there was no evidence of increased risk of cardiovascular thrombotic events associated with celecoxib compared with either conventional NSAIDs or placebo.

► The results of this pooled analysis of data from randomized controlled trials of celecoxib failed to demonstrate a statistically significant increased risk for

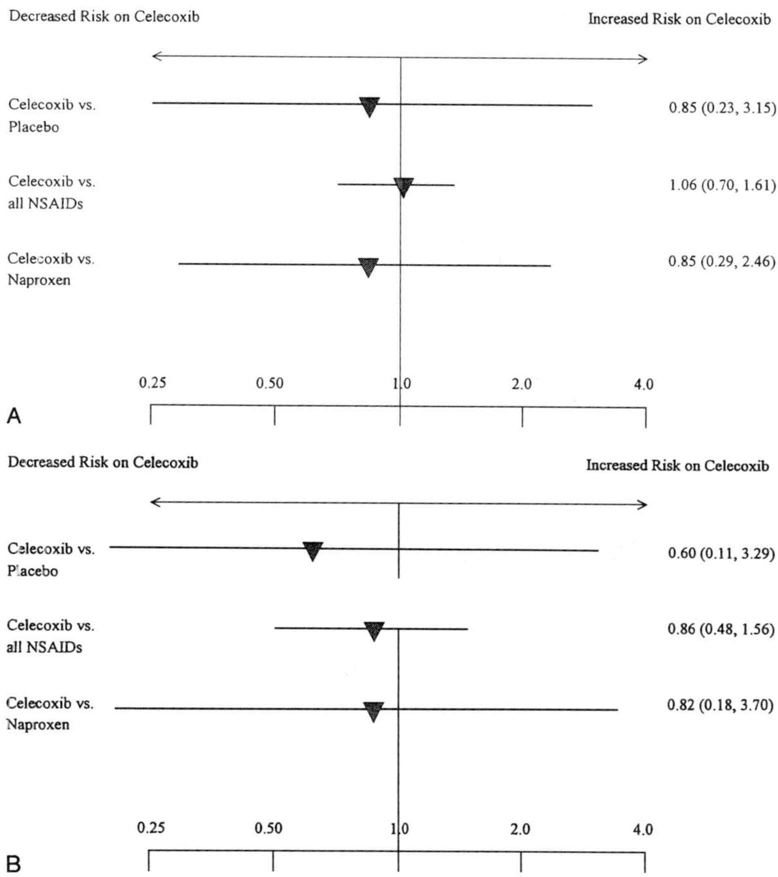

FIGURE 1.—Pooled analysis of Antiplatelet Trialists Collaboration end points by trial type: relative risks (*triangles*) and 2-sided 95% confidence intervals (*bars*) for celecoxib vs placebo, all NSAIDs, and naproxen. **A**, All patients; **B**, aspirin nonusers. (Reprinted from the American Journal of Cardiology, courtesy of White WB, Faich G, Borer JS, et al: Cardiovascular thrombotic events in arthritis trials of the cyclooxygenase-2 inhibitor celecoxib. *Am J Cardiol* 92:411-418. Copyright 2003, with permission from Excerpta Medica Inc.)

serious cardiovascular thrombotic events defined by the Antiplatelet Trialists Collaborative end point among patients randomly assigned to celecoxib compared with those randomized to placebo, all nonselective NSAIDs, and naproxen only. While the numbers of patients enrolled in the trials were large, the person-years of exposure, particularly in the placebo and naproxen groups, were small, contributing to wide confidence intervals. Nonetheless, the results fail to demonstrate an increased risk of serious cardiovascular thrombotic events in patients randomly assigned to celecoxib compared with naproxen, in contrast to results of pooled analyses that demonstrated an increased risk of such events in patients randomized to rofecoxib compared with naproxen.[1] Inferences drawn from such comparisons need to be limited, however, because of differences in patient characteristics, design of the individual trials, and differences in dosing of the COX-2 selective inhibitors in the trials, among other reasons. The appropriate way to compare different drugs within a class is in "head-to-head" randomized controlled trials; such data are not available for the outcome of serious cardiovascular thrombotic events.

M. C. Hochberg, MD

Reference

1. Konstam MA, Weir MR, Reicin A, et al: Cardiovascular thrombotic events in controlled, clinical trials of rofecoxib. *Circulation* 104:R15-R23, 2001.

Effect of a Topical Herbal Cream on the Pain and Stiffness of Osteoarthritis: A Randomized Double-Blind, Placebo-Controlled Clinical Trial

McKay L, Gemmell H, Jacobson B, et al (Pharmaceutical Research, Park City, Utah; Internatl Research Consortium, Tulsa, Okla; Oklahoma State Univ, Stillwater)

J Clin Rheumatol 9:164-169, 2003 5–21

Background.—Natural agents, such as capsaicin, have been shown to provide relieve for patients with osteoarthritis (OA). An equivalence trial of a homeopathic SRL gel containing comfrey, poison ivy, and marsh tea in homeopathic tinctures has been reported to be as effective and as well tolerated as the nonsteroidal anti-inflammatory gel. The efficacy of an herbal ointment was compared with a placebo ointment for relief of the pain and stiffness of osteoarthritis.

Methods.—This double-blind, randomized, placebo-controlled clinical trial involved 11 patients in an active group and 8 patients in a placebo group. All the patients were selected from attendees to an arthritis clinic, and their selection was based on American College of Rheumatology criteria.

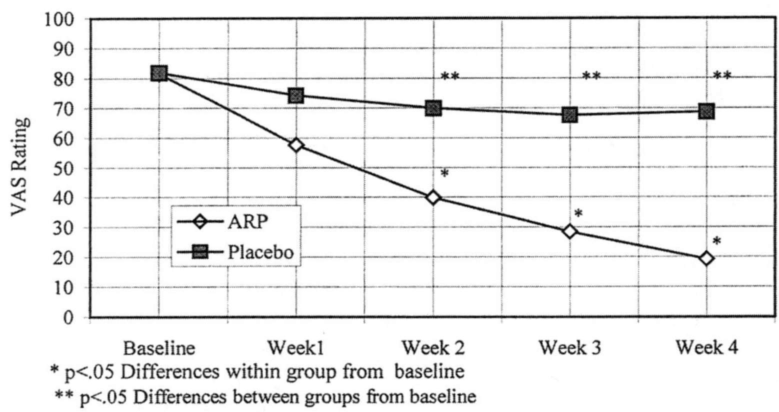

FIGURE 1.—Pain visual analog score(*VAS*) between active and placebo ointments. (Courtesy of McKay L, Gemmell H, Jacobson B, et al: Effect of a topical herbal cream on the pain and stiffness of osteoarthritis: A randomized double-blind, placebo-controlled clinical trial. *J Clin Rheumatol* 9:164-169, 2003.)

The herbal ointment and control ointment contained small amounts of capsaicin and menthol and were similar when applied. Subjects were graded on their levels of pain and stiffness for a 1-week no-treatment baseline. The subjects then applied the herbal or sham ointment to the involved joint(s) for 28 consecutive days and recorded their levels of pain and stiffness daily on visual analog scales.

Results.—There were significant differences between the active and placebo groups for pain and stiffness compared with the baseline phase with the fourth week (Fig 1).

Conclusions.—This study found that an herbal ointment was effective in relieving the pain and stiffness of osteoarthritis without adverse effects. This treatment may have a role as an adjunct to standard drug therapy if its effectiveness is confirmed in future studies.

► There is increasing interest in the use of complementary and alternative medicine, now called integrative medicine, among both patients and practitioners for the management of pain in patients with OA.[1,2] This small (19 patient) short-term (4 week) trial demonstrated greater pain relief in patients who applied a topical herbal cream compared with those who applied a "placebo" cream. The amount of improvement in pain and stiffness was large and much greater than that seen in other trials of rubefacients[3] as well as trials of nonsteroidal anti-inflammatory drugs of similar duration; this suggests the possibility of bias from unblinding of the participants in the treatment group. Nonetheless, topical agents may be useful in the management of patients with localized OA, especially if the patients are "risk averse" or have contraindications to systemic therapies.

M. C. Hochberg, MD

References

1. Eisenberg DM, Davis RB, Ettner SL, et al: Trends in alternative medicine use in the United States, 1990-97. *JAMA* 280:1569-1575, 1998.
2. Hochberg MC: Multidisciplinary integrative approach to treating knee pain in patients with osteoarthritis. *Ann Intern Med* 139:781-783, 2003.
3. Mason L, Moore RA, Edwards JE, et al: Systematic review of efficacy of topical rubefacients containing salicylates for the treatment of acute and chronic pain. *BMJ* 328:995, 2004.

Treatment With Licofelone Prevents Abnormal Subchondral Bone Cell Metabolism in Experimental Dog Osteoarthritis

Lajeunesse D, Martel-Pelletier J, Fernandes JC, et al (Centre Hospitalier de l'Université de Montréal)

Ann Rheum Dis 63:78-83, 2004 5–22

Background.—Subchondral bone modifications are now believed to be linked intimately to the progression of cartilage erosion in osteoarthritis. Licofelone is a combined 5-lipoxygenase and cyclooxygenase inhibitor.

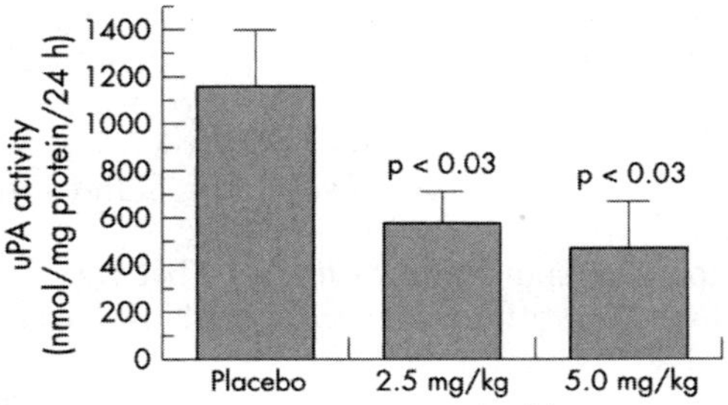

FIGURE 3.—Evaluation of urokinase plasminogen activator (*uPA*) activity in dog osteoblasts. Dogs were treated with placebo or with 2.5 mg/kg or 5 mg/kg licofelone for 8 weeks before the preparation of primary osteoblast cell cultures. Confluent primary dog osteoblasts were incubated for their last 2 days of culture in the presence of Ham's F12/Dulbecco's modified Eagle's medium (DMEM) without serum containing 1% insulin-transferrin-selenium (ITS) mix. uPA activity was determined on aliquots of conditioned media using a chromogenic substrate. Values are the mean (SEM) of 7 cell cultures for each group. (Courtesy of Lajeunesse D, Martel-Pelletier J, Fernandes JC, et al: Treatment with licofelone prevents abnormal subchondral bone cell metabolism in experimental dog osteoarthritis. *Ann Rheum Dis* 63:78-83, 2004. Reprinted with permission from the BMJ Publishing Group.)

Whether licofelone treatment modifies bone cell metabolism in long-term in vitro subchondral osteoblast cell cultures was determined.

Methods.—The effects of licofelone were assessed in vivo in experimental dog osteoarthritis. In group 1, the placebo group, the anterior cruciate ligament of the right knee was sectioned, and no active treatment given. In groups 2 and 3, licofelone, 2.5 or 5 mg/kg daily by mouth, respectively, was given for 8 weeks beginning the day after sectioning of the anterior cruciate ligament of the right knee. Primary osteoblast cell cultures were prepared from the subchondral bone plate. The animals were then assessed for levels of phenotypic markers, urokinase plasminogen activator (uPA), and insulin-like growth factor-I (IGF-I). Prostaglandin E_2 (PGE_2) and leukotriene B_4 levels were also determined.

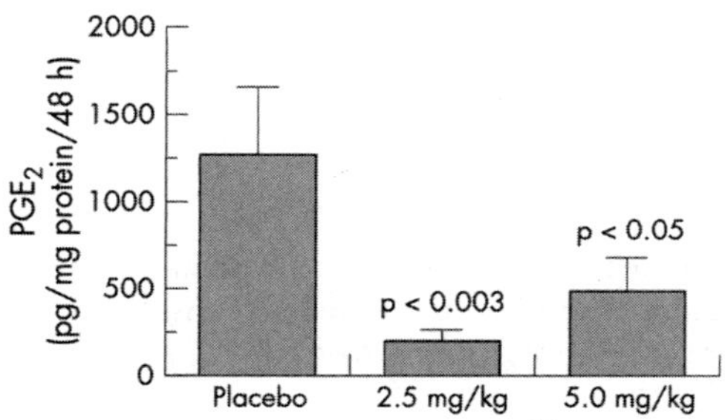

FIGURE 5.—Evaluation of prostaglandin E_2 (PGE_2) levels in dog osteoblasts. The same experimental protocol as in Figure 3 was performed. PGE_2 was determined on aliquots by a selective enzyme-linked immunosorbent assay (ELISA). Values are the mean (SEM) of 7 cell cultures for each group. (Courtesy of Lajeunesse D, Martel-Pelletier J, Fernandes JC, et al: Treatment with licofelone prevents abnormal subchondral bone cell metabolism in experimental dog osteoarthritis. *Ann Rheum Dis* 63:78-83, 2004. Reprinted with permission from the BMJ Publishing Group.)

Findings.—The 3 groups did not differ significantly in alkaline phosphatase activity or osteocalcin release from osteoblast cell cultures, under basal or $1,25(OH)_2D_3$ induction. In contrast, licofelone treatment reduced uPA and IGF-I levels in osteoblast cell cultures. Licofelone markedly reduced PGE_2 levels, which were still increased in the placebo group. A relationship was demonstrated between treatment with licofelone and either the reduction in the size of lesions on tibial plateaus or the levels of PGE_2, uPA, or IGF-I (Figs 3 and 5).

Conclusions.—In this experimental model, licofelone prevented or delayed abnormal metabolism of subchondral osteoblasts. Licofelone decreased PGE_2 concentrations after long-term osteoblast cell cultures, suggesting that the decrease in uPA and IGF-I concentrations is at least partially linked to this decrease.

► Licofelone is a dual 5-lipoxygenase and nonselective cyclooxygenase inhibitor that is currently in phase III development for treatment of osteoarthritis. Previous work by this group has shown that licofelone treatment reduced the size of cartilage lesions in dogs with experimental osteoarthritis after sectioning of the anterior cruciate ligament.[1] This study demonstrates that osteoblasts, derived from primary bone cell cultures from tibial plateaus of licofelone-treated animals in the above-referenced study, synthesized less uPA and PGE_2 than did osteoblasts from placebo-treated animals (Figs 3 and 5). The authors suggest that these and other changes in metabolic function of osteoblasts are related to the changes in morphology in the subchondral bone plate seen in the licofelone-treated animals and may explain, in part, the effects on development of cartilage lesions in the experimental model of osteoarthritis. Studies in humans with osteoarthritis are awaited to determine whether this drug has disease-modifying properties.

M. C. Hochberg, MD

Reference

1. Jovanovic DV, Fernandes JC, Martel-Pelletier J, et al: The in vivo dual inhibition of cylcooxygenase and lipoxygenase by ML-3000 reduces the progression of experimental osteoarthritis: Suppression of collagenase-1 and interleukin-1 beta synthesis. *Arthritis Rheum* 44:2320-2330, 2001.

Inhibition of Interleukin-1β–Stimulated Production of Matrix Metalloproteinases by Hyaluronan via CD44 in Human Articular Cartilage

Julovi SM, Yasuda T, Shimizu M, et al (Kyoto Univ, Japan)

Arthritis Rheum 50:516-525, 2004 5–23

Background.—Matrix metalloproteinases (MMPs) are zinc-containing, calcium-dependent proteinases that collectively degrade all components of the extracellular matrix. MMPs are thought to be important in the chondrolytic processes that contribute to the degenerative changes in osteoarthritic cartilage. Hyaluronan is a major component of synovial fluid and cartilage matrix, and it plays a central role in joint lubrication. It is now widely used in the treatment of osteoarthritis by intra-articular administration into affected joints. The mechanism of the inhibitory action of hyaluronan on interleukin-1β (IL-1β)–stimulated production of MMPs in human articular cartilage was investigated.

Methods.—IL-1β was added to normal and osteoarthritic human articular cartilage in explant culture to stimulate MMP production. Articular cartilage was incubated or preincubated with a clinically used form of 800-kd hyaluronan to assess its effect on IL-1β–induced MMPs. Levels of secreted MMPs 1, 3, and 13 in conditioned media were detected by immunoblotting, and intracellular MMP synthesis in chondrocytes was evaluated by immunofluorescence microscopy. Penetration of hyaluronan into cartilage tissue and its binding to CD44 were analyzed by fluorescence microscopy with fluoresceinated hyaluronan. The mechanism of action of hyaluronan was investigated by blocking experiments with anti-CD44 antibody.

Results.—Treatment and pretreatment with 800-kd hyaluronan at 1 mg/mL caused significant suppression of IL-1β–stimulated production of MMPs 1, 3, and 13 in both the normal and osteoarthritic cartilage explant cultures. On fluorescence histocytochemistry hyaluronan was shown to penetrate cartilage tissue and to localize in the pericellular matrix around chondrocytes. The hyaluronan blocking experiments showed the association of hyaluronan with chondrocytes was mediated by CD44. Preincubation with anti-CD44 antibody, which suppressed IL-1β–stimulated MMPs, reversed the inhibitory effect of hyaluronan on MMP production induced by IL-1β in both normal and osteoarthritic cartilage.

Conclusions.—It appears that the IL-1β–stimulated production of MMP-1, MMP-3, and MMP-13 is effectively inhibited by hyaluronan; findings that are supportive of the clinical use of hyaluronan in the treatment of osteoarthritis. The action of hyaluronan on IL-1β may involve the direct interaction between hyaluronan and CD44 on chondrocytes.

► Hyaluronic acid (HA) binds to the CD44 cell surface receptor on synoviocytes and articular chondrocytes. While systematic reviews and meta-analyses demonstrate that intra-articular administration of hyaluronates is associated with reduction in pain in patients with knee osteoarthritis (OA),[1,2] it is unclear whether there is a disease-modifying effect of these agents. This group studied human femoral head cartilage from patients with OA and controls in vitro and found that HA reduced IL-1β–stimulated synthesis of MMP-1, MMP-3, and MMP-13 in both normal and OA cartilage. This effect was mediated by binding of HA to the CD44 receptor on chondrocytes. These data suggest that intra-articular HA preparations could have disease-modifying effects mediated by reduction in cartilage matrix catabolism stimulated by IL-1β.

M. C. Hochberg, MD

References

1. Lo GH, LaValley M, McAlindon T, et al: Intra-articular hyaluronic acid in treatment of knee osteoarthritis: A meta-analysis. *JAMA* 290:3115-3121, 2003.

2. Wang C-T, Lin J, Chang C-J, et al: Therapeutic effects of hyaluronic acid on osteoarthritis of the knee: A meta-analysis of randomized controlled trials. *J Bone Joint Surg* 86-A:538-545, 2004.

Osteoporosis

LEAD ARTICLE

The Effects of Strontium Ranelate on the Risk of Vertebral Fracture in Women With Postmenopausal Osteoporosis

Meunier PJ, Roux C, Seeman E, et al (Edouard Herriot Hosp, Lyons, France; Reneé Descartes Univ, Paris; Univ of Melbourne, Australia; et al)
N Engl J Med 350:459-468, 2004 5–24

Introduction.—Prevention of fractures is the primary focus of antiosteoporotic treatment. Strontium ranelate is a new orally active agent that stimulates the formation of new bone tissue and reduces bone resorption both in vitro and in animal experiments. The safety of strontium ranelate and its efficacy against vertebral fracture when administered orally at a dose of 2 g/day for 3 years was evaluated in postmenopausal women with osteoporosis and a history of vertebral fracture.

Methods.—Between November 1996 and July 1998, women were recruited from 72 centers in 11 European countries and Australia in the Spinal Osteoporosis Therapeutic Intervention trial, a randomized, double-blind, placebo-controlled, phase III trial. A total of 1649 postmenopausal women

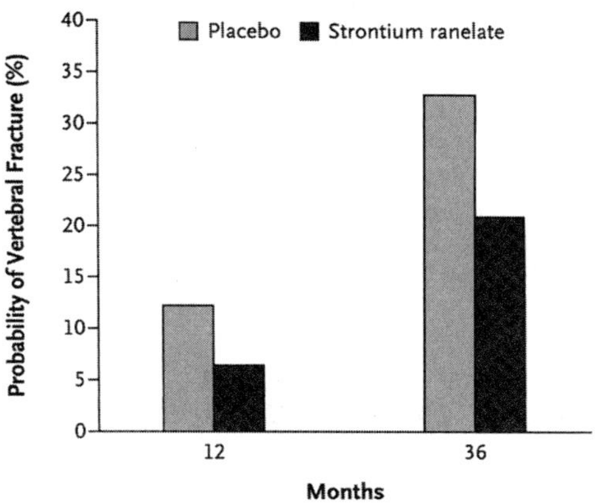

FIGURE 2.—Proportion of patients in intention-to-treat population who had 1 or more new vertebral fractures, assessed by semiquantitative method. Analysis at 12 months was restricted to patients with assessable radiographs at baseline and at month 12 (686 patients in the strontium ranelate group and 699 in the placebo group). Relative risk of fracture in treatment group at 12 months was 0.51 (95% confidence interval, 0.36 to 0.75; $P < .001$). Analysis for 3-year period was restricted to patients with assessable radiographs at baseline and after baseline (719 patients in strontium ranelate group and 723 in placebo group). Relative risk of fracture over 36-month period was 0.59 (95% confidence interval, 0.48 to 0.73; $P < .001$). (Courtesy of Meunier PJ, Roux C, Seeman E, et al: The effects of strontium ranelate on the risk of vertebral fracture in women with postmenopausal osteoporosis. *N Engl J Med* 350:459-468.)

with osteoporosis (low bone mineral density [BMD]) and at least 1 vertebral fracture were randomly assigned to receive 2 g of oral strontium ranelate/day or placebo for 3 years. Calcium and vitamin D supplements were administered to both groups before and after the intervention. Vertebral radiographs were obtained annually and measurements of BMD were performed every 6 months.

Results.—New vertebral fractures occurred in fewer patients in the strontium ranelate group compared with control subjects. There was a risk reduction of 49% in the first year of treatment and 41% during the 3-year evaluation period (relative risk, 0.59; 95% confidence interval, 0.48-0.73) (Fig 2). Strontium ranelate increased BMD at 36 months by 14.4% in the lumbar spine and 8.3% in the femoral neck ($P < .001$ for both comparisons). No significant between-group differences were observed in the incidence of serious adverse events.

Conclusion.—The treatment of postmenopausal osteoporosis with strontium ranelate produces early and sustained decreases in the risk of vertebral fractures.

► Strontium ranelate is an oral agent that both reduces bone resorption and stimulates bone formation.[1] This study presents data from the phase III trial that tested efficacy for vertebral fracture prevention in postmenopausal women with prevalent vertebral fractures and osteoporosis. There was a significant 41% reduction in risk of a new vertebral fracture over a 3-year period in the group that received strontium ranelate compared with placebo. The reduction in risk of nonvertebral fractures did not reach statistical significance; however, the study was not powered for this outcome. Robust increases in bone mineral density were noted at the lumbar spine, femoral neck, and total hip. Changes in bone turnover markers confirmed reduction in bone resorption and increases in bone formation among strontium ranelate treated patients compared with those who received placebo. This agent expands the armamentarium of drugs that reduce the risk of new vertebral fractures in postmenopausal women with osteoporosis; however, like raloxifene, there is no evidence at present that this antifracture efficacy extends to nonvertebral fractures.[2]

M. C. Hochberg, MD

References

1. Marie PJ, Amman P, Boivin G, et al: Mechanisms of action and therapeutic potential of strontium in bone. *Calcif Tissue Int* 69:121-129, 2001.
2. Ettinger B, Black DM, Mitlak BH, et al: Reduction of vertebral fracture risk in postmenopausal women with osteoporosis treated with raloxifene: Results from a 3-year randomized clinical trial. *JAMA* 282:637-645, 1999.

Diagnosis and Epidemiology

Genetic Predisposition for Adult Lactose Intolerance and Relation to Diet, Bone Density, and Bone Fractures

Obermayer-Pietsch BM, Bonelli CM, Walter DE, et al (Karl-Franzens Univ, Graz, Austria)

J Bone Miner Res 19:42-47, 2004 5–25

Background.—In adult lactase deficiency the intestinal cells lose the ability to cleave lactose into glucose and galactose because of a physiologic decline in lactase phlorizin hydrolase (LPH) activity that occurs after the age of weaning. Study in Finnish families (among others) of the DNA variants of the *LPH* gene region has indicated a strong association between a −13910 T/C variant (LCT) and intestinal biopsy findings plus biochemically verified lactase deficiency. The effects of this dimorphism on calcium supply, bone density, and osteoporotic fractures among elderly women were explored.

Methods.—A polymerase chain reaction–based assay was used to determine the LCT genotypes TT, TC, and CC in 258 postmenopausal women. These genotypes were then matched to milk intolerance, nutritional calcium intake, intestinal calcium absorption, bone mineral density (BMD), and fractures (other than vertebral).

Results.—Significant differences in BMD were noted with the various genotypes (Fig 1). The TT group had the highest BMD and the CC group had the lowest. The incidence of nonvertebral fracture was significantly higher in the CC group, with an increasing but not significant gene-dose effect toward

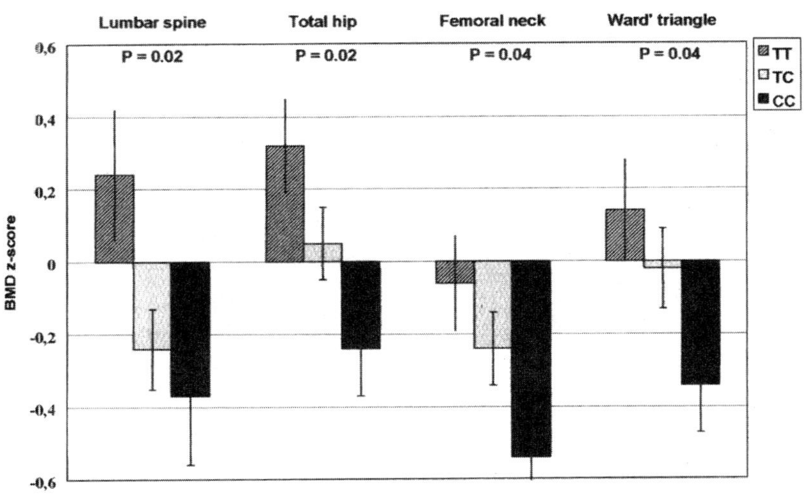

FIGURE 1.—Age-adjusted measurements of BMD expressed as Z-scores at lumbar spine, total hip, femoral neck, and Ward's triangle according to LCT genotypes in 258 postmenopausal women. Individuals with genotype CC (*dark bars*) had significantly lower BMD Z-scores than other genotypes. (Courtesy of Obermayer-Pietsch BM, Bonelli CM, Walter DE, et al: Genetic predisposition for adult lactose intolerance and relation to diet, bone density, and bone fractures. *J Bone Miner Res* 19:42-47, 2004. Reprinted with permission from the American Society for Bone and Mineral Research.)

the CC and TC genotypes (Fig 2). In one model the percentage of the variance of BMD explained by the $LCT_{(T/C-13910)}$ genotype was 4% at the total hip; for the CC genotype, it was 2.3% at the femoral neck and Ward's triangle. This model also attributed 14% to body weight and 2.5% to height. By genotype alone, genotypes CC and TC accounted for 3% of the lumbar spine bone density and 10% including weight. Other unknown factors contributing to the whole variance of BMD must be assumed to be operative. Calcium intake also differed significantly between the genotype groupings, with the CC group having a 55% decline compared with the TT group. Women in the CC group showed the highest aversion to milk and milk products, although dislike of milk's taste was similar among the 3 groups. No significant differences in intestinal calcium absorption equivalents were found. Known lactose intolerance was present in 27% of the CC group, 7% of the TT group, and 3% of the TC group. Subjects with the CC genotype had significantly lower calcium intake from milk and had slight body weight losses over the preceding 5 years compared with a body weight increase in other women.

Conclusions.—The $LCT_{(T/C-13910)}$ polymorphism was linked to subjective intolerance of milk, reduced intake of calcium through milk consumption, and reduced BMD at the hip and lumbar spine. These individuals may have an increased susceptibility to bone fractures. In efforts to detect persons at risk for lactose malabsorption and osteoporosis, a genetic test of lactase deficiency may prove helpful.

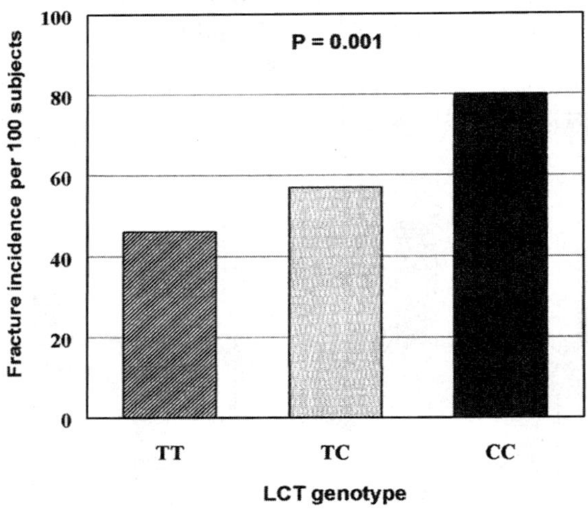

FIGURE 2.—Fracture incidence per 100 subjects in postmenopausal women according to LCT genotypes. Individuals with genotype CC (*dark bars*) had significantly higher nonvertebral fracture incidence (*P = .001) than TC (*shaded bars*) and TT (*dashed bars*) genotypes, showing increasing gene-dose effect toward these genotypes. (Courtesy of Obermayer-Pietsch BM, Bonelli CM, Walter DE, et al: Genetic predisposition for adult lactose intolerance and relation to diet, bone density, and bone fractures. *J Bone Miner Res* 19:42-47, 2004. Reprinted with permission from the American Society for Bone and Mineral Research.)

▶ The syndrome of lactose intolerance, which includes mild to severe abdominal symptoms after milk consumption occurring in persons with lactase deficiency, is common in adult whites and African Americans in the United States and in Southeast Asians. Recently, a −13910 T/C variant in the *LPH* gene has been identified that correlates with lactase deficiency.[1] These authors examined DNA from 258 postmenopausal women enrolled in a study of osteoporosis. Age-adjusted BMD was significantly lower and fracture incidence was higher in women with the homozygous C/C genotype. Only a minority of individuals with the C/C genotype had known lactose intolerance. These data identify a new genetic marker for low BMD and increased fracture risk, probably related to decreased calcium intake from milk products in adulthood. Persons who have lactose intolerance or report abdominal symptoms related to consumption of dairy products should be considered at risk for osteoporosis.

M. C. Hochberg, MD

Reference

1. Enattah NS, Sahi T, Savilahti E, et al: Identification of a variant associated with adult-type hypolactasia. *Nat Genet* 30:233-237, 2002.

Soluble RANKL and Risk of Nontraumatic Fracture

Schett G, Kiechl S, Redlich K, et al (Univ of Vienna; Univ Clinic of Innsbruck, Austria; Bruneck Hosp, Italy; et al)

JAMA 291:1108-1113, 2004 5–26

Background.—The receptor activator of nuclear factor κB ligand (RANKL) is necessary for osteoclast and possibly osteoblast activation. It may also be a key link between bone formation and resorption. The association between serum levels of RANKL and the risk of nontraumatic fracture were investigated.

Methods.—All fractures occurring between 1990 and 2000 in 906 participants in a prospective, population-based trial in Bruneck, Italy, were recorded. One hundred fifteen traumatic fractures and 31 nontraumatic fractures occurred. Serum RANKL and osteoprotegerin levels were assessed in 1990, 1995, and 2000, in addition to bone metabolism characteristics and lifestyle.

Findings.—Levels of RANKL were comparable in men and women and did not correlate with age, menopausal status, lifestyle characteristics, or data from bone US at the heel. However, RANKL significantly predicted nontraumatic fracture. A pooled logistic regression analysis indicated a 10.0 and 3.9 relative risk of nontraumatic fracture in the lowest and middle versus the highest tertile for RANKL, respectively. Patients in the highest tertile had a low risk of fracture even when they had other predisposing factors. Women aged 60 years or older in the lowest tertile had a 5-year rate of nontraumatic fracture that was greater than 7%.

Conclusions.—A low RANKL level independently predicts nontraumatic fracture. This is consistent with the hypothesis that RANKL plays an important role in human bone turnover. If confirmed by further research, RANKL levels may become relevant in evaluating fracture risk.

▶ RANKL, a protein with structural homology to tumor necrosis factor, stimulates osteoclastogenesis and induces osteoclast activation. Its interaction with the transmembrane receptor RANK is competitively inhibited by the decoy receptor osteoprotegerin. These investigators measured RANKL levels in archived fasting serum specimens and correlated serum RANKL levels with risk of fracture. Persons in the lowest third of the serum RANKL distribution (≤0.80 pmol/L) had the highest rate and risk of nontraumatic fractures, even after adjustment for multiple potential confounders. While these results are provocative, they are based on only 31 "nontraumatic" fractures and "the nature and causality of the relationship between RANKL and fracture risk...are speculative at this time." Furthermore, there was no relationship between serum RANKL levels and broadband US attenuation or speed of sound (measured with heel US) or bone turnover markers. However, those in the lowest third of RANKL distribution did have higher mean levels of parathyroid hormone than those in the other groups. The results are surprising and need to be confirmed in other observational studies.

M. C. Hochberg, MD

Statin Use, Clinical Fracture, and Bone Density in Postmenopausal Women: Results From the Women's Health Initiative Observational Study

LaCroix AZ, Cauley JA, Pettinger M, et al (Fred Hutchinson Cancer Research Ctr, Seattle; Univ of Pittsburgh, Pa; George Washington Univ, Washington, DC; et al)

Ann Intern Med 139:97-104, 2003 5–27

Background.—Several large multicenter trials have established the long-term efficacy and safety of 3-hydroxy-3-methylglutaryl coenzyme A (HMG-CoA) reductase inhibitors, or statins, for the prevention of coronary events in both men and women. Recent studies have also shown that statins stimulate bone formation in vitro and in vivo. In early epidemiologic studies, findings showed a lower risk for hip fracture among statin users than among nonusers. However, subsequent studies have produced mixed results. The association of statin use with the incidence of hip, lower arm or wrist, and other clinical fractures and with baseline levels of bone density was evaluated.

Methods.—The Women's Health Initiative Observational Study was a prospective study conducted in 40 clinical centers in the United States. A total of 93,716 postmenopausal women aged 50 to 79 years were enrolled in the study, which compared rates of hip, lower arm or wrist, and other clinical fractures among 7846 statin users and 85,870 nonusers over a median

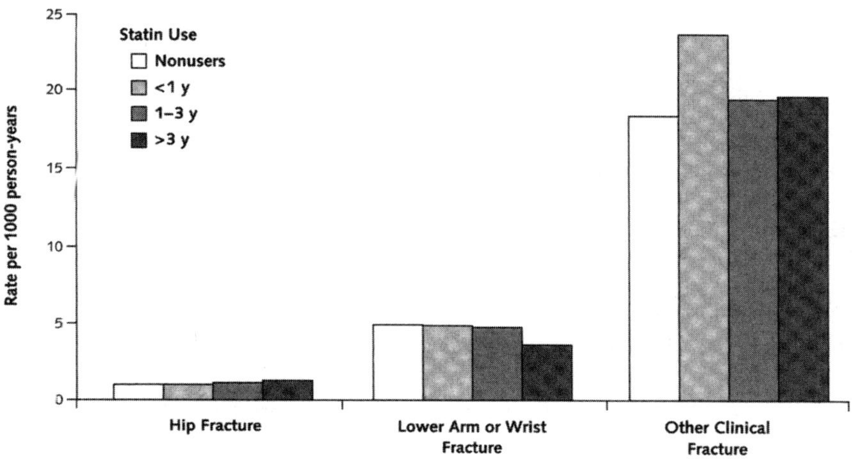

FIGURE.—Age-adjusted rates of fracture per 1000 person-years according to duration of statin use among postmenopausal women aged 50 to 79 years in the Women's Health Initiative Observational Study. (Courtesy of LaCroix AZ, Cauley JA, Pettinger M, et al: Statin use, clinical fracture, and bone density in postmenopausal women: Results from the Women's Health Initiative Observational Study. *Ann Intern Med* 139:97-104, 2003.)

follow-up of 3.9 years. In 6442 women enrolled at 3 clinical centers, baseline levels of total hip, posterior-anterior spine, and total-body bone density measured by dual-energy x-ray absorptiometry were compared on the basis of statin use.

Results.—Statin users and nonusers were found to have similar age-adjusted rates of hip, lower arm or wrist, and other clinical fractures, regardless of the duration of statin use (Figure). There was no statistically significant difference in bone density levels between statin users and nonusers at any skeletal site after adjustment for age, ethnicity, body mass index, and other factors.

Conclusion.—The Women's Health Initiative Observational Study found that statin use did not improve fracture risk or bone density. The use of statins for the prevention or treatment of osteoporosis is not supported by the cumulative evidence.

▶ Previous observational studies have generated conflicting results concerning the risk of fractures in patients receiving statins.[1] These authors analyzed data from more than 90,000 postmenopausal women enrolled in the Women's Health Initiative Observational Study. There were many systematic differences in statin users compared with nonusers in this observational cohort. After adjusting for these potential confounders, there was no association between statin use and risk of hip, wrist, or other clinical fracture. These results do not support the use of statins for fracture risk reduction in postmenopausal women. Nonetheless, randomized controlled trials would be needed to definitely demonstrate or exclude an effect.

M. C. Hochberg, MD

Reference

1. Bauer DC, Mundy GR, Jamal SA, et al: Use of statins and fracture: Results of 4 prospective studies and cumulative meta-analysis of observational studies and controlled trials. *Arch Intern Med* 164:146-152, 2004.

Pathophysiology/Mechanisms of Action

Estrogen Deficiency Induces Bone Loss by Increasing T Cell Proliferation and Lifespan Through IFN-γ-Induced Class II Transactivator

Cenci S, Toraldo G, Weitzmann MN, et al (Emory Univ, Atlanta, Ga; San Raffaele Scientific Inst, Milan, Italy; Washington Univ, St Louis)
Proc Natl Acad Sci U S A 100:10405-10410, 2003 5–28

Background.—Estrogen deficiency leads to osteoporosis. Tumor necrosis factor α (TNF) is a cytokine that increases the production and activity of osteoclastogenic elements and induces various cytokines that mediate bone loss after ovariectomy. With more T cells in the bone marrow, TNF production is enhanced. The effect of estrogen deficiency on the generation and death of cytokine-producing T cells was investigated.

Methods.—Female mice aged 12 weeks were sham operated or ovariectomized. T cells from the spleen, lymph node, and bone marrow; B cells from the spleen; and macrophages from the bone marrow were purified and subjected to various assessments. Included were antigen-presenting cell (APC) assay; major histocompatibility complex class II expression; T-cell proliferation, activation, and apoptosis; measures of T-cell and cytokine production; and reverse transcriptase real-time polymerase chain reaction assay. The mice underwent bone mineral density (BMD) and bone histology tests at baseline and 2 and 4 weeks after surgery.

Results.—Ovariectomy increased the activation of T cells and the lifespan of activated T cells. As a result, there were more T cells present. APC activity was determined to be critical to the process by which ovariectomy increases T-cell proliferation and lifespan. Increased APC activity and decreased activation-induced cell death produced by ovariectomy was accomplished by augmented interferon-γ (IFN-γ) production. Ovariectomy specifically upregulates T helper 1 (T_H1) IFN-γ production in vivo, leading to an increase in class II transactivator (CIITA). One possible mechanism is the stimulation of IFN-γ secretion through enhanced macrophage production of the IFN-γ–inducing cytokines interleukin (IL)-12 and IL-18. In testing mice that were IFN-γ receptor $(\text{IFN-}\gamma\text{R})^{-/-}$ to see the relevance of IFN-γ–induced CIITA in ovariectomy-induced T-cell expansion and bone loss, it was found that $\text{IFN-}\gamma\text{R}^{-/-}$ mice are protected from ovariectomy-induced immune alterations, T-cell expansion, and bone loss.

Conclusions.—The bone loss that results from estrogen deficiency after ovariectomy depends on the ability to expand the number of T cells that produce TNF. An in vivo estrogen deficiency leads to T-cell expansion by enhancing the proliferation and lifespan of T cells. Both these operate by the IFN-γ–mediated induction of CIITA in macrophages and T cells. Thus, ovariectomy produces T-cell expansion and bone loss through APC-induced activation of T cells and IFN-γ signaling by inducing the critical mediator CIITA.

► It turns out that bone loss after surgical menopause (at least in mice) is an inflammatory immune-mediated process.[1,2] Estrogen deficiency leads to IFN-γ–mediated induction of major histocompatability complex class II expression in macrophages and T cells in the bone marrow with T-cell expansion due to increased proliferation and decreased apoptosis. The increased number of TNF-producing T cells leads to stimulation of osteoclast formation and increased bone turnover and bone loss. These data provide evidence of a link between estrogen deficiency and the immune system and bone loss and suggest the possibility of new therapeutic targets for postmenopausal osteoporosis on the one hand and autoimmune disease on the other.

M. C. Hochberg, MD

References

1. Manologas SC, Kousteni S, Jilka RL: Sex steroids and bone. *Recent Prog Horm Res* 57:385-409, 2002.
2. Pfeilschifter J, Koditz R, Pfohl M, et al: Changes in proinflammatory cytokine activity after menopause. *Endocr Rev* 23:90-119, 2002.

THERAPIES

Effects of Estrogen Plus Progestin on Risk of Fracture and Bone Mineral Density: The Women's Health Initiative Randomized Trial

Cauley JA, for the Women's Health Initiative Investigators (Univ of Pittsburgh, Pa; et al)
JAMA 290:1729-1738, 2003 5–29

Introduction.—In the Women's Health Initiative trial of estrogen plus progestin therapy, the women assigned to active treatment had fewer fractures. It was hypothesized that the relative risk reduction of estrogen plus progestin on fractures differs according to risk factors for fractures.

Methods.—A randomized controlled trial was conducted between September 1993 and July 2002, in which 16,608 postmenopausal women aged 50 to 79 years with an intact uterus at baseline were recruited at 40 US centers. Follow-up was an average of 5.6 years. Participants were randomly assigned to receive either conjugated equine estrogen, 0.625 mg/d, plus medroxyprogesterone acetate, 2.5 mg/d, in 1 tablet or placebo. The primary outcome measures were all verified osteoporotic fracture events that occurred from enrollment to trial discontinuation (July 7, 2002); bone mineral density, measured in a subset of 1024 women at baseline and years 1 and 3; and a global index, created to summarize the balance of risks and benefits to test whether the risk-benefit profile varied across tertiles of fracture risk.

Results.—Fractures occurred in 833 women (8.6%) in the estrogen plus progestin group and 896 women (11.1%) in the placebo group (hazard ratio [HR], 0.76; 95% confidence interval [CI], 0.69-0.83). In subgroup analyses, active treatment reduced the risk of hip fracture by 60% in women with baseline calcium intake of more than 1200 mg/d and not among women with lower calcium intake (P for interaction = .02). There was no evidence that the efficacy of active treatment differed according to any risk factors for fractures, including age, body mass index, smoking, history of falls, calcium intake, personal and family history of fractures, and past use of hormones. Estrogen plus progestin decreased the rate of fractures to a similar extent in women at low, medium, and high risk of fracture.

Conclusion.—Estrogen plus progestin increases bone mineral density and decreases the risk of fractures in healthy postmenopausal women. The reduced risk of fracture attributed to estrogen plus progestin appeared to be present in all subgroups. When considering the effects of hormone therapy on other important disease outcomes in a global model, there was no net benefit, even in women considered to be at high risk of fracture.

► The Women's Health Initiative trial of combined estrogen and progestin therapy found a significant reduction in hip, vertebral, and total fractures in treated participants compared with those randomly assigned to placebo.[1] This article updates those results and examines fracture risk reduction by baseline characteristics of participants. Combined hormone therapy reduced risk of hip fracture by 34%; significant treatment-by-subgroup interaction was noted for only total calcium intake at baseline, as there was significant hip fracture reduction in the group that consumed 1200 mg or more of calcium per day but not in those who consumed less than 1200 mg calcium per day. No evidence of treatment-by-subgroup interaction was noted for reduction in total fractures. These data confirm that combined estrogen and progestin therapy significantly reduces the risk of fracture in postmenopausal women, irrespective of most baseline characteristics. Despite these results, such therapy cannot be routinely recommended because of adverse health effects (increase in risk of serious cardiovascular thrombotic events and breast cancer) and the availability of alternative efficacious therapies (ie, nitrogen-containing bisphosphonates) for women with osteoporosis.

M. C. Hochberg, MD

Reference

1. Writing Group for the Women's Health Initiative Investigators: Risks and benefits of estrogen plus progestin in healthy postmenopausal women: Principal results from the Women's Health Initiative randomized controlled trial. *JAMA* 288:321-333, 2002.

Exogenous Testosterone or Testosterone With Finasteride Increases Bone Mineral Density in Older Men With Low Serum Testosterone

Amory JK, Watts NB, Easley KA, et al (Emory Univ, Atlanta, Ga; Univ of Cincinnati, Ohio; Univ of Washington, Seattle)

J Clin Endocrinol Metab 89:503-510, 2004 5–30

Background.—In older men, testosterone therapy may improve bone mineral density (BMD) and decrease fracture risk. Older men with low serum testosterone levels may especially benefit from such treatment. However, concerns have been raised about the effects of testosterone therapy on the prostate. Whether the combination of testosterone and finasteride, a 5α-reductase inhibitor, would increase BMD without damaging the prostate was evaluated in older men.

Methods.—Seventy men aged 65 years or older with a serum testosterone level of less than 12.1 nmol/L on 2 occasions were studied. The participants were randomly assigned to testosterone enanthate, 200 mg IM every 2 weeks with placebo pills (testosterone-only); testosterone enanthate, 200 mg, every 2 weeks with 5 mg F daily (T+F); or placebo injections and pills (placebo). Fifty men finished the 36-month treatment. Serial measures of lumbar spine and hip BMD were obtained by dual x-ray absorptiometry. Prostate-specific antigen (PSA) and prostate size were assessed at baseline and during treatment.

Findings.—Intent-to-treat analysis showed that testosterone therapy for 36 months (both alone and combined with finasteride) increased BMD at the lumbar spine and hip. Significant BMD increases were also evident in the intertrochanteric and trochanteric regions of the hip. After 6 months of treatment, urinary deoxypyridinoline levels declined significantly compared with baseline levels in the testosterone-only and T+F groups. No significant reductions were seen in the placebo group. During the 36 months of treatment, PSA increased significantly from baseline in the testosterone-only group. Although prostate volume increased in all groups during the study, the increase was significantly lower in the T+F group than in the other 2 groups.

Conclusions.—Testosterone therapy alone or combined with finasteride increases vertebral and hip BMD over a 36-month period in older men with lower serum testosterone. Dihydrotestosterone does not appear to be essential to the benefits of testosterone on BMD in men. Concomitant administration of finasteride with testosterone appears to attenuate the effects of testosterone therapy on prostate size and PSA. This combined approach may decrease the chance of prostate-related complications in older men receiving testosterone therapy.

► Both alendronate and teriparatide are FDA approved for the treatment of men with osteoporosis. There have been few studies, however, of the effect of testosterone replacement on BMD in older men with low serum testosterone levels. This study enrolled patients with low testosterone levels; however, the vast majority did not have osteoporosis. There was a progressive increase in BMD in the patients who received testosterone over the 36-month study period and this correlated with increases in serum total and bioavailable testosterone and estradiol concentrations. Testosterone replacement, given in conjunction with finasteride (for safety reasons: ie, less prostate growth and no increases in PSA levels), can be considered as a treatment to increase BMD in older men with low serum testosterone levels who do not have osteoporosis. Until fracture data are available for testosterone replacement therapy, only alendronate and teriparatide should be used for treatment of older men with osteoporosis.

M. C. Hochberg, MD

Oral Daily Ibandronate Prevents Bone Loss in Early Postmenopausal Women Without Osteoporosis

McClung MR, for the Oral Ibandronate Study Group (Oregon Osteoporosis Ctr, Portland; et al)

J Bone Miner Res 19:11-18, 2004 5–31

Background.—More strategies are needed to manage patients most at risk for postmenopausal osteoporosis. The efficacy, tolerability, and optimal dose of oral daily ibandronate in preventing bone loss in postmenopausal women were reported.

Methods.—Six hundred fifty-three women were enrolled in the multicenter, double-blind, randomized, placebo-controlled trial. All had been postmenopausal for at least 1 year. Their mean bone mineral density (BMD) T-score exceeded −2.5 at the lumbar spine. Based on time since menopause and baseline lumbar spine BMD, women were assigned to 1 of 4 strata. Patients received calcium, 500 mg daily, plus placebo or ibandronate, 0.5, 1, or 2.5 mg once a day. Treatment lasted for 2 years.

Findings.—After 2 years of treatment, ibandronate resulted in a dose-related, sustained maintenance or increase in BMD at the lumbar spine and hip. There was also a dose-related decrease in bone turnover rate. The best nominal increases in spinal and hip BMD occurred with the 2.5-mg dose. Compared with placebo, this dose produced significant BMD gains at 6 months and all subsequent time points at the spine and hip.

Conclusions.—Oral daily ibandronate effectively maintains or increases BMD at the spine and hip in postmenopausal women without osteoporosis. The treatment also normalizes bone turnover. Ibandronate appears to be effective in early as well as later stages of bone loss in postmenopausal women.

► Ibandronate is a potent nitrogen-containing bisphosphonate that has recently been approved by the Food and Drug Administration for the treatment and prevention of osteoporosis in postmenopausal women; as of July 2004, it has not been marketed in the United States. This article presents data from a phase II/III dose-ranging trial for prevention of bone loss in postmenopausal women without osteoporosis. Oral daily ibandronate at a dose of 2.5 mg once daily prevented bone loss at the lumbar spine and hip sites, and was associated with mean reductions of about 40% and 35% in markers of bone resorption and formation, respectively. While ibandronate, as well as other nitrogen-containing bisphosphonates, is safe and efficacious for this indication, it is still unclear which, if any, women without osteoporosis should receive pharmacologic treatment over and above calcium and vitamin D supplementation.

M. C. Hochberg, MD

Oral Weekly Ibandronate Prevents Bone Loss in Postmenopausal Women

Tankó LB, for the Oral Ibandronate Group (Ctr for Clinical and Basic Research A/S, Ballerup and Vejle, Denmark; et al)

J Intern Med 254:159-167, 2003 5–32

Background.—Bisphosphonates have a high affinity for mineralized tissues, resist enzymatic degradation, and strongly inhibit osteoclast-mediated bone resorption, leading to interest in using them to prevent or treat postmenopausal osteoporosis. Low oral availability and concern over gastrointestinal safety have prompted strict dosing guidelines. Ibandronate is a biphosphonate currently being investigated for treating or preventing osteoporosis. A phase II/III study was undertaken to evaluate the efficacy, safety, and dose-response data obtained with once-weekly oral ibandronate in preventing bone loss among postmenopausal women and to determine a dose suitable for use in bone loss prevention efforts.

Methods.—Participants were drawn from the primary care units of 14 osteoporosis centers and included 630 women in 4 strata based on the length of time since menopause and baseline bone mineral density (BMD). Within these strata, women were randomly designated to receive either once-weekly ibandronate in doses of 5, 10, or 20 mg/week or placebo for 24 months. The relative changes from baseline in spine and hip BMD on dual energy x-ray absorptiometry were noted, as were the biochemical markers of bone turnover, including serum and urinary C-telopeptide of collagen type 1, osteocalcin, and alkaline phosphatase, measured by enzyme immunoassays.

Results.—Five hundred thirty-nine patients completed the 24-month study. Among the women receiving ibandronate, dose-dependent increases in spine and hip BMD were noted (Fig 1). After 6 months there were statistically significant differences between the placebo group and those receiving 10 and 20 mg of ibandronate. After 24 months the differences between those receiving 20 mg of ibandronate and placebo were 4.0 for the relative changes in spine BMD and 2.7% for hip BMD. The increase in spine and hip BMD was found in women 1 to 3 years after menopause as well as in those more than 3 years postmenopausal. Osteopenic women in the early group had statistically significant increases in hip BMD in all the dose groups, but the hip BMD increases in normal women did not reach statistical significance. Osteopenic women in the later group also had statistically significant increases in hip BMD with the 10- and 20-mg doses of ibandronate. Both the resorption and formation biochemical markers showed declines in women receiving ibandronate that were dose dependent. Among women receiving 20 mg of ibandronate, regardless of their stratum, the 24-month measure-

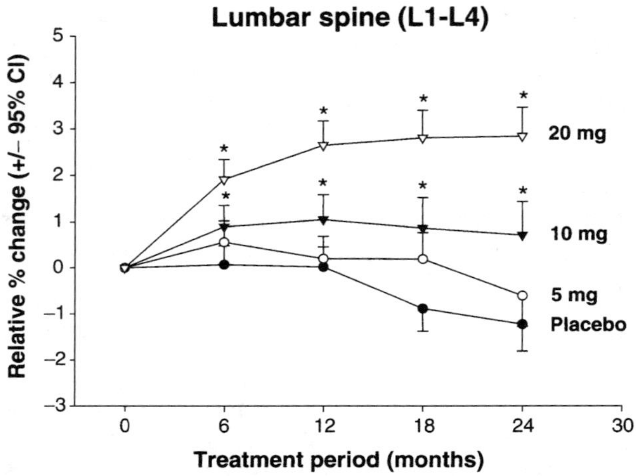

FIGURE 1.—Mean relative change (±95% confidence interval) in BMD at lumbar spine induced by different doses of once-weekly oral ibandronate treatment in postmenopausal women. *$P < .05$ vs placebo at same time point. (Courtesy of Tankó LB, for the Oral Ibandronate Group: Oral weekly ibandronate prevents bone loss in postmenopausal women. *J Intern Med* 254:159-167, 2003. Reprinted by permission of Blackwell Publishing.)

ments showed significant suppression of all the biochemical markers of bone turnover. The oral once-weekly ibandronate therapy was well tolerated at each of the 3 doses, with a safety profile resembling that of placebo.

Conclusions.—Once-weekly dosing with 20 mg of oral ibandronate was effective and safe in preventing osteoporosis in these postmenopausal women. Bone loss from both the hip and the spine was prevented, and the effect was noted regardless of the time that had elapsed since menopause.

▶ Ibandronate is a potent nitrogen-containing bisphosphonate that has recently been approved by the Food and Drug Administration for the treatment and prevention of osteoporosis in postmenopausal women. As of July 2004 it has not been marketed in the United States. This study presents data from a phase II/III dose-ranging trial for prevention of bone loss in postmenopausal women without osteoporosis. Oral ibandronate at a dose of 20 mg once weekly prevented bone loss at the lumbar spine and total hip and was associated with mean reductions of approximately 40% and 10% in markers of bone resorption and formation, respectively. While ibandronate, as well as other nitrogen-containing bisphosphonates, is safe and efficacious for this indication, it is still unclear which, if any, women without osteoporosis should receive pharmacologic treatment over and above calcium and vitamin D supplementation.

M. C. Hochberg, MD

Intravenous Ibandronate Injections Given Every Three Months: A New Treatment Option to Prevent Bone Loss in Postmenopausal Women

Stakkestad JA, for the Ibandronate Intravenous Study Group (CECOR AS, Haugesund, Norway; et al)

Ann Rheum Dis 62:969-975, 2003 5–33

Background.—Ibandronate, a highly potent nitrogen-containing bisphosphonate, has been under investigation for the treatment and prevention of postmenopausal osteoporosis. The efficacy, safety, and dose response of 3 doses of ibandronate, given intermittently by IV injection every 3 months, were investigated for the prevention of postmenopausal osteoporosis.

Methods.—Six hundred twenty-nine postmenopausal women were enrolled in the multicenter, double-blind, placebo-controlled study. The participants were stratified by time since menopause and baseline lumbar spine bone mineral density (BMD) and randomly assigned to receive IV ibandronate, 0.5, 1, or 2 mg, or placebo every 3 months. Daily calcium supplementation was provided to all the women.

Findings.—After 1 year of treatment, there was a dose-dependent gain in mean lumbar spine BMD from baseline. The increases were 2.5% in patients receiving 2 mg, 2.6% in those receiving 1 mg, and 2.8% in those receiving 0.5 mg of ibandronate (Fig 2). Women in the placebo group had a BMD loss of 2.4%. The highest BMD increases were documented in women with osteopenia taking 2 mg of ibandronate. All 3 doses of ibandronate at the hip produced significantly better increases in BMD than placebo. The greatest increases were in women with osteopenia receiving the 2-mg dose. Ibandronate suppressed bone turnover markers in a concomitant, dose-dependent manner compared with placebo. Injections were well tolerated.

Conclusions.—This is the first study to demonstrate the efficacy and tolerability of intermittent IV injections of a bisphosphonate in preventing bone loss in women early in postmenopause. Intermittent IV ibandronate in-

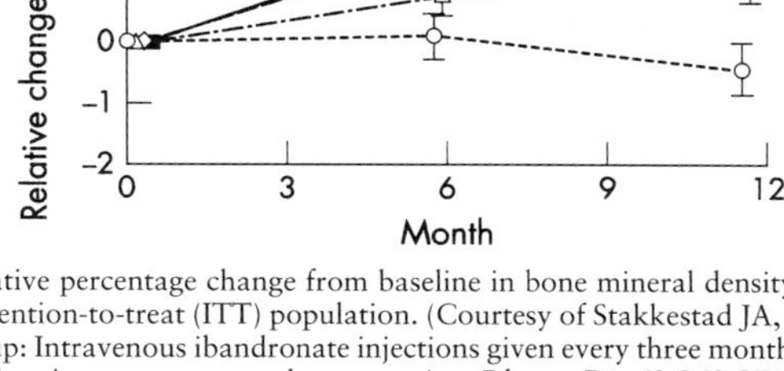

FIGURE 2.—Relative percentage change from baseline in bone mineral density (BMD) at the lumbar spine (L1-4) in the intention-to-treat (ITT) population. (Courtesy of Stakkestad JA, for the Ibandronate Intravenous Study Group: Intravenous ibandronate injections given every three months: A new treatment option to prevent bone loss in postmenopausal women. *Ann Rheum Dis* 62:969-975, 2003. Reprinted with permission of the BMJ Publishing Group.)

jections appear to be an effective, convenient alternative to oral selective estrogen receptor modulators and estrogen replacement treatment.

▶ Ibandronate is a potent nitrogen-containing bisphosphonate that has recently been approved by the Food and Drug Administration for the treatment and prevention of osteoporosis in postmenopausal women; as of July 2004, it has not been marketed in the United States. This article presents data from a phase II/III dose-ranging trial for prevention of bone loss in postmenopausal women without osteoporosis. All doses of IV ibandronate prevented bone loss at the lumbar spine (Fig 2) and total hip; maximal separation from placebo occurred in the group that received 2.0 mg every 3 months. The acute-phase reaction characterized by myalgias that is commonly seen with IV administration of bisphosphonates was noted in one fifth of patients receiving 2.0 mg every 3 months and resulted in withdrawal of 2.5% of subjects in this group. If one decides to treat postmenopausal women without osteoporosis for the "indication" of preventing bone loss, there seems little advantage to giving ibandronate IV every 3 months compared with giving it or other approved bisphosphonates (eg, alendronate, risedronate) orally once weekly. The exception would be for women with contraindications to orally administered bisphosphonates.

M. C. Hochberg, MD

Recombinant Human Parathyroid Hormone (1-34) [Teriparatide] Improves Both Cortical and Cancellous Bone Structure

Jiang Y, Zhao JJ, Mitlak BH, et al (Univ of California, San Francisco; Eli Lilly and Co, Indianapolis, Ind)

J Bone Miner Res 18:1932-1941, 2003 5–34

Background.—A large, randomized, double-blind, multicenter study (the Fracture Prevention Trial) was initiated to compare the efficacy of recombinant human parathyroid hormone(1-34) (rhPTH[1-34]; teriparatide) with that of placebo in postmenopausal women. The effects of this treatment on cancellous and cortical bone in a subset of women enrolled in that trial were investigated after a mean treatment of 19 months.

Methods.—Fifty-one paired iliac crest bone biopsy specimens were analyzed. Specimens were obtained from 19 women receiving placebo, 18 receiving 20 μg of teriparatide, and 14 receiving 40 μg of teriparatide. Two-dimensional histomorphometry and 3-dimensional micro-CT (μCT) were used in the analysis. In the data analysis, data for both teriparatide groups were pooled.

Findings.—Two-dimensional histomorphometric analyses demonstrated that teriparatide significantly increased cancellous bone volume. Median changes were a 14% increase in the teriparatide group and a 24% decrease in the placebo group. Teriparatide also reduced marrow star volume by 16%, compared with a 112% increase with placebo. Teriparatide treatment was unrelated to osteomalacia or woven bone. No significant changes were seen in mineral appositional rate or wall thickness. Three-dimensional cancellous and cortical bone structural analyses indicated that teriparatide significantly reduced the cancellous structure model index by 12% (compared with a 7% increase with placebo) and increased cancellous connectivity density by 19% (compared with a 14% decrease with placebo). In addition, teriparatide increased cortical thickness by 22%, compared with 3% with placebo.

Conclusions.—Teriparatide in the treatment of postmenopausal osteoporosis significantly increases cancellous bone volume and connectivity, improves trabecular morphology, and increases cortical bone thickness. Such changes should improve biomechanical competence.

▶ Teriparatide (rhPTH[1-34]) has been shown to be effective for treatment of postmenopausal women with osteoporosis[1] and is approved by the Food and Drug Administration. This study reports the changes in bone remodeling and trabecular and cortical bone microarchitecture in paired iliac crest bone biopsy specimens from 51 patients analyzed using 2-dimensional histomorphometry and 3-dimensional μCT. Trabecular volume, cortical thickness, and trabecular connectivity density increased significantly in the teriparatide-treated patients. Importantly, no osteomalacia or woven bone was noted in biopsy specimens of teriparatide-treated patients. These findings confirm the short-term safety of teriparatide and provide data to support improvement in bone quality with this agent.

M. C. Hochberg, MD

Reference

1. Neer RM, Arnaud CD, Zanchetta JR, et al: Effect of parathyroid hormone (1-34) on fractures and bone mineral density in postmenopausal women with osteoporosis. *N Engl J Med* 344:1434-1441, 2001.

Efficacy and Safety of Human Parathyroid Hormone-(1–84) in Increasing Bone Mineral Density in Postmenopausal Osteoporosis

Hodsman AB, Hanley DA, Ettinger MP, et al (Univ of Western Ontario, London, Canada; Univ of Calgary, Alta, Canada; Regional Osteoporosis Ctr of South Florida and Radiant Research, Stuart; et al)

J Clin Endocrinol Metab 88:5212-5220, 2003 5–35

Background.—In women with osteoporosis, daily subcutaneous injections of N-terminal analogs of parathyroid hormone (PTH) increase bone mass and reduce fractures. The efficacy and safety of human PTH-(1–84) in the treatment of postmenopausal osteoporosis were investigated.

Methods.—Two hundred six women were enrolled in the double-blind, placebo-controlled trial. Patients were randomly assigned to receive PTH (50, 75, or 100 μg) or placebo for 12 months by daily subcutaneous self-injection.

Findings.—Treatment with PTH induced increases in lumbar spine bone mineral density (BMD) that were time and dose related. The 100-μg dose resulted in a significant 2% increase in BMD at 3 months and 7.8% at 12 months. The anabolic effects of PTH in the lumbar spine were underestimated by BMD, as bone area increased significantly. In the first 6 months of treatment with the 100-μg dose of PTH, the total hip BMD declined nonsignificantly, but this trend reversed in the second 6 months. Bone turnover markers rose during the first 6 months and were maintained at increased levels through the second 6 months. Compliance with the protocol ranged from 95% to 98%. Patients generally tolerated the treatment well. Dose-related incidences of transient hypercalcemia were documented. However, only 1 person in the 100-μg group was withdrawn from the study because of repeated hypercalcemia.

Conclusions.—Daily treatment with full-length PTH for 12 months induced significant dose-dependent increases in lumbar spine BMD. Minimal, nonsignificant changes occurred at sites containing a higher proportion of cortical bone. Thus, full-length PTH appears to be effective and safe in the treatment of postmenopausal osteoporosis.

▶ Teriparatide (recombinant human PTH-[1–34]) has been shown to be effective for treatment of postmenopausal women with osteoporosis[1] and is approved by the Food and Drug Administration. This study reports results of a 12-month phase II dose-ranging study of recombinant "full-length" PTH-(1–84) given subcutaneously in women with postmenopausal osteoporosis. There was a dose-dependent increase in lumbar spine bone mineral content and BMD; furthermore, patients with the lowest BMD at entry had the greatest percent increase in BMD during treatment. Dose-related adverse events included nausea, fatigue, hypercalciuria, and transient hypercalcemia. Phase III trials of recombinant "full-length" PTH-(1–84) to assess antifracture efficacy are in progress, and results are eagerly anticipated.

M. C. Hochberg, MD

Reference

1. Neer RM, Arnaud CD, Zanchetta JR, et al: Effect of parathyroid hormone (1-34) on fractures and bone mineral density in postmenopausal women with osteoporosis. *N Engl J Med* 344:1434-1441, 2001.

The Effects of Parathyroid Hormone and Alendronate Alone or in Combination in Postmenopausal Osteoporosis

Black DM, for the PaTH Study Investigators (Univ of California, San Francisco; et al)

N Engl J Med 349:1207-1215, 2003 5–36

Background.—The use of antiresorptive drugs is an established practice for the prevention of osteoporotic fractures in patients with osteoporosis. Studies have shown that nitrogen-containing bisphosphonates, such as alendronate and risedronate, reduce the risk of fracture and increase bone mineral density by suppressing bone resorption. Unlike bisphosphonates, parathyroid hormone is anabolic when administered intermittently for osteoporosis. Tested was the hypothesis that concurrent administration of alendronate and parathyroid hormone would increase bone density more than the use of either agent alone.

Methods.—A total of 238 postmenopausal women not using bisphosphonates were enrolled in this study. All of the women had low bone mineral density at the hip or spine as determined by a T score of less than −2.5 or a T score of less than −2.0 with an additional risk factor for osteoporosis. The women were randomly assigned to daily treatment with parathyroid hormone (100 μg, 119 women), alendronate (10 mg, 60 women) or both (59 women) and were followed up for 12 months. Dual-energy x-ray absorptiometry and quantitative CT were used to assess bone mineral density at the spine and hip. Markers of bone turnover were measured in fasting blood samples.

Results.—An increase in the bone mineral density at the spine was manifest in all treatment groups, and there was no significant difference in the increase between the parathyroid hormone group and the combination therapy group. The volumetric density of the trabecular bone at the spine was significantly increased in all groups; however, the increase in the parathyroid hormone group was nearly twice that in the other groups. Bone formation was significantly increased in the parathyroid hormone group but not in the combination-therapy group. Bone resorption decreased in the combination-therapy group and the alendronate group.

Conclusion.—No evidence of synergy between parathyroid hormone and alendronate was found in this study. However, changes in the volumetric density of trabecular bone, the cortical volume at the hip, and levels of markers of bone turnover provide evidence that the concurrent use of alendronate may reduce the anabolic effects of parathyroid hormone. There is a need for longer-term studies of fractures to determine whether and how antiresorptive drugs can be optimally used in conjunction with parathyroid hormone therapy.

► Both alendronate and teriparatide are effective for treatment of postmenopausal women and men with osteoporosis. There is much interest in the potential use of combinations of these antiresorptive and anabolic agents in clinical practice. This study reports data from the first year of a 2-year study comparing changes in bone mineral density and bone turnover between patients randomly assigned to alendronate alone (10 mg once daily), recombinant human parathyroid hormone (1-84) alone (100 μg subcutaneously once daily), or both in combination. Changes in bone mineral density at the lumbar spine did not differ significantly between the groups; however, patients receiving parathyroid hormone alone had significantly greater reduction in bone mineral density at both the total hip and distal one third of the radius than patients in the alendronate alone or combination groups. Volumetric bone mineral density, measured by CT, showed significantly greater increases in lumbar spine trabecular bone but greater decreases in hip cortical bone in patients randomly assigned to parathyroid hormone alone than those in the combination or alendronate alone groups. It is difficult to draw meaningful conclusions from these data as there is considerable controversy about the role of changes in bone mineral density as a surrogate end point for fracture risk reduction[1,2]; this study was not designed to measure fracture risk reduction between the groups. Furthermore, it is impossible to generalize from these results to the common clinical situation that requires the physician to decide whether to initiate therapy with parathyroid hormone in a patient who has previously received or is currently receiving an oral bisphosphonate.

M. C. Hochberg, MD

References

1. Hochberg MC, Greenspan S, Wasnich RD, et al: Changes in bone density and turnover explain the reductions in incidence of non-vertebral fractures that occur during treatment with anti-resorptive agents. *J Clin Endocrinol Metab* 87:1586-1592, 2002.
2. Delmas PD, Seeman E: Changes in bone mineral density explain little of the reduction in vertebral or nonvertebral fracture risk with anti-resorptive therapy. *Bone* 34:599-604, 2004.

Growth Hormone Replacement in Adults and Bone Mineral Density: A Systematic Review and Meta-analysis

Davidson P, Milne R, Chase D, et al (Univ of Southampton, England)
Clin Endocrinol (Oxf) 60:92-98, 2004 5–37

Background.—Growth hormone (GH) deficiency in adults is characterized by reduced bone mineral density (BMD) as well as symptoms of depression and anxiety, low energy, increased weight, and impaired cardiac func-

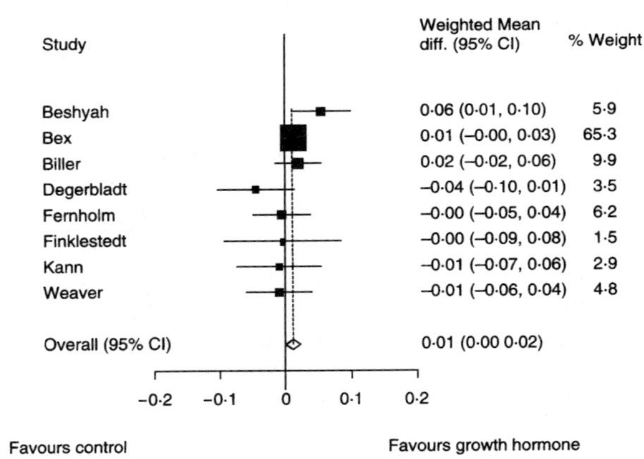

FIGURE 2.—Weighted mean difference of BMD in GH-treated group against no active treatment at 6 months. (Courtesy of Davidson P, Milne R, Chase D, et al: Growth hormone replacement in adults and bone mineral density: A systematic review and meta-analysis. *Clin Endocrinol [Oxf]* 60:92-98, 2004. Reprinted by permission of Blackwell Publishing.)

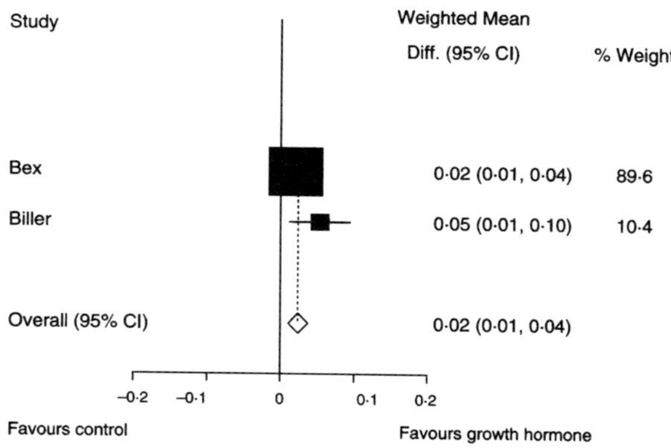

FIGURE 3.—Weighted mean difference of BMD in GH-treated group against no active treatment at 18 months. (Courtesy of Davidson P, Milne R, Chase D, et al: Growth hormone replacement in adults and bone mineral density: A systematic review and meta-analysis. *Clin Endocrinol [Oxf]* 60:92-98, 2004. Reprinted by permission of Blackwell Publishing.)

tion. The effects of GH replacement on BMD in affected patients have not been established. A systematic review of randomized studies comparing GH with no active treatment in patients with GH deficiency was conducted.

Methods.—Electronic databases were searched, and articles, abstracts, and conference proceedings to March 2002 were identified. Two independent reviewers extracted data. Data from individual studies were combined by fixed effects model meta-analysis by using weighted mean difference of change in BMD at the lumbar spine and other sites.

Findings.—Eighteen studies including a total of 700 patients were identified from the search. Maximum follow-up ranged from 12 weeks to 24 months. The quality of reporting of study design and findings was judged to be poor. After trials with insufficient data were excluded, 10 trials with a total of 458 participants were included in the meta-analysis. The mean change in BMD at the lumbar spine with GH treatment was 0.01 g/cm^2 after 6 and 12 months, 0.02 g/cm^2 after 18 months, and 0.03 g/cm^2 after 24 months (Figs 2 and 3). These changes were significant. However, they were small and may have been influenced by bias.

Conclusions.—GH replacement appears to have a small effect on BMD in adults with GH deficiency. The clinical significance of these effects is uncertain.

► The authors reviewed 18 trials of human GH replacement that included 700 patients with adult GH deficiency. Data pooled across 8 studies showed only minimal differences from placebo in change in lumbar spine BMD after 6 and 18 months that are probably not of clinical importance (Figs 2 and 3). No significant differences were noted at the femoral neck. The take-home message is that there is no basis from this meta-analysis to support the use of GH to increase BMD in older adults.[1]

M. C. Hochberg, MD

Reference

1. Isley WL: Growth hormone therapy for adults: Not ready for prime time. *Ann Intern Med* 137:190-196, 2002.

Prevention and Treatment of Glucocorticoid-Induced Osteoporosis: A Comparison of Calcitriol, Vitamin D Plus Calcium, and Alendronate Plus Calcium

Sambrook PN, Kotowicz M, Nash P, et al (Univ of Sydney, Australia; Univ of Melbourne, Geelong, Australia; Nambour Gen Hosp, Sunshine Coast, Australia; et al)

J Bone Miner Res 18:919-924, 2003 5–38

Background.—High-dose corticosteroid therapy is used to treat many medical conditions. However, this treatment is associated with rapid bone loss from sites such as vertebrae. Compression fractures can occur within months. Bisphosphonate or active vitamin D analog treatment may decrease bone loss and the risk of fracture in patients receiving glucocorticoids. The efficacy of alendronate, calcitriol, and simple vitamin D in treating and preventing glucocorticoid-induced bone loss was compared in a randomized, multicenter, open-label study.

Methods and Findings.—One hundred ninety-five patients beginning or continuing glucocorticoids were randomly assigned to receive calcitriol, 0.5 to 0.75 μg/d; simple vitamin D (ergocalciferol), 30,000 IU weekly, plus cal-

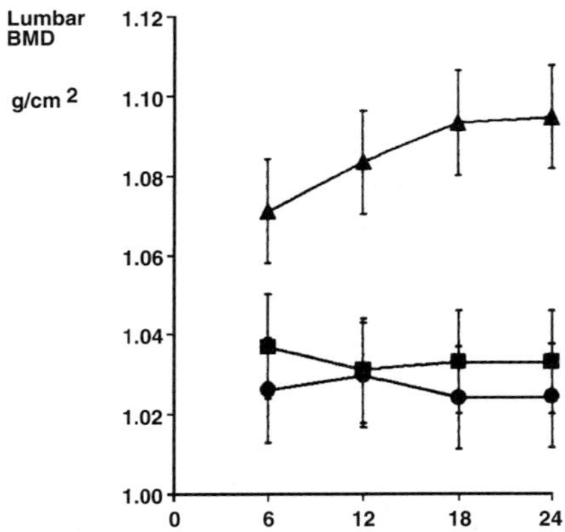

FIGURE 1.—Adjusted mean bone mineral density (*BMD*) at the lumbar spine (g/cm^2) at 6, 12, 18, and 24 months. These means are adjusted from the analysis of covariance for those factors and covariates included in the model for the primary efficacy analysis (ie, baseline BMD, center, prior duration of corticosteroid treatment, dose of corticosteroid at baseline, and cumulative dose of corticosteroid treatment 0-1 year). The SED between means is shown as the *error bars* in the graph of means; error bars are used to compare between different treatment groups. If the error bars do not overlap by more than 2 SEDs, the means are significantly different by $P < .05$. Alendronate (*solid triangles*), calcitriol (*solid squares*), and ergocalciferol *(solid circles)*. (Courtesy of Sambrook PN, Kotowicz M, Nash P, et al: Prevention and treatment of glucocorticoid-induced osteoporosis: A comparison of calcitriol, vitamin D plus calcium, and alendronate plus calcium. *J Bone Miner Res* 18:919-924, 2003, with permission from the American Society for Bone and Mineral Research.)

cium carbonate, 600 mg daily; or alendronate, 10 mg/d, plus calcium carbonate, 600 mg daily. After 2 years of treatment, the mean lumbar bone mineral density increased by 5.9% with alendronate, decreased 0.5% with ergocalciferol, and decreased by 0.7% with calcitriol (Fig 1). Treatment groups did not differ significantly in bone mineral density change at the femoral neck. A gain of 0.9% occurred with alendronate, and losses of 3.2% and 2.2% were seen with ergocalciferol and calcitriol, respectively. Lumbar bone loss varied by whether patients were beginning treatment or receiving chronic glucocorticoid treatment. A significant interaction effect between treatment and prior glucocorticoid use was documented. New vertebral fractures occurred in 6 calcitriol recipients, 1 ergocalciferol recipient, and no alendronate recipients.

Conclusions.—Simple vitamin D and calcitriol do not appear to differ in their effects on glucocorticoid-induced bone loss; however, alendronate was superior to both simple vitamin D and calcitriol.

▶ This randomized active-comparator controlled trial found that patients randomized to alendronate plus calcium had significant increases in lumbar spine bone mineral density (Fig 1) and fewer incident vertebral deformities compared with those randomized to either calcitriol alone or ergocalciferol plus calcium. Upper gastrointestinal side effects were similar across groups, but hypercalcemia only occurred in those groups that received calcitriol or vitamin D plus calcium. These results support the use of bisphosphonates for the prevention and treatment of glucocorticoid-induced osteoporosis.[1]

M. C. Hochberg, MD

Reference

1. American College of Rheumatology Ad Hoc Committee on Glucocorticoid-Induced Osteoporosis: Recommendations for the prevention and treatment of glucocorticoid-induced osteoporosis. *Arthritis Rheum* 44:1496-1503, 2001.

Glucocorticoid-Induced Osteoporosis

Promotion of Osteoclast Survival and Antagonism of Bisphosphonate-Induced Osteoclast Apoptosis by Glucocorticoids

Weinstein RS, Chen J-R, Powers CC, et al (Univ of Arkansas, Little Rock)
J Clin Invest 109:1041-1048, 2002 5–39

Background.—Glucocorticoids inhibit osteoblastogenesis and increase osteoblast apoptosis, thereby depressing bone formation. The role of bone resorption in the initial rapid phase of bone loss that characterizes glucocorticoid-induced osteoporosis is not known. Also unknown is why bisphosphonates are effective in treating this condition.

Methods and Findings.—In murine osteoclast cultures, it is reported that glucocorticoids prolonged baseline survival of osteoclasts. They also antagonized bisphosphonate-induced caspase activation and apoptosis by a glucocorticoid receptor–mediated action. The number of cancellous osteoclasts rose, although osteoclast progenitor numbers declined. The expected proapoptotic effect of bisphosphonates on osteoclasts was abrogated in mice given both glucocorticoids and bisphosphonates, as evidenced by maintenance of osteoclast numbers and loss of bone density. However, the administration of bisphosphonate prevented glucocorticoid-induced osteoblast apoptosis.

Conclusions.—Early bone loss with glucocorticoid excess is a result of the extension of the life span of preexisting osteoclasts. Bisphosphonates cannot prevent this effect. Thus, the early benefits of these agents can be attributed partly to prolongation of osteoblast life span.

▶ Bisphosphonates are recommended for the prevention and treatment of glucocorticoid-induced osteoporosis.[1] The mechanism of action of bisphosphonates in this condition has been largely ascribed to their antiresorptive effects mediated by osteoclast apoptosis. This study examined the mechanism of both glucocorticoid and bisphosphonate action in a murine-model of acute glucocorticoid-induced osteoporosis. Contrary to expectations, dexamethasone completely blocked the proapoptotic effects of alendronate on osteoclasts in vitro by inhibiting alendronate-induced activation of caspase-3 and caspase-9. In mice treated with prednisolone, alendronate administration decreased bone turnover, manifest by reduced osteoclast number, and prevented glucocorticoid-induced osteoblast apoptosis. Indeed, these authors suggest that the beneficial effects of bisphosphonates in glucocorticoid-induced osteoporosis are due to their prolongation of osteoblast life span. Stay tuned for further developments in understanding the pathophysiology of this important side effect of glucocorticoids and the molecular mechanisms of the interventions used to prevent or treat it, or both.

M. C. Hochberg, MD

Reference

1. American College of Rheumatology Ad Hoc Committee on Glucocorticoid-Induced Osteoporosis: Recommendations for the prevention and treatment of glucocorticoid-induced osteoporosis. *Arthritis Rheum* 44:1496-1503, 2001.

Bone Density Threshold and Other Predictors of Vertebral Fracture in Patients Receiving Oral Glucocorticoid Therapy

Van Staa TP, Laan RF, Barton IP, et al (Univ of Southampton, England; Univ Med Centre, Nijmegen, The Netherlands; Procter & Gamble Pharmaceuticals, Egham, England; et al)

Arthritis Rheum 48:3224-3229, 2003 5–40

Background.—Oral glucocorticoids (GCs) are commonly used to treat a variety of inflammatory and allergic illnesses. The predictors of vertebral fractures were determined in patients receiving oral GC treatment.

Methods.—Data from 2 randomized clinical studies similar in method but differing in inclusion criteria were analyzed. A total of 306 patients participated in the studies. Cox regression with forward selection was used to iden-

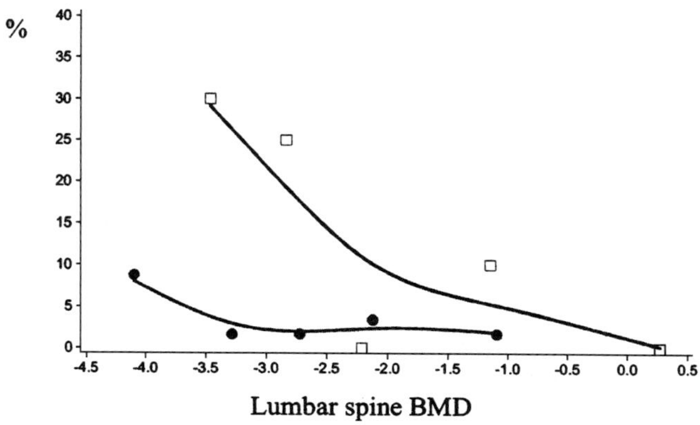

FIGURE 1.—Incidence of vertebral fracture in patients receiving glucocorticoids (GCs) (*open squares*) compared with nonusers of GCs (*solid circles*), by baseline lumbar spine bone mineral density (*BMD*). The individual data points correspond to the incidence in subgroups of the GC user and nonuser populations, as based on quintiles of baseline BMD. The *solid line* is a curve representing smoothing of these individual estimates. (Courtesy of Van Staa TP, Laan RF, Barton IP, et al: Bone density threshold and other predictors of vertebral fracture in patients receiving oral glucocorticoid therapy. *Arthritis Rheum* 48:3224-3229, 2003. Reprinted by permission of John Wiley & Sons, Inc.)

tify predictors of vertebral fracture in the placebo group. An analysis of bone mineral density (BMD) threshold included a comparison of the 1-year fracture risk in postmenopausal women receiving placebo in the GC trials with that in postmenopausal women not taking GCs in 3 additional studies.

Findings.—In the placebo group, significant predictors of incident fracture were baseline lumbar spine BMD and daily GC dose. The BMD threshold analysis demonstrated that patients receiving GCs, compared with non-GC users, were younger, had a higher BMD at baseline, and had fewer prevalent fractures. However, the fracture risk was greater in GC users than in nonusers, the adjusted relative risk being 5.67 (Fig 1). The fracture risk was increased in GC users regardless of whether osteoporosis was present.

Conclusions.—Daily but not cumulative GC dose appears to be a strong predictor of vertebral fracture in patients receiving GCs. At comparable levels of BMD, postmenopausal women taking GCs have a markedly higher risk of fracture than women not taking GCs.

► The authors performed a *post hoc* analysis of data from the risedronate prevention and treatment studies in GC-induced osteoporosis and found that baseline lumbar spine BMD and daily GC dose were independent predictors of risk of new vertebral fractures in patients randomized into the placebo groups. Of greater interest was the comparison of data from postmenopausal women enrolled in these trials with that from postmenopausal women who were randomized to placebo in the 3 risedronate pivotal trials. This latter analysis showed that postmenopausal women receiving GCs had an almost 6-fold higher adjusted risk of incident vertebral fractures and that this risk was independent of lumbar spine BMD (Fig 1). These results provide additional evidence for the deleterious effects of GCs on bone quality independent of their recognized effects on BMD, and provide further support for the American College of Rheumatology recommendations for prevention and treatment of GC-induced osteoporosis.[1]

M. C. Hochberg, MD

Reference

1. American College of Rheumatology Ad Hoc Committee on Glucocorticoid-Induced Osteoporosis: Recommendations for the prevention and treatment of glucocorticoid-induced osteoporosis. *Arthritis Rheum* 44:1496-1503, 2001.

Inhaled and Nasal Corticosteroid Use and the Risk of Fracture

Suissa S, Baltzan M, Kremer R, et al (McGill Univ, Montreal, Quebec, Canada)
Am J Respir Crit Care Med 169:83-88, 2004 5–41

Background.—Inhaled and nasal corticosteroids (INCSs) increase the rate of bone resorption and have prompted concerns about an increased risk of fracture with their long-term use. Whether the risk of fracture is increased by long-term INCS use was prospectively investigated.

Methods.—The study included patients 65 years old or more who filled a prescription for at least 1 respiratory medication from 1988 through 2001. All subjects were followed up for 4 or more years to determine the incidence of hip or upper-extremity fracture. The use and dosage of INCSs were compared between the 9624 cases with a new fracture during the study (69% women; mean age, 81 years) and the 191,622 age-matched control subjects who did not have a fracture during the study.

Results.—The cases and the control subjects did not differ significantly in their current use of inhaled corticosteroids (31.9% vs 30.7%; adjusted risk ratio [RR], 0.97) or nasal corticosteroids (4.4% vs 4.7%; RR, 0.92). None of the dosages of nasal corticosteroids was associated with a significantly increased risk of fracture. However, every 1000-μg increase in the daily dose of inhaled corticosteroids was associated with a 12% increase in the rate of upper-extremity fracture (but not hip fracture). Among subjects followed for 8 or more years, inhaled corticosteroid doses of more than 2000 μg/d were significantly associated with an increased rate of hip fracture (RR, 1.61).

Conclusion.—Even after 4 years of daily use, INCSs at the conventional dosages were not associated with an increased risk of hip or upper-extremity fracture in elderly patients with respiratory disease. The risk of fracture increased only with long-term use of high-dose inhaled corticosteroids. These findings support the safety of long-term INCS use in elderly patients at the currently recommended dosages.

► Prior epidemiologic studies were inconclusive regarding the association between use of inhaled corticosteroids and an increased risk of fracture. This study, which uses data from a large population-based cohort of the elderly in Quebec, demonstrated a dose-related increase in the risk of hip and upper-extremity fractures among users of inhaled corticosteroids (6% increased risk per 1000 µg increase in daily dose) but no relation for nasal corticosteroids. These data suggest that elderly patients using high doses of inhaled corticosteroids should receive prophylaxis or treatment for glucocorticoid-induced osteoporosis to reduce their increased risk of fracture.[1]

M. C. Hochberg, MD

Reference

1. American College of Rheumatology Ad Hoc Committee on Glucocorticoid-Induced Osteoporosis: Recommendations for the prevention and treatment of glucocorticoid-induced osteoporosis. *Arthritis Rheum* 44:1496-1503, 2001.

6 Regional Pain Syndromes, Non-Articular Musculoskeletal Disorders, and Fibromyalgia

Introduction

I have been culling the literature on this topic for the readers of the YEAR BOOK since 1997. For those of us who are professional students of the social constructedness of disease and the process of medicalization, the exercise of culling this literature is rewarded in enlightenment. The current yield is particularly gratifying.

Most diseases are both *real*—they cause pain and suffering—and *socially constructed*—their particular formulation reflects the social and historical context in which they are made. Alcoholism is an example of a disorder that society has codified as a disease, rather than the result of prostacycline. Medicalization occurs whenever a set of social problems is reformulated as a medical problem. This entails labeling as a disease with the presumption of some underlying pathobiology upon which therapy can be based. The social construction of the regional musculoskeletal disorders so as to medicalize regional musculoskeletal pain has become entrenched in the western mind over the past 50 years, and is now a precept of western medicine. It is clear that this dialectic advantages many in the enterprise it underpins, but very few if any people with regional disorders who choose to be patients. I have developed this theme in 2 monographs published in 2004: "The Last Well Person" (McGill-Queens University Press) examines the process of medicalization and the 3rd Edition of Occupational Musculoskeletal Disorders

(Lippincott Williams & Wilkins) examines the clinical ramifications as they relate to the regional musculoskeletal disorders.

This chapter is replete with object lessons. Take the lead article, which sounds the death knell for spinal fusion for regional back pain, and *pari passu* the "discal herniations" hypothesis. We have witnessed nearly 70 years of escalating surgical zeal and inventiveness before we witnessed surgeons with the courage to systematically put the underlying premise to the test. Read the paper by Englund et al (Abstract 6–27) and ask whether you would submit to a meniscectomy, regardless of the technique. The meniscal hypothesis for knee pain is joining the discal hypothesis for back pain in ignominy.

The notion of "wear and tear arthritis" is tottering on the edge of the archives. Spector and his colleagues are adding their analyses of the Chingford cohort and the British twin registry to that of others (Abstracts 6–2 and 6–3) to challenge this social construction. The ramifications are substantial in terms of culpability, liability, and biomechanics. And they are substantial in terms of removing one of the greatest health hazards facing a worker with a regional musculoskeletal disorder which all ascribe to the physical demands of work, namely escalating illness and disabling pain which is recalcitrant even to the interventions tested in many of the papers I have chosen for commentary.

As many of the papers in this chapter bear witness, regional musculoskeletal disorders are not diseases. They are intermittent and remittent predicaments of life for everyone. As such they join heartache and heartburn and headache and the like. To be well is not to be spared. To be well is to have the wherewithal to cope effectively till remission provides succor, and the episode fades from memory. Rather than potions, manipulations, and aggressive care, those who lack such wherewithal need empathic assistance. That will require a revision of the social construction that avoids medicalization.

Nortin M. Hadler, MD

Lead Article

Randomized Clinical Trial of Lumbar Instrumented Fusion and Cognitive Intervention and Exercises in Patients With Chronic Low Back Pain and Disc Degeneration

Brox JI, Sørensen R, Friis A, et al (St Olav's Hosp, Trondheim, Norway; Ullevaal Univ, Oslo, Norway; Univ North Norway, Tromso; et al)

Spine 28:1913-1921, 2003 6–1

Introduction.—Lumbar fusion rates have greatly increased during the past 20 years; rates vary from country to country among individual surgeons, and among small and large geographic regions. Only 1 randomized trial is known to have assessed the effectiveness of lumbar fusion. According to the Swedish Lumbar Spine Study, lumbar fusion is better than continuing physiotherapy and care by the family physician. The effectiveness of lumbar-instrumented fusion was compared with that of cognitive intervention and exercises in patients with chronic low back pain and disc degeneration in a single, blind, randomized investigation.

Methods.—The study included 64 patients, 25 to 60 years old, with low back pain of more than 1-year duration and evidence of disc degeneration at L4-L5 or L5-S1 or both at radiographic examination who were randomly selected to undergo either lumbar fusion with posterior transpedicular screws and postoperative physiotherapy, or cognitive intervention and exercises. The cognitive intervention included a lecture to give the patient an understanding that ordinary physical activity would not harm the disc and a recommendation to use the back and bend it. These lectures and recommendations were augmented by 3 daily physical therapy sessions for 3 weeks. The primary outcome measure was the Oswestry Disability Index.

Results.—At 1 year follow-up, 97% of patients, including 6 who had either not attended treatment or changed groups, were evaluated. The Oswestry Disability Index was significantly decreased from 41 to 26 after surgery, versus 42 to 30 after cognitive intervention and exercises. The mean between-group difference was 2.3 (−6.7-11.4; $P = .33$). Improvements in back pain, use of analgesics, emotional distress, life satisfaction, and return to work were not different between the fusion and conventional groups. Fear-avoidance beliefs and fingertip-floor distance were decreased more after nonoperative treatment. Lower limb pain was decreased more after surgery. The success rate was 70% after surgery and 76% after cognitive intervention and exercises. The incidence of early complications was 18% in the surgical group.

Conclusion.—Equal improvement was observed in patients with chronic low back pain and disc degeneration who underwent either lumbar fusion or cognitive intervention and exercises.

► Bravo! The legacy of the spine surgeons of the mid-20th century is an *idée fixe*. Backache is to be considered a surgical challenge. Countless patients with chronic back pain have been subjected to surgical violence in the past 50 years. Countless patients were to be disappointed in the outcome. The surgical community seemed less inclined to question their *idée fixe* than to question their technique. Laminectomies were no match, so they added spinal fusion using various bone grafts. That proved disappointing, so they substituted various forms of hardware for the bony fusing. That is also proving disappointing, so the trend is to implant an "artificial disc." All of this is going on without a single well-designed randomized controlled trial (RCT). If spine surgery were a pharmaceutical, it would never be licensed. However, all regulatory agencies apply no such test—only whether the materials to be used are safe and pure.

Along come these courageous Norwegian surgeons. This is as well designed an RCT for fusing hardware as one could hope for. It should drive a stake through the *idée fixe*. Furthermore, it should call a halt to any and all innovative spine surgery (and any other form of elective surgery) that has not passed regulatory muster by virtue of compelling scientific support.

I can dream.

N. M. Hadler, MD

Axial Pain

Predictors of Back Pain in a General Population Cohort

Kopec JA, Sayre EC, Esdaile JM (Univ of British Columbia; Arthritis Research Ctr of Canada, Vancouver, BC)

Spine 29:70-78, 2004 6–2

Introduction.—Predictors of back pain in the general population are not well delineated. Most prior trials have focused on specific occupational groups and used a cross-sectional or case–control design. Prediction models for back pain in the general male and female household populations were examined.

TABLE 4.—Predictors of Back Pain Among Males in the National Population Health Survey

Variable	*N*	OR	95% CI
Age group (yr)			
18-24	609	0.61	0.30, 1.24
25-44	1,934	1.31	0.74, 2.31
45-64	1,211	1.60	0.92, 2.80
65+*	722	1.00	
Self-rated health			
Excellent*	1,188	1.00	
Very Good	1,781	1.78	1.21, 2.63
Good	1,110	1.75	1.13, 2.69
Fair	312	1.96	1.00, 3.84
Poor	85	3.39	0.26, 43.92
Usual daily activity†			
Sitting*	885	1.00	
Walking or standing	1,940	1.59	1.11, 2.28
Lifting light loads	858	1.61	1.03, 2.51
Heavy work	511	1.84	1.14, 2.99
Gardening/yard work‡			
None*	2,181	1.00	
< 3 hours/month	920	0.62	0.40, 0.94
≥ 3 hours/month	1,094	0.55	0.38, 0.80
Chronic stress index (0-100)§			
Interquartile range	NA	1.25	1.05, 1.49
Height (cm)∥			
Inter–quartile range	NA	1.24	1.04, 1.49

*Reference category.

†Usual daily activity (including work habits) had 4 categories: (1) usually sit during the day and do not walk about very much; (2) stand or walk about quite a lot during the day but do not have to carry or lift things very often; (3) usually lift or carry light loads or have to climb stairs or hills often; and (4) do heavy work or carry very heavy loads.

‡Amount of time spent gardening or doing yard work was estimated from questions asking how many times the respondent engaged in such activities and how much time they spent on average on each occasion.

§Chronic stress index was composed of 15 true/false items measuring activity overload, financial difficulties, child-related stress, and problems with relationships in day-to-day encounters. The score (adjusted for the number of questions applicable) was treated as a continuous variable and converted to a 0-100 scale. The OR was calculated for the interquartile range (20 points).

∥Height was a continuous variable measured in centimeters. The OR was calculated for the interquartile range (10 cm).

Abbreviations: NA, Not applicable; *OR*, odds ratio.

(Courtesy of Kopec JA, Sayre EC, Esdaile JM: Predictors of back pain in a general population cohort. *Spine* 29(1):70-78, 2004.)

Methods.—Longitudinal data from the first and second cycles (1994-1995 and 1996-1997) of the Canadian National Population Health Survey was reviewed. All 11,063 residents aged 18 years and older who reported no back problems in the 1994-1995 National Population Health Survey cycle were evaluated. Potential predictors of chronic back pain were categorized into 9 groups and entered into stepwise logistic regression models. Bootstrap methods were used to determine the final models and evaluate their predictive power.

Results.—The overall incidence of back pain was 44.7 per 1000 person-years; this was higher in women (47.0/1000 person-years) versus men (42.2/1000 person-years). In men, significant predictors of back pain included: age (peak effect in 45-64 years), height, self-rated health, usual pattern of activity (particularly heavy work), yard work or gardening (negative association), and general chronic stress (Table 4). In women, significant predictors were as follows: self-reported restrictions in activity, being diagnosed with arthritis, personal stress, and history of psychologic trauma in childhood or adolescence.

Conclusion.—Overall health and psychosocial factors are important predictors of back pain in both men and women. Other risk factors vary between genders.

► Many western countries have undertaken surveys similar to the Canadian National Population Health Survey, and many are coming up with results similar to those presented in this article. I still have not convinced many of the epidemiologists involved in this work to adopt a more stringent vocabulary. These surveys have little to do with the incidence of back pain, but much to do with the incidence of memorable back pain. This article is assessing the incidence of memorable persistent back pain. After all, the cohort is surveyed biennially as to "long-term" back pain that had "lasted or were expected to last 6 months or longer" during the last 2 years.

The data analysis, as is true of all multivariate analyses, focuses on all associations that jump out of the initial screening. Realize that for many variables there is no hint of an association, such as all sorts of sporting activities. If one chooses to spend hours each week gardening, one is less likely to recall persistent back pain (Table 4). But skiing, volleyball, weight lifting, yoga, tennis, and the like do not increase the likelihood of recalling persistent backache.

Back pain is more likely to be memorable when life is treating one poorly, Furthermore, one's sense of wellness in general is at risk (Table 4). When will we ever learn to hear the chief complaint as surrogate in this fashion?

N. M. Hadler, MD

Risk Factors for Progression of Lumbar Spine Disk Degeneration: The Chingford Study

Hassett G, Hart DJ, Manek NJ, et al (St Thomas' Hosp, London; Whipps Cross Hosp, London)

Arthritis Rheum 48:3112-3117, 2003 6–3

Introduction.—There are few data concerning the natural history of lumbar spine disk degeneration and related risk factors. The radiographic progression of lumbar spine disk degeneration was followed during a 9-year period in a population-based inception cohort of females from the Chingford Study population, a well-described prospective longitudinal cohort of 1003 females seen annually since 1988.

Methods.—A total of 796 paired lumbar spine radiographs were interpreted by a single reader for anterior osteophytes (AO) and disk space narrowing (DSN) using the Lane atlas at each lumbar disk space (L1-5). Disk degeneration was defined using thresholds of AO and DSN grade 1+ in 1 or more vertebrae (L1-5) for each participant. Progression was considered to be an increase in grade in an affected y-1 vertebra. Potential risk factors were evaluated using odds ratios and 95% confidence intervals adjusted for age, body mass index (BMI), and other potential confounders in logistic regression models.

Results.—Mean participant age at baseline was 53.8 years and mean BMI was 25.4 kg/m^2. Progression rates for AO and DSN were 4%/annum and 3%/annum, respectively. The progression of DSN was predicted by age, back pain, and radiographic hip and knee osteoarthritis (OA); progression of AO was predicted by age and radiographic hip OA, with borderline significance for BMI over 30 kg/m^2. No significant effects were observed for smoking, physical activity, hormone replacement therapy use, multiparity, or hand OA.

Conclusion.—This is the first population-based longitudinal investigation to evaluate progression of the individual radiographic characteristics of AO and DSN in lumbar spine disk degeneration. Progression rates of 3% to 4% per annum were observed, in conjunction with important risk factors for progression, including age, back pain, and radiographic OA at the hip and knee.

The Association of Body Mass Index and Osteoarthritis of the Knee Joint: An Examination of Genetic and Environmental Influences

Manek NJ, Hart D, Spector TD, et al (St Thomas' Hosp, London)

Arthritis Rheum 48:1024-1029, 2003 6–4

Introduction.—There is considerable evidence that genetic factors have an important role in the determination of osteoarthritis. Twin trials have estimated that up to 65% of the population variance of OA can be attributed to genetic factors. Obesity, or high body mass index (BMI), also has a strong genetic basis. It is possible that there is a positive link between BMI and knee

OA due to shared genetic determinants of these 2 traits. The genetic and environmental influences on the known relationship between BMI and knee OA were examined using adult twin data.

Methods.—Bilateral knee radiographs from 785 pairs of healthy female twins with a mean age of 54.5 years from the St. Thomas' Hospital Adult Twin Registry (261 monozygotic [MZ] and 524 dizygotic [DZ] twin pairs) were reviewed. Tibiofemoral knee OA was graded using the Kellgren and Lawrence (K/L) scoring system on an ordinal scale of 0-4. The presence of knee OA was considered to be a K/L grade of 2 or greater on either side of the knee joint. Body weight and height were measured. Participants were stratified into quartiles of BMI. Cross-trait cross-twin association of BMI and knee OA was evaluated using logistic regression to determine whether genetic or environmental influences explain the BMI-knee OA link. The genetic (heritability) and environmental contributions to each of the measures were estimated via path modeling.

Results.—A strong correlation was seen between high BMI and the presence of knee OA (odds ratio [OA], 3.9 for highest versus lowest quartile of BMI; $P = .0001$). The heritability of knee OA was 50.4% (95% CI, 34-62%); BMI was 55.7% (95% CI, 35-72%). Cross-train cross twin associations did not significantly vary from unity in either the MZ or DZ twin pairs, suggesting that shared genetic influences were not likely to explain the association. Path modeling demonstrate that the model containing additive genetic factors, common environmental factors, and unique environmental factors had the best fit to the data overall. The shared genetic path between BMI and knee OA could be excluded without deterioration in the fit of the model.

Conclusion.—The strong correlation between high BMI and knee OA is not likely to be mediated by shared genetic factors. It appears that environmental modification of BMI can influence knee OA.

► The Chingford study is the British answer to the Framingham cohort from a rheumatological point of view. More than 1000 women have been followed with annual clinical and radiographic examinations for 15 years. The cohort has reached an average age of 55. It requires such a cohort to probe for subtle predispositions to degenerative spine disease. By this age, degenerative changes are ubiquitous. Furthermore, we know from analysis of the large British and Finnish twin studies that nearly all the propensity to degenerative lumbar spine disease is inherited. So, this paper is reporting on an analysis of other, minor factors.

It's important to realize what was not found. Whether the women were sedentary at home or at work did not influence the progression of their inherited spinal osteoarthritis. Neither did their BMI. Clearly we need to expunge the notion of "wear and tear" arthritis from our preconceptions and from our teachings.

It's important to realize what was found. The progression of lumbosacral degenerative joint disease is more marked in women who have degenerative hip and knee disease but not women who have hand OA (which associates with hip OA but not knee OA). Perhaps the polyarticular involvement causes the afflicted women to be more likely to recall their backache. It is clear that when one inherits a propensity toward spinal OA, one is inheriting a propensity to OA elsewhere but not everywhere. Different joints have differing biology.

Furthermore, the fact that BMI does not influence the genetic predisposition to OA at the spine (and hip), does not mean it has no influence elsewhere. That is the point of the second paper, another contribution from the analysis of the British twin study mentioned above. Weight gain would not be expected to influence the progression of radiographic spine or hip OA, but it might predispose to radiographic knee OA. However, even this association is complex. It is clear that there are several patterns of knee OA that are not associated with tibiofemoral cartilage loss and therefore not with biomechanical instability. Furthermore, the association of knee OA and knee pain is remarkably inconsistent and minor. Perhaps the increasing BMI affects knee OA through metabolic rather physical factors.

N. M. Hadler, MD

The Pathogenesis of Schmorl's Nodes

Peng B, Wu W, Hou S, et al (304th Hosp, Beijing, China)
J Bone Joint Surg Br 85-B:879-882, 2003 6–5

Background.—It has been widely assumed that Schmorl's nodes represent the herniation of the nucleus pulposus through the cartilaginous end plate into the body of a vertebra. Included in the hypotheses of their origin and pathogenesis are developmental factors, degenerative conditions, and pathologic processes, such as infection, neoplasia, and trauma. However, these hypotheses have not been critically examined. The histologic features of specimens of Schmorl's nodes and the corresponding images from conventional radiographs, MRI studies, and CT scans were analyzed.

Methods.—The pathogenesis of Schmorl's nodes was determined in 12 surgical specimens obtained from 10 patients (8 males, 2 females), 14 to 61 years old (mean age, 34 years), with severe low back pain, with or without leg pain. The mean duration of pain from onset to first presentation was 3.5 years, and all of the patients denied a history of lumbar injury. In addition to conventional radiography and CT of the lumbar spine in all patients, 5 patients underwent MRI evaluation. Three patients underwent diskography of 5 intervertebral spaces with Schmorl's nodes just before radiologic examination, and in all 3 patients, the pain was reproduced during injection of contrast material.

Results.—CT scans demonstrated round, often multiple cystic lesions with indistinct sclerotic margins beneath the cartilaginous end plate. These findings are similar to the changes typically seen in CT images of osteonecrosis. Histologic examination of en bloc slices through Schmorl's nodes provided clear evidence of subchondral osteonecrosis. Fibrosis was found beneath the end plate, within the marrow cavities along with the disappearance of fat cells. Osteocytes within bone trabeculae were dead or had disappeared.

Conclusions.—Schmorl's nodes may be the result of ischemic necrosis beneath the cartilaginous end plate, and the herniation into the vertebral body is a secondary process.

► Schmorl, Heine, and others in the Heidelberg pathology school fathered modern skeletal pathology 80 years ago. Schmorl's nodes are common and are commonly seen in adolescents. They are incidental findings on imaging studies, predominating in the lower dorsal spine. No one has been postulating that they are a cause of backaches. I am horrified that these authors from Beijing could not only mobilize such an inference but, literally, operate on it. They extirpated the nodes and fused the spine. Heaven help us.

The histopathology caused them to publish their experience and, I presume, allowed the editors and "peer reviewers" of this distinguished journal see their way clear to publishing the series.

Most thinking about Schmorl's nodes relates to a fracture of the end plate with herniation of the nucleus of pulposus into the subchondral bone. Applying axial force to necropsy specimens can cause this lesion (and never lateral herniation). Thus, the thinking has been that the nodes occur because of such forces in individuals with weak end plates. It turns out that the weakness is a consequence of focal avascular necrosis.

These patients still should not have been operated on for Schmorl's nodes. The pathophysiologic insight was not worth it.

N. M. Hadler, MD

Chronic Pain and Poor Self-Rated Health

Mäntyselkä P, Turunen JHO, Ahonen RS, et al (Univ of Kuopio, Finland)

JAMA 290:2435-2442, 2003 6–6

Introduction.—Recent studies have focused on the impact of chronic pain on daily living. Self-rated health is an important indicator of both morbidity and mortality. Little is known concerning the association between chronic pain and self-rated health in the general population. A population-based investigation of persons 15 to 74 years old was performed in Finland to assess the prevalence of chronic pain and its impact on self-rated health.

Methods.—A questionnaire survey was conducted during the spring of 2002 in an age- and sex-stratified population sample of 6500 persons. The response rate was 71% (4542 respondents) after exclusion of participants with unobtainable data (n = 38). Chronic pain was defined as pain with a minimum duration of 3 months and was graded by frequency as follows: (1) at most, once weekly; (2) several times per week; and (3) daily or continuously. On the basis of a 5-item questionnaire on self-rated health, participants were classified as having good, moderate, or poor health. Multinomial logistic regression analysis was used to evaluate the determinants of health. Analysis included sex, age, education, working status, chronic disease, and mood. The primary outcome measures were perceived chronic pain graded by frequency and self-rated health status.

Results.—The prevalence of any chronic pain was 35.1%; for chronic daily pain, it was 14.3%. The incidence of moderate self-rated health was 26.6%; for poor health, it was 7.6%. For moderate self-rated health among persons with chronic pain at most once weekly versus those with no chronic pain, the adjusted odds were 1.36 (95% confidence interval [CI], 1.05-1.76); several times per week, 2.41 (95% CI, 1.94-3.00); and daily, 3.69 (95% CI, 2.97-4.59). The odds for poor self-rated health were having chronic pain at most once per week, 1.16 (95% CI, 0.65-2.07); several times per week, 2.62 (95% CI, 1.76-3.90); and daily, 11.82 (95% CI, 8.67-16.10).

Conclusion.—Chronic pain is independently associated with low self-rated health in the general population.

Neck and Shoulder Pain in 70- to 79-Year-Old Men and Women: Findings From the Health, Aging and Body Composition Study

Vogt MT, Simonsick EM, Harris TB, et al (Univ of Pittsburgh, Pa; Natl Inst on Aging, Baltimore, Md; Natl Inst on Aging, Bethesda, Md; et al)

Spine J 3:435-441, 2003 6–7

Introduction.—The cumulative lifetime incidence of neck and shoulder pain is similar to that of low back pain (about 66% to 71%). Musculoskeletal pain in the cervicobrachial region is an important problem among adults of working age. Little is known concerning the impact of this discomfort in the elderly population. A cross-sectional investigation was conducted to (1) ascertain the incidence of neck and shoulder pain in a well-functioning elderly cohort; (2) identify factors linked with the pain; (3) evaluate the pattern of coexisting joint pain; and (4) assess the impact of this pain on physical functioning.

Methods.—African-American and white men and women, 70 to 79 years old, participated in the Health, Aging, and Body Composition (Health ABC) investigation. Between April 1997 and June 1998, 3075 men and women participating in the Health ABC study completed an initial home interview and clinical examination. Data were obtained concerning musculoskeletal pain, medical history, depressive symptomatology, and physical function. Physical performance measures were conducted.

Results.—Neck pain of 1 month or more duration was reported by 11.9% of participants; 18.9% reported shoulder pain. White women had the highest incidence of neck pain (15.4%); African-American women had the highest incidence of shoulder pain (24.3%). The correlates of both neck and shoulder pain were female sex, no education beyond high school, poorer self-related health, depressive symptomatology, and a medical history of arthritis, heart attack, and angina. Increasing severity of both neck and shoulder pain was linked with an increased incidence of joint pain at other sites and with poor functional capacity. Measures of physical performance involving the upper extremity were also reduced.

Conclusion.—Neck and shoulder pain, either alone or in conjunction with pain in other joints, has a marked influence on the function and well-being of older adults.

Function and Back Symptoms in Older Adults

Edmond SL, Felson DT (Univ of Medicine and Dentistry New Jersey/SHRP, Newark; Boston Univ)

J Am Geriatr Soc 51:1702-1709, 2003 6–8

Introduction.—Increasing functional loss and dependency are characteristic of the elderly years. Few trials have evaluated the contribution of back symptoms to overall physical disability in older adults, even though the incidence of back symptoms is high in this population. The correlation between back symptoms and limitations was assessed in 9 specific functional activities in a cross-sectional investigation.

Methods.—This trial was conducted as part of the Framingham Heart Study, a population-based trial performed on a representative sample of community-living residents of Framingham, Massachusetts. A total of 1007 surviving members of the original cohort who participated in the 22nd Biennial Examination in 1992-1993 were evaluated. The age range was 70 to 100 years. Participants were asked whether they experienced pain, aching, or stiffness in their back on most days and whether they had difficulty performing 9 specific functional skills. The proportion of functional limitations attributable to back symptoms and the proportion of limitations that participants with these limitations attributed to back symptoms were evaluated.

Results.—A total of 26.6% of participants reported pain, aching, or stiffness in at least 1 of 3 back areas. For most functional activities, limitations were at least twice as prevalent among participants with back symptoms as among participants without back symptoms. A moderate to strong relationship was observed between back symptoms and functional limitations, particularly among women. The multiply-adjusted odds ratios were highest for difficulty standing in one place for about 15 minutes, pushing or pulling a large object, and walking half a mile. Among participants with back symptoms, 43% to 63% of limitations in activities were caused by back symptoms. Overall, back symptoms were so prevalent that 18% to 34% of all functional limitations were attributable to back symptoms.

Conclusion.—Back symptoms are responsible for a large percentage of functional limitations in older adults, particularly in women.

Prevalence of Lower Extremity Pain and Its Association With Functionality and Quality of Life in Elderly Women in Australia

Chen J, Devine A, Dick IM, et al (Univ of Western Australia, Perth)

J Rheumatol 30:2689-2693, 2003 6–9

Introduction.—Musculoskeletal conditions are an important cause of physical limitations and disability in elderly individuals. The prevalence of these conditions is expected to increase markedly as the population ages. Functional impairment and musculoskeletal disability are frequently underestimated or overlooked when elderly patients see their physician for other reasons. The prevalence of self-reported lower extremity pain and the impact on functionality and quality of life were assessed in a population-based investigation of elderly women in Western Australia.

Methods.—A total of 1486 women (6.2% of 24,800 women) older than 70 years in Perth, Australia, were recruited. An index of relative socioeconomic disadvantage was determined via postcode. Self-reported lower extremity pain at the hip, knee, and foot was obtained by questionnaire. The incidence of lower extremity pain was classified into 5 groups. Mobility was ascertained by the Timed Up and Go Test (TUG). The quality of life was determined via the Medical Outcome Study Short Form 36 (SF-36) summary statistics: physical and mental component scores (PCS and MCS).

Results.—The prevalence of women reporting any hip, knee, or foot pain was 39%, 52%, and 34%, respectively. Fourteen percent of the cohort experienced pain at all sites, and 28% had no pain. No age difference was present between the various pain groups. Women with more pain were heavier and had higher body mass index (BMI) scores. At all lower limb sites, women with more frequent pain had decreased mobility and a lower quality of life, as determined by TUG, PCS, and MCS. For the TUG test, important determinants in stepwise regression were age, BMI, knee pain, and hip pain. For the SF-36 PCS, important predictors were age, socioeconomic disadvantage, BMI, and foot, knee, and hip pain. For the SF-36, MCS, socioeconomic disadvantage, and foot pain were important predictors.

Conclusion.—The prevalence of lower extremity pain in elderly women in Australia is high. Lower extremity pain significantly diminishes both physical and mental aspects of the quality of life and mobility. More aggressive intervention in those most disabled by lower extremity pain is recommended.

► There is a consistent and compelling message emerging from these 4 articles (Abstracts 6–6 to 6–9) and an extensive corollary literature. The West is taking pride in its longevity. However, a substantial number of the elderly in the West are living longer absent joie de vivre. However, it is a feature of the culture that discourages that realization and disallows that complaint. The complaint that is acceptable is a somatic complaint, and in recent centuries, it is the complaint of musculoskeletal pain. A third of the elderly are hurting all the time. More than hurting, they feel awful and tend to live life under a pall. They will not outlive their blithe birth cohort. They are leaning on canes by their graveside. That is the implication of the article in *JAMA* (Abstract 6–6).

The 3 other articles are in the tradition of western medicine. What is hurting? And what is wrong with what is hurting? Hence, there is an article on persistent pectoral girdle pain in the elderly (Abstract 6–7), another on back pain in the elderly (Abstract 6–8), and a third on lower extremity pain in the elderly (Abstract 6–8). All point out that the elderly in pain function less well. All point out that the elderly in pain feel awful. All are suggesting interventions for the pain and interventions to compensate for the functional compromise in the particular anatomical region. All are missing the forest for the trees.

A third of the elderly are living under a pall. They can express their distress only in somatic terms, and the culture hears best the complaint of musculoskeletal pain. If life were not so bleak, perhaps they could cope more effectively. Will we ever be able to hear that complaint and act on it?

N. M. Hadler, MD

Cost Effectiveness of Physiotherapy, Manual Therapy, and General Practitioner Care for Neck Pain: Economic Evaluation Alongside a Randomised Controlled Trial

Korthals-de Bos IBC, Hoving JL, van Tulder MW, et al (VU Univ Med Centre, Amsterdam; Erasmus Univ, Rotterdam, The Netherlands)

BMJ 326:911-914, 2003 6–10

Introduction.—Neck problems are not life threatening yet do cause pain and stiffness that often result in use of health care resources, absenteeism from work, and disability. Many conservative interventions are available for treating neck pain, including analgesics prescribed by general practitioners, physiotherapy, and manual therapy. Information from randomized controlled trials concerning the effectiveness of these treatments is scarce. The cost-effectiveness of physiotherapy, manual therapy, and care by a general practitioner for patients with neck pain was examined.

Methods.—A total of 183 patients with neck pain for at least 2 weeks were recruited by 42 general practitioners and were randomly assigned to treatment with either manual therapy (spinal mobilization), physiotherapy (primarily exercise), or general practitioner care (counseling, education, drugs) in 60, 59, and 64 patients, respectively. The clinical outcomes included perceived recovery, intensity of pain, functional disability, and quality of life. Both direct and indirect costs were measured with the use of cost diaries that were kept by patients for 1 year. Differences in mean costs between groups, the cost-effectiveness, and cost utility ratios were assessed by applying nonparametric bootstrapping methods.

Results.—The manual therapy group experienced quicker improvement than did the physiotherapy group and the general practitioner care group up to 26 weeks; the differences were negligible by 52 weeks' follow-up. The total cost of manual therapy was significantly different from that of physiotherapy and general practitioner care (about one third the cost; $P = .01$; $P =$

.55 for general practitioner care vs physiotherapy). The cost-effectiveness ratios and the cost utility ratios revealed that manual therapy was less costly and more effective than physiotherapy or general practitioner care.

Conclusion.—Manual therapy (spinal mobilization) is more effective and less costly in treating neck pain than is physiotherapy or care given by a general practitioner.

▶ When will we come to understand the difference between *treatment* and *treatment act*?

Treatments are particular interventions, the modalities of therapeusis, if you will. For those who practice manual therapy (there are many forms, many of which are sectarian), the modality is the application of force to musculoskeletal structures. For physiotherapy (again the menu of modalities is extensive), the modality in this study was some sort of exercise. The general practitioners were instructed to spend 10 minutes each fortnight to educate, encourage, reassure, and, maybe, prescribe acetaminophen or an NSAID. We have very little data that any of these modalities will alter the natural history of neck pain of 2 weeks' duration.

The treatment acts are a human event. The patient is enveloped in the personality, language, and convictions of the therapist. The patient learns idioms of distress so that the narrative of illness is forever changed. In Amsterdam in the late 1990s, the manual therapy treatment act was cost-effective in provoking a narrative of perceived improvement. I suspect, as is the case elsewhere, that the cost-effectiveness will seem more problematic when it is shown that these patients are predisposed to returning for another manual therapy treatment act whenever they have their next regional musculoskeletal disorder.

N. M. Hadler, MD

Rapid Magnetic Resonance Imaging vs Radiographs for Patients With Low Back Pain: A Randomized Controlled Trial

Jarvik JG, Hollingworth W, Martin B, et al (Univ of Washington, Seattle; Minor and James Clinic PLLC, Seattle; Virginia Mason Med Ctr, Seattle; et al)

JAMA 289:2810-2818, 2003 6–11

Introduction.—Faster MRI scanning has made MRI a potential cost-effective replacement for radiographs in patients with low back pain. Whether rapid MRI scanning results in outcomes superior to that of radiographic evaluations or a cost-effective alternative is not known. The clinical outcomes and economic consequences of replacing spine radiographs with rapid MRI for primary care patients was examined in a randomized controlled trial.

Methods.—A total of 380 patients 18 years or older whose primary physicians had ordered radiographs for evaluation of their low back pain were evaluated between November 1998 and June 2000 at 1 of 4 imaging centers (a university-based teaching program, a non–university-based teaching program, and 2 private clinics). Patients were randomly assigned to receive lumbar spine evaluation by either rapid MRI or radiography. The primary outcome measure was back-related disability, determined by the modified Roland Questionnaire. The secondary outcome measures were the Medical Outcomes Study 36-Item Short-Form Health Survey (SF-36), pain, preference scores, satisfaction, and costs.

Results.—Measures of functional disability were obtained in 337 patients (89%) at a 12-month follow-up. The mean back-related disability modified Roland score for the 170 patients who received radiographic evaluation was 8.75 compared with 9.34 for the 167 patients who underwent rapid MRI evaluation (mean difference, −0.59; 95% CI, −1.69-0.87). The mean differences for secondary outcome measures were not statistically significant: pain bothersomeness (0.07; 95% CI, −0.88-1.22), pain frequency (0.12; 95% CI, −0.69-1.37), SF-36 subscales of bodily pain (1.25; 95% CI, −4.46-4.96), and physical functioning (2.73; 95% CI, −4.09-6.22). Ten patients in the rapid MRI group compared with 4 in the radiographic group underwent lumbar surgery (risk difference, 0.34; 95% CI, −0.06-0.73). The mean cost of the rapid MRI was $2380 compared with $2059 for the radiographic strategy (mean difference, $321; 95% CI, −$1100-$458).

Conclusion.—Rapid MRI and radiography produced nearly identical outcomes for patients with low back pain. Both physicians and patients preferred rapid MRI to radiography, yet this practice may offer little additional benefit to patients and may increase the cost of care because patients who undergo rapid MRI are more likely to undergo a spinal operation.

► The following comment is abstracted from Hadler NM: MRI for regional back pain: Need for less imaging, better understanding. *JAMA* 289:2863-2865, 2003.

Introduction.—The Jarvik and colleagues article reported that substituting rapid MRI neither saved money nor led to improved clinical outcomes. The use of rapid MRI increased costs because it predisposed patients to undergo surgical intervention. This randomized controlled trial adds to the ranks of illusionary appealing innovations. The importance of defining the anatomy of the lumbosacral spines of patients with regional back pain is questioned.

Less Imaging, Better Understanding.—Imaging the spine has been the practice of medical practitioners and the expectation of their patients for generations. Although imaging may not facilitate a return to well-being, it does contribute to patient satisfaction. Is this a valuable outcome or does it contribute to the persistence of illness? Imaging does not serve as a diagnostic modality in patients with regional back pain; rather, it is 1 element in a complex treatment act that endows patients with unfounded notions of pathophysiology. When a patient complains that "My back hurts," it may mean "My back hurts, but I'm really here because I can't cope with this episode right now." Almost everyone is repeatedly challenged by self-limiting regional musculoskeletal disorders that occur without extraordinary provocation. The accepted notion that back pain is the manifestation of underlying disease is flawed. Most theories suggest that something, somewhere in or near or about the back, has gone terribly wrong, yet no theory concerning regional back pain has withstood scientific testing. It seems that the role of imaging is to bolster the notion that back pain is nothing more than the symptom of an underlying disease. This social construct nurtures an immense treating enterprise far more than it benefits the patient. Few modalities have any demonstrable effectiveness.

Conclusion.—It is important for both practitioners and patients to abandon the thinking that back pain is the symptom of an underlying disease. Imaging bolsters this notion, is costly, and can factor into an increased incidence of surgical intervention. Patients may do better by managing back pain themselves and perhaps using some lay advice rather than becoming primary care patients. Patients may fare better if they would state, "I can't cope with this backache" when seeking care.

Consultation and the Outcome of Shoulder-Neck Pain: A Cohort Study in the Population

Badcock LJ, Lewis M, Hay EM, et al (Univ of Keele, Stoke-on-Trent, England; Staffordshire Rheumatology Centre, Stoke-on-Trent, England)
J Rheumatol 30:2694-2699, 2003 6–12

Background.—Shoulder pain is a common experience, affecting from 7% to 34% of adults at any given time. A number of studies have contradicted the commonly held view that shoulder pain is a benign and self-limiting problem. However, data from general practitioners in the United Kingdom have suggested that only a minority of individuals with shoulder pain seek health care at any one time. The effectiveness or influence of consultation on clinical outcomes and health status is unclear. Randomized controlled trials are considered to provide the most reliable guide to efficacy, but observational studies of outcomes in a broader sample of patients can provide an overall view of the influence of health care. The association between primary care consultation and subsequent outcomes in a cohort of patients with shoulder-neck pain was investigated.

Methods.—The study group was identified by questionnaires mailed to 4002 adults randomly selected from the register of 1 family practice. Research subjects were asked to shade areas of pain on a blank mannequin and to provide demographic details and scales of pain, anxiety, and depression. For the next 2 years, general practitioner consultations for shoulder and neck problems were determined with the use of the practice database. Persistence of pain and the degree of disability specific to the shoulder, as well as general health status, were assessed by survey at 2 years' follow-up.

Results.—A total of 224 respondents with unilateral shoulder-neck pain at baseline were included in the study. Of these patients, 47 (21%) consulted their general practitioners for shoulder-neck pain over the 2 years of the study (Table 2). Of these 47 consultations, 36 (77%) reported shoulder-neck pain at follow-up, which was a percentage that was higher than that for participants who did not have consultations (Table 3). Among all research subjects with persistent shoulder-neck pain, consulters were more likely than nonconsulters to have shoulder-related disabilities at follow-up. Consulters were also found to have more pain and lower levels of physical functioning

TABLE 2.—Baseline Factors Associated With GP Consultation for Shoulder or Neck Pain Among 224 Research Subjects With Unilateral Shoulder-Neck Pain at Baseline Assessment

	Total Number of Adults	No. (%) Who Consulted	RR* (95% CI)
Age			
18-54†	108	22 (20)	1.0
55-75	116	25 (22)	1.1 (0.6, 1.8)
Sex			
Females†	113	25 (22)	1.0
Males	111	22 (20)	0.9 (0.5, 1.5)
Employment status			
Not employed†	98	24 (25)	1.0
Employed	126	23 (18)	0.7 (0.4, 1.2)
Non-manual‡	60	10 (17)	0.7 (0.4, 1.3)
Manual‡	63	12 (19)	0.8 (0.4, 1.4)
Current pain score§			
Mild†	126	23 (18)	1.0
Severe	92	23 (25)	1.4 (0.8, 2.3)
Duration of pain			
< 3 months†	85	15 (18)	1.0
≥ 3 months	133	32 (24)	1.4 (0.8, 2.4)
Psychological distress‖			
No†	134	26 (19)	1.0
Yes	90	21 (23)	1.2 (0.7, 2.0)
Co-morbidity			
No†	60	17 (28)	1.0
Yes	164	30 (18)	0.6 (0.4, 1.1)

*Crude risk ratios.

†Reference category for risk ratio analysis.

‡Categories were defined according to the Standard Occupational Classification, ONS 1991. Percentages are total of those 123 research subjects who reported being employed and who filled-in their job description at baseline assessment.

§ Current pain score dichotomy was based on the following cutoff: 1-5, mild; 6-10, severe.

‖HAD categories were based on the following cutoff: 0-7, no psychological distress; ≥8, psychological distress.

Abbreviations: GP, General practitioner; *HAD*, Hospital Anxiety and Depression Scale.

(Courtesy of Badcock LJ, Lewis M, Hay EM, et al: Consultation and the outcome of shoulder-neck pain: A cohort study in the population. *J Rheumatol* 30:2694-2699, 2003.)

TABLE 3.—Association Between GP Consultation for Shoulder or Neck Problems and Persistent Shoulder–Neck Pain at Follow-up Among 224 Adults With Shoulder-Neck Pain at Baseline

	Persistent Pain			
	Yes	No	RR* (95% CI)	RR† (95% CI)
GP consultation				
No‡	101 (57%)	76 (43%)	1.0	1.0
Yes	36 (77%)	11 (23%)	1.3 (1.1, 1.6)	1.3 (0.8, 1.8)

*Crude risk ratios.

†Risk ratio adjusted for age, sex, employment status, current pain severity, duration of pain, psychological distress, and co-morbid musculoskeletal pain at baseline, and GP consultation during follow-up for URTI.

‡Reference category for statistical analysis.

Abbreviations: GP, General practitioner; *URTI*, upper respiratory tract infection.

(Courtesy of Badcock LJ, Lewis M, Hay EM, et al: Consultation and the outcome of shoulder-neck pain: A cohort study in the population. *J Rheumatol* 30:2694-2699, 2003.)

at follow-up than were nonconsulters, as measured on the Medical Outcome Study Short Form-36.

Conclusions.—Among research subjects with shoulder-neck pain, the relatively few individuals who sought consultation with a primary care practitioner had no better outcomes in terms of pain and disability than did those individuals who did not seek consultation. These findings call into question the current influence of medical care on the natural history of shoulder-neck pain.

▶ I have been writing for 20 years about the forces that drive a person who is coping with a regional musculoskeletal predicament to choose to be a patient with a regional musculoskeletal illness.[1] Those forces are difficult to discern in epidemiologic studies, as is apparent in Table 2. They relate to perceptions of the intensity of pain by each individual, tempered by the psychosocial context in which the pain is suffered. There is a difference between pain and suffering. Epidemiology is a field of study that evaluates the behavior of groups of people and attempts to discern common threads and capture those threads with a statistic. Fortunately, no statistical model is a match for the heterogeneity that is life and the individual differences that make people so interesting. Table 2 is missing something special about each individual that cannot be captured by applying a single measure. Each person has an idiosyncratic reason to choose to be a patient. The task for the physician is to recognize the idiosyncrasy and address it.

However, that is not what is happening. The physicians are focusing on the painful region and not the suffering patient. The outcome is dismal (Table 2). As I've said for backaches,[2] these people would do better not telling their physicians they were hurting unless their physicians can hear that they are suffering also.

N. M. Hadler, MD

References

1. Hadler NM: *Occupational Musculoskeletal Disorders*, ed 3. Philadelphia, Lippincott Williams & Wilkins, 2004.
2. Hadler NM: MRI for regional back pain. Need for less imaging, better understanding. *JAMA* 289:2863-2865, 2003.

Patient Characteristics Associated With Opioid Versus Nonsteroidal Anti-inflammatory Drug Management of Chronic Low Back Pain

Breckenridge J, Clark JD (Veterans Affairs Palo Alto Health Care System, Calif; Stanford Univ, Palo Alto, Calif)

J Pain 4:344-350, 2003 6–13

Introduction.—Opioids are the mainstay for a wide variety of moderate and severe pain. Only limited data are available concerning the use of opioids in chronic pain states. There are many guidelines for the prescription of opioids for chronic nonmalignant pain. However, it is not clear which factors are involved when providers initiate and maintain opioid therapy. Patient characteristics associated with the treatment of chronic low back pain with opioids versus nonsteroidal anti-inflammatory drugs (NSAIDs) were examined in 2 groups of patients with chronic low back pain.

Methods.—Medical records of 2 groups of 100 patients each were reviewed to obtain and tabulate health care utilization factors and demographic, medical, and psychological information. Group N patients received long-term NSAID therapy for pain management, and group O received long-term opioids. The identities of the specific analgesics were determined.

Results.—Regression analysis identified 4 variables closely associated with the use of opioids for treatment of back pain in preference to NSAIDs alone: age, depression, personality disorder, and history of substance abuse. Pain intensity was not predictive of opioid use.

Conclusion.—Analgesia is not likely to be the only reason patients with chronic pain take opioids. Physicians ultimately decide which drug is prescribed, but there are patient characteristics that affect drug choices. Management with alternative therapies may have failed for patients who take opioids. Patients with psychiatric disorders may be less likely to respond to alternative therapies. Patients with depression, substance abuse, and personality disorders may present themselves in such a manner that they appear to be in need of more help, which could result in more aggressive therapy in the form of opioids. All these factors are linked to poor coping skills.

► There is a "pain" lobby. These are staunch advocates of the plight of patients suffering from pain. Thanks to their efforts, medicine has learned how to be more effective in treating such patients. If the pain is palliated with opiates, the suffering is relieved. There have been major advances in improving the lot of patients with postoperative pain and patients with pain from metastatic cancers. Because of the advocacy and the success in these 2 settings, pain scores are now to be considered another vital sign like blood pressure, pulse rate, and temperature and are to be recorded by regulatory fiat.

However, the success in these clinical arenas does not generalize readily to other areas of clinical medicine. There are patients who are stricken with suffering *and* pain, not suffering *from* pain. In these clinical circumstances, treating the pain will not alleviate the suffering completely, if at all, and will leave the patient at the mercy of the complications of analgesic therapy, without the benefits. For that reason, rheumatologists uniformly have found that opiates seldom advantage patients with RA whose pain is but a component of their illness experience. For that reason, rheumatologists eschew opiates for elderly patients with knee, hip, or shoulder pain in the setting of osteoarthritis. Pain scores are incomprehensible to these patients and, therefore, are useless as indicators for management. When asked about their pain scores, patients with RA are likely to respond with "which joint?" or "when?"

Patients with chronic low back pain are seldom "patients;" they are usually claimants in medicolegal contests regarding disability determination. That is almost certainly true of the veterans sampled from the Stanford's affiliated Veteran's Administration Hospital and described in this article. Those prescribed opiates were suffering an illness confounded by psychosocial adversities and challenges. These psychosocial confounders certainly color their experience of illness, if not dominate the experience. Treating them with opiates makes no sense and has never proven effective in returning them to well-being.

N. M. Hadler, MD

Prolotherapy Injections, Saline Injections, and Exercises for Chronic Low-Back Pain: A Randomized Trial

Yelland MJ, Glasziou PP, Bogduk N, et al (Univ of Queensland, Brisbane, Australia; Univ of Newcastle, Australia)

Spine 29:9-16, 2004 6–14

Introduction.—The premise of prolotherapy is that low-back pain results from weakened ligaments, and that these ligaments can be strengthened by injection into them of irritant proliferant solutions. The efficacy of a prolotherapy injection and exercise protocol in the treatment of chronic nonspecific low-back pain was examined in a randomized, controlled trial with 2-by-2 factorial design, triple-blinded for injection status, and single-blinded for exercise status.

Methods.—A total of 110 participants with nonspecific low-back pain with an average 14-year duration were randomized to undergo repeated prolotherapy (20% glucose/0.2% lignocaine) or normal saline injections into tender lumbo-pelvic ligaments and randomized to perform either flexion/extension exercises or normal activity during a 6 month evaluation period. The primary outcome measures were pain intensity (VAS) and disability scores (Roland-Morris) at 2.5, 4, 6, 12, and 24 months.

Results.—Follow-up was achieved in 96% and 80% of patients at 12 months and 2 years, respectively. Ligament injections with exercises and normal activity produced significant and sustained decreases in pain and disability throughout the trial. No attributable effect was identified for prolotherapy injection over saline injection, or for exercises over normal activity. At 12-month follow-up, the proportions achieving over a 50% decrease in pain from baseline by injection group were glucose-lignocaine: 0.46 versus saline: 0.36. By activity group, these proportions were exercise: 0.41 versus normal activity: 0.39. Corresponding proportions for > 50% decrease in disability were glucose-lignocaine: 0.42 vs saline 0.36 and exercise: 0.36 versus normal activity: 0.38. There were no between-group differences in any of these measures.

Conclusion.—In chronic nonspecific low-back pain, significant and sustained decreases in pain and disability are observed with ligament injections, irrespective of the solution injected or the concurrent use of exercises.

► This is a reasonably well done trial. I am always concerned about design issue when the intervention is potentially painful, as is prolotherapy, which often requires adjuvant analgesia. The study population is remarkable—a hundred middle-aged adults whose prior decade of life was colored by persistent low-back pain. Prolotherapy was no better than placebo injections, or an exercise regimen, or leaving them alone. This is neither surprising nor particularly interesting.

However, the paper is interesting and, for me, disconcerting. The authors point out that the patients they injected tended to have an important degree of palliation whether injected with a sclerosant or saline. Therefore, they advocate injection therapy. It harkens to an earlier, less enlightened age when physicians prescribed placebos. I cannot countenance such a therapeutic posture. Firstly, I cannot countenance "fooling" a patient. Secondly, I doubt that placebo therapy works twice—what are you going to do for an encore?

No. For me the take-home message is that participation in the trial, even in one of the placebo limbs, was associated with a diminished need to perceive the pain as intense. This may be simply a function of time, but I surmise it is a function of the interactions with the investigative team that altered the perception. There must be a way to do that without fooling the patient.

N. M. Hadler, MD

Effectiveness of Dynamic Muscle Training, Relaxation Training, or Ordinary Activity for Chronic Neck Pain: Randomised Controlled Trial

Viljanen M, Malmivaara A, Uitti J, et al (Tampere Regional Inst of Occupational Health, Finland; Natl Research and Development Centre for Welfare and Health, Helsinki; Urho Kaleva Kekkonen Inst for Health Promotion Research, Tampere, Finland; et al)

BMJ 327:475-477, 2003 6–15

Background.—About 67% of adults have neck pain at some time in their lives. Because the underlying pathologic mechanism of this condition is unknown, treatments are directed toward pain relief. The efficacy of dynamic muscle training and relaxation training was investigated for chronic neck pain.

Methods.—Three hundred ninety-three office workers with chronic nonspecific neck pain were enrolled in the randomized controlled study at 5 occupational centers in Finland. All participants were women (mean age, 45 years). The women were assigned to 12 weeks of dynamic muscle training or relaxation, plus 1 week of reinforcement training 6 months after baseline, or to a control group that performed ordinary activities.

Findings.—At follow-up 3, 6, and 12 months later, the 3 groups did not differ in their neck pain intensity (Figure). Measures of neck disability and sick leave also did not differ. The training groups had significant increases in range of motion for cervical rotation and lateral flexion compared with the control group, but this was not relevant clinically. Participants in the training groups reported better subjective recovery.

Conclusions.—Neither dynamic muscle training nor relaxation training lessens pain intensity or neck disability in female office workers with chronic

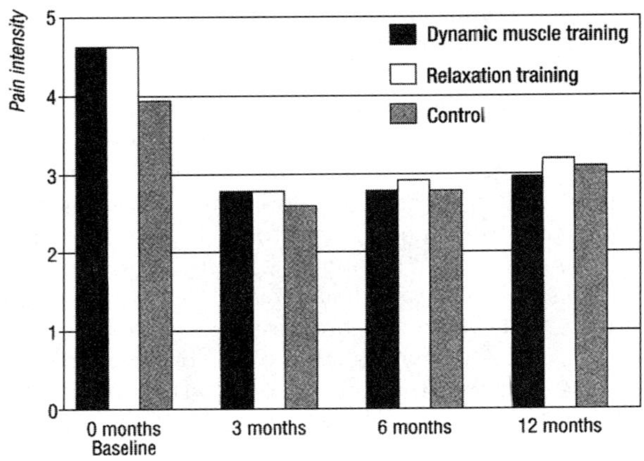

FIGURE.—Intensity of neck pain at baseline and follow-up after dynamic muscle training, relaxation training, or ordinary activity. (Courtesy of Viljanen M, Malmivaara A, Uitti J, et al: Effectiveness of dynamic muscle training, relaxation training, or ordinary activity for chronic neck pain: Randomised controlled trial. *BMJ* 327:475-477, 2003, with permission from the BMJ Publishing Group.)

neck pain. The slight improvement in cervical range of motion in the training groups did not seem to be clinically important.

► This group of Finnish investigators is world-class. They are whipping a dead horse, and I suspect that, at some level, they are doing so intentionally. This study represents considerable effort. It is beautifully designed. Is the implication that these women are better off left alone? After all, the results (see Fig) document that neither training their muscles nor their mind did them any good.

No one should be surprised. There is a wealth of data, including pioneering studies by Steve Linton in Sweden, supporting the premise that regional musculoskeletal complaints in workers are surrogate complaints. Yes, they have neck discomfort, as do we all intermittently throughout the year. Most of us most of the time find some way to carry on until the discomfort remits, and the episode fades rapidly from memory. When people need to seek professional help, more often than not, the issue is less the pain and more the aspects of life that thwart coping. For workers, those aspects are often embedded in the psychosocial context of working and not in the physical demands of tasks.

If there is a successful intervention, it relates to work architecture rather than spinal or cerebral anatomy.

N. M. Hadler, MD

Active Intervention in Patients With Whiplash-Associated Disorders Improves Long-term Prognosis: A Randomized Controlled Clinical Trial

Rosenfeld M, Seferiadis A, Carlsson J, et al (Göteborg Univ, Sweden)

Spine 28:2491-2498, 2003 6–16

Introduction.—Whiplash-associated disorders (WAD) account for a large proportion of medical injuries. A recent trial assessing the long-term effects of WAD resulting from a motor vehicle accident (MVA) reported that 55% of participants had residual sequelae 17 years later. The long-term efficacy of active versus standard intervention in patients with WAD was prospectively assessed, along with the importance of early versus delayed initiation of intervention.

Methods.—The study included 97 patients who were randomly selected to an intervention in which frequent active cervical rotation was used complemented by evaluation and treatment, according to McKenzie's principles or to a standard intervention consisting of initial rest, recommended soft collar, and graded self-mobilization. To assess the time factor, interventions were either made within 96 hours or delayed 14 days from the MVA. The effects of the 2 interventions and the time factor on pain intensity, cervical range of motion (ROM), and sick leave were evaluated at 6 months and 3 years. The cervical ROM at 3 years was also compared with that of matched, unexposed individuals.

Results.—Pain intensity and sick leave were significantly less in the active versus the standard intervention group ($P < .05$). Delaying intervention by 2 weeks did not impact the outcome variables. At 3 years, only patients who received early active intervention had total cervical ROM similar to that of matched unexposed persons.

Conclusion.—Active intervention is more effective than standard intervention in decreasing pain intensity and sick leave and in retaining or regaining total ROM in patients with WAD. Active intervention can be performed as home exercises, initiated and supported by appropriately educated health professionals.

Low Back Pain After Traffic Collisions: A Population-Based Cohort Study

Cassidy JD, Carroll L, Côté P, et al (Univ of Alberta, Edmonton, Canada; Univ of Toronto)

Spine 28:1002-1009, 2003 6–17

Introduction.—In the occupational setting, low back injury is insured by workers' compensation. It provides no-fault insurance benefits to injured workers. Employers are not held liable for injuries, and claimants are not eligible for pain and suffering benefits. In the setting of traffic injury, most jurisdictions allow claimants who are not at fault to receive payment for pain and suffering (tort law). However, concern has been expressed that compensation for pain and suffering may be detrimental to recovery. The effect of changing from tort to no-fault insurance on the incidence and prognosis for collision-associated low back pain was assessed in a population-based, incidence cohort.

Methods.—An incidence cohort of 4473 low back pain injury claims was formed between July 1, 1994 and December 31, 1995 in the Canadian Province of Saskatchewan. On January 1, 1995, the public insurance system changed from a tort system to a no-fault system that eliminated compensation for pain and suffering. The incidence of claims and the time-to-claim closure were determined before and after this change. Prognostic models were created using baseline and follow-up data.

Results.—The 6-month incidence of claims decreased from 256 to 175 per 100,000 after the change in insurance systems. The median time-to-claim closure diminished from 505 days for tort claims to 210 days and 216 days for claims made during the first and second 6 months, respectively, of the no-fault period. Improvement in bodily pain and physical functioning and the absence of depressive symptoms were linked with faster claim closure. High pain intensity, female sex, full-time employment, concentration problems, and lawyer involvement early in the claim process delayed claim closure.

Conclusion.—The incidence and prognosis of low back pain caused by traffic injury is affected by many factors, including the type of compensation system. Findings from this investigation suggest that biopsychosocial factors are important determinants of prognosis.

► WAD is a classic example of a social construction. This is a concept that is "common sense," but the basis for the credibility is inferential reasoning rather than serious scientific testing, and the basis for the consensus is advocacy by a cadre of effective believers. Social constructions are part of the fabric of life—and always will be. Society advances when social constructions are identified and tested. WAD has been in the public arena for some time. Only recently have we been made to realize that there is more than 1 public arena. It turns out that there are countries where the consequences of rear-end collisions are transient and self-limited, and others where a significant minority of the people in the car that is struck (seldom is this the fate of occupants of the car that does the striking) go on to a prolonged and complex chronic pain state in the absence of demonstrable damage. Such is rarely the fate of motor vehicle accident victims in Lithuania,[1,2] Greece,[3] or Germany[4], whereas it is commonplace in Canada, Switzerland and the United States. It was argued that these differences reflected the differences in tort systems. After all, Swedes who choose not to pursue litigation following rear-end collisions suffer no long-term consequences compared to Swedes who sue regardless of the violence of the collision.[5] However, the "evil tort" argument was tenuous until the studies from Saskatchewan.[6] When Saskatchewan went to a no-fault system that eliminated awards for pain and suffering, the incidence of WAD plummeted with no demonstrable long-term health consequences.[7] The article by Cassidy et al (Abstract 6–17) is another observation derived from the Saskatchewan experience. WAD is a social construction that plays out in the recesses of the medicolegal enterprise.[8]

Once that is realized, it is possible to return to the biomechanical data without preconception[9] and to speak of the biopsychosocial models of illness. That is the approach taken by the British multidisciplinary team in their recent publication "The Whiplash Book,"[10] which debunks the WAD social construction in a fashion that allows the patient to avoid a litigious vortex. However, the patient will not be well served unless the treating physicians are willing to act on this science. Recently, the Cochrane Collaboration has undertaken a systematic review of the literature that bears on the treatment modalities afforded patients with WAD.[11] The Cochrane Collaboration is an international collaboration of health service researchers, funded by many sources including the National Institutes of Health, that undertake to collect, select for quality, and synthesize the literature on many clinical topics. The WAD literature is notably lacking in high-quality studies. However, there is enough to suggest that patients with neck pain following putative "whiplash" trauma who have suffered no demonstrable tissue damage should avoid rest and collars and pursue active interventions, notably "maintain usual activities." The Cochrane Collaboration reached that conclusion before the article by Rosenfeld et al (Abstract 6–16) appeared. The conclusion is based on sounder science, thanks to this article.

N. M. Hadler, MD

References

1. Schrader H, Obelieniene D, Bovim G, et al: Natural evolution of late whiplash syndrome outside medicolegal context. *Lancet* 347:1207-1211, 1996.
2. Obelieniene D, Schrader H, Bovim G, et al: Pain after whiplash—a prospective controlled inception cohort study. *J Neurol Neurosurg Psychiatry* 66:279-283, 1999.
3. Partheni M, Constantoyannis C, Ferrari R, et al: A prospective cohort study of the outcome of acute whiplash injury in Greece. *Clin Exp Rheumatol* 18:67-70, 2000.
4. Bonk A, Ferrari R, Giebel GD, et al: A prospective randomized controlled outcome study of two trials of therapy for whiplash injury. *J Musculoskeletal Pain* 8:123-132, 2000.
5. Berglund AA, Alfredsson L, Cassidy JD, et al: The association between exposure to a rear-end collision and future neck or shoulder pain: a cohort study. *J Clin Epidem* 53:1089-1094, 2000.
6. Cassidy JD, Carroll L, Cote P, et al: Effect of eliminating compensation for pain and suffering on the outcome of insurance claims for whiplash injury. *N Engl J Med* 342:1179:1186, 2000.
7. Berglund A, Alfredsson L, Jensen I, et al: The association between exposure to a rear-end collision and future health complaints. *J Clin Epidemiol* 54:851-856, 2001.
8. Malleson A: *Whiplash and Other Useful Illnesses.* Montreal, McGill-Queen's University Press, 2002.
9. Ferrari R, Russell AS: The engineering of whiplash: A clinician's work is never done. *Arthritis Care Res* 13:443-455, 2000.
10. Waddell G, Burton K, McClune T: *The Whiplash Book*. London, The Stationery Office, 2001.
11. Verhagen AP, Peeters GGM, de Bie RA, et al: Conservative treatment for whiplash, in *The Cochrane Library*, vol. 4, Oxford: Update Software. 2001.

Does Early Intervention With a Light Mobilization Program Reduce Long-term Sick Leave for Low Back Pain: A 3-Year Follow-up Study

Hagen EM, Grasdal A, Eriksen HR (Hedmark Central Hosp, Ottestad, Norway; Univ of Bergen, Norway)

Spine 28:2309-2316, 2003 6–18

Introduction.—Most patients with back pain will recover quickly, regardless of the treatment approach. For those with long-lasting back pain, uncertainty remains regarding the optimum treatment. The longer a patient is off from work because of low back pain (LBP), the greater the risk of chronic pain and the lower the chance of ever returning to work. The long-term clinical and economic effects of a light mobilization program on the duration of sick leave was investigated in patients with subacute LBP.

Methods.—Four hundred fifty-seven patients placed on sick leave for 8 to 12 months for LBP were randomly assigned to either an intervention or control group (237 and 220 patients, respectively). The intervention group was evaluated at a spine clinic and was given information and advice concerning staying active. Control subjects were not examined at the spine clinic. They were treated within the primary health care system.

Results.—During a 3-year observation period, the intervention group had significantly fewer days of sickness compensation than did control subjects (125.7 vs 169.6 days per person). This difference was primarily because of a more rapid return to work during the first year. No significant differences were observed during the second and third years. The risk of a recurrence of LBP was not increased because of an early return to work. At 6-months' follow-up, the only significant between-group difference was in the use of stretching and walking to cope with LBP in the intervention group versus in the control group. This effect diminished over time. At 12-months' follow-up, the only significant between-group difference was in the use of stretching. Economic returns of the intervention were calculated in measures of increases in the net present value of production for society because of the decrease in the number of days sick leave was taken. The net benefits accumulated over 3 years of treating the 237 patients in the intervention group totaled about $2822 per person.

Conclusion.—In patients with subacute LBP, a short and simple early intervention of physical examination, information, reassurance, and encouragement to engage in as normal physical activity as possible yielded economic gains for society. The effect was observed only during the first year after the intervention. The initial gain obtained during the first year did not produce increased costs or risks of a recurrence.

► Introduction.—Norway, population 4.3 million, is a resource-advantaged, relatively homogeneous, highly progressive nation that has provided its citizenry with a comprehensive social security program for more than half a century. The Norwegian Royal Ministry of Health and Social Affairs has been reevaluating this system for the past decade. Discussed are insights into the limitations of this program in the provision for workers with a chronic disabling regional backache.

Workers and Regional Back Pain.—Norwegian workers with disabling regional backache can take sickness absence without financial penalty. The cost of the first 2 weeks of regional backache is assumed by the employer, then by the National Insurance Administration thereafter. About 85% of workers return to work within 2 weeks. The greatest effort at reform is focused on workers who have not returned to work by the end of 2 to 3 months. About one third of these never return to work. About 10 years ago, the National Insurance Administration started underwriting full wages for workers with disabling regional back pain who returned to modified duties at the job site. To date, there has been no more effective intervention. A multidisciplinary intervention designed to educate and reassure the worker may influence only a small number of workers still disabled at 2 months who were otherwise destined for long-term disability. Workers are persons who are gainfully employed; persons with chronic disabling regional backache are actually insurance claimants. Persons with insurmountable regional backache in Norway are distinctive in that "life inside the workplace and outside the workplace succors them not . . . they have multiple somatic symptoms and are usually tired and worn out."

Conclusion.—For persons with disabling backache, a goal of return to work may be too narrow a public health goal and "likely to prove iatrogenic in its pursuit."

N. M. Hadler, MD

Graded Activity for Low Back Pain in Occupational Health Care: A Randomized Controlled Trial

Staal JB, Hlobil H, Twisk JWR, et al (VU Univ, Amsterdam; Univ Hosp Maastricht, The Netherlands; Body@Work Research Ctr, Amsterdam)

Ann Intern Med 140:77-84, 2004 6–19

Introduction.—Some workers with low back pain miss work for several days to weeks and are at risk for more permanent disability. To decrease the individual and socioeconomic burden associated with this burden, effective intervention strategies are needed in occupational health care settings that promote both safe and rapid return to work. The effectiveness of a behavior-oriented graded activity program compared with usual care was assessed in a single-blind, randomized, controlled, trial in an occupational health services center of an airline company in The Netherlands.

Methods.—A total of 134 workers absent from work because of low back pain were randomly assigned to either graded activity or to usual care. Graded activity is a physical exercise program that is based on operant conditioning behavioral principles to augment a quick return to work. Patients were followed for the number of absence from work because of low back pain, functional status (Roland Disability Questionnaire), and severity of pain (1-point numerical scale).

Results.—The median number of days of absence from work during a 6-month follow-up was 58 days in the graded activity group and 87 days in the usual care group. After randomization, graded activity was effective after 50 days of absence from work (hazard ratio, 1.9 [95% CI, 1.2-3.2]; *P* = .009). The graded activity group was more effective in improving functional status and pain, compared with the usual care group; differences were small and not statistically significant.

Conclusion.—Graded activity was more effective versus usual care in decreasing the number of days of absence from work because of low back pain.

► This article needs to be contrasted with Abstract 3–21. Why does "graded activity" seem to be helpful for KLM employees at Schiphol Airport whereas the Norwegian experience with a multidisciplinary approach was dismal? Both studies recruited workers on sick leave for more than a month for work-related back pain. Perhaps the Dutch emphasis on physical modalities was the secret. Perhaps KLM workers are more advantaged in terms of salary or work architecture than the more general sample of Norwegian workers. Perhaps the distinctive nature of the Dutch social insurance scheme ("injury" is not at issue in determining benefits) produces less impedance to returning to work. I suspect the answer to the difference lies in notions such as these. After all, there are very few reports describing this degree of success in returning workers disabled from back pain to the workforce.

N. M. Hadler, MD

Tumor Necrosis Factor-α Monoclonal Antibody, Infliximab, Used to Manage Severe Sciatica

Karppinen J, Korhonen T, Malmivaara A, et al (Oulu Univ, Finland; Finnish Inst of Occupational Health, Helsinki; Orton Hosp, Helsinki)

Spine 28:750-754, 2003 6–20

Background.—Sciatica has traditionally been blamed on compression of nerve roots or dorsal root ganglions by the herniated nucleus pulposus (HNP), but inflammatory factors have now been identified. Tumor necrosis factor-α (TNF-α) is active in HNP-induced nerve root damage. Exogenous TNF α produces neuropathologic changes similar to those produced by the nucleus pulposus (NP). An NP-induced porcine nerve conduction block can be reversed with etanercept. Infliximab is used to manage RA and similar chronic conditions. Its efficacy and safety when given as a single IV infusion to patients with severe sciatica coming for surgical treatment were evaluated.

Methods.—Infliximab was given to 10 patients with disk herniation–induced severe sciatica. The IV dosage was 3 mg/kg over 2 hours. Outcomes were evaluated after 1 hour, 1 week, 2 weeks, 1 month, and 3 months. The historical data on 62 patients who received saline solution in a trial of periradicular infiltration for sciatica were compared with the outcomes for the

10 patients. A painless state was defined as a decrease of more than 75% in leg pain from baseline.

Results.—Both groups had a decline of leg and back pain of about 50% after 1 hour (Table 2). Sixty percent of the infliximab group and 16% of the control subjects reported a painless state after 2 weeks. At 1 month, a painless state was reported by 70% of the infliximab group but by only 27% of the control subjects. After 3 months, 90% of the infliximab group and 46% of the control subjects reported painlessness. The improvements in the infliximab group in terms of leg pain and back-related disability were significantly better than those seen in control subjects. All patients taking infliximab were able to return to work after 1 month, but 38% of control subjects

TABLE 2.—Outcomes of Patients With Sciatica Receiving IV Infliximab or Periradicular Infiltration of Isotonic Saline (Historical Controls) at Follow-up Assessments

	IV Infliximab (n = 10)	Periradicular Saline (n = 62)	Change From Baseline‡	
			IV Infliximab	Periradicular Saline
Baseline				
Leg pain	80 ± 18	76 ± 19		
Back pain	76 ± 18	60 ± 25		
Oswestry	43 ± 21	44 ± 15		
SLR	46 ± 8	54 ± 17		
Schober	3.9 ± 1.4	4.6 ± 1.4		
One hour*				
Leg pain	39 ± 28	43 ± 29	−51	−43
Back pain	39 ± 28	29 ± 27	−49	−52
One week†				
Leg pain	26 ± 21		−68	
Back pain	30 ± 19		−61	
Two weeks				
Leg pain	19 ± 20	57 ± 32	−76	−25
Back pain	20 ± 15	38 ± 28	−74	−37
Oswestry	15 ± 10	35 ± 18	−65	−20
SLR	69 ± 17	66 ± 21	+50	+22
Schober	5.1 ± 1.0	4.6 ± 1.2	+31	±0
One Month				
Leg pain	18 ± 19	47 ± 32	−78	−38
Back pain	19 ± 17	32 ± 28	−75	−47
Oswestry	15 ± 9	30 ± 17	−65	−32
SLR	74 ± 18	70 ± 21	+61	+30
Schober	5.1 ± 1.0	4.6 ± 1.4	+31	±0
Three months				
Leg pain	10 ± 16	37 ± 35	−88	−51
Back pain	16 ± 18	24 ± 28	−79	−60
Oswestry	7 ± 6	24 ± 20	−84	−45
SLR	82 ± 16	79 ± 17	+78	+46
Schober	5.5 ± 0.9	5.1 ± 1.3	+41	+11

Note: Outcomes include leg and back pain (mm on 100-mm visual analog scale), Oswestry Disability (%), SLR (°), and modified Schober (cm). Values are presented as means ± SD.

*n = 8 and 61 in the infliximab and periradicular saline groups, respectively.

†Only in the infliximab group.

‡Percentage change from baseline values. Negative values indicate improvement in symptoms, except for SLR and Schober, and positive values indicate lesser restriction or better mobility.

Abbreviation: SLR, Straight leg raising test.

(Courtesy of Karppinen J, Korhonen T, Malmivaara A, et al: Tumor necrosis factor-α monoclonal antibody, infliximab, used to manage severe sciatica. *Spine* 28(8):750-754, 2003.)

were still taking sick leave. Surgery was not required for any of the patients taking infliximab within the 3 months of follow-up, but 9 of the control subjects had surgery during this time. No adverse drug reactions or adverse effects of infliximab were reported.

Conclusions.—The use of IV infliximab provided dramatic, immediate, and effective pain relief for 70% to 90% of the patients with severe sciatica. The effect was maintained for 3 months, and no adverse drug effects occurred. All patients were able to return to work within 1 month, and none required surgery.

► I never would have thought about using TNF-α antagonists for sciatica, but, apparently, TNF-α plays a role in disk-mediated nerve damage and resultant symptoms. Yes, the study was open; yes, the numbers were small; but the results were very impressive: 50% pain reduction in 1 hour, 60% of patients pain free in 2 weeks, and 90% pain free at 3 months, and all patients in the infliximab-treated group were back at work by 1 month. I almost can't wait to see the data from a proper trial.

R. S. Panush, MD

Upper Extremity Pain

A Randomized Comparative Study of Short Term Response to Blind Injection Versus Sonographic-Guided Injection of Local Corticosteroids in Patients With Painful Shoulder

Naredo E, Cabero F, Beneyto P, et al (Severo Ochoa Hosp, Madrid)
J Rheumatol 31:308-314, 2004 6–21

Background.—Patients with painful shoulder are often given local injections of long-acting corticosteroids. The efficacy and effectiveness of these injections have been questioned, but the problem may relate to the placement of the steroid. High-frequency US is generally available, safe, and easy to use as a guide for musculoskeletal fluid aspiration, infiltration, or biopsy. The effectiveness of sonographically guided local corticosteroid injection in patients with periarticular shoulder disorders in contrast to the results of blind injection was investigated.

Methods.—Forty-one consecutive patients with painful shoulder were studied, none of whom had previous trauma or chronic inflammatory arthritis or had previously received physiotherapy or local steroid injections. Group 1 included 20 patients who received a blind subacromial injection of 20 mg triamcinolone. Group 2 consisted of 21 patients who received the triamcinolone injection under sonographic guidance. Documentation included shoulder abnormalities and placement of the steroid after injection as determined on US. Clinical assessments were made 5 days before and 6 weeks after the injection.

Results.—Initially, the 2 groups were similar in all aspects. After 6 weeks, group 2 had a significantly greater improvement in Shoulder Function Assessment (SFA) and visual analogue scale (VAS) scores in comparison to group 1. Patients in group 1 experienced a mean decline in the VAS score of

7.1, while those in group 2 had a mean decline of 34.9. After 6 weeks, 1 group 2 and 7 group 1 patients had a worse VAS score. Five patients in group 2 had a worse SFA score. Ten patients in group 1 and 2 in group 2 had nocturnal pain 6 weeks after injection.

Impaired active shoulder motion was present in 20 group 1 and 9 group 2 patients at 6 weeks. Nonsteroidal antiinflammatory drugs were taken by 12 patients in each group. One patient in group 1 had a mild increase in pain after injection, but this was seen in none of the group 2 patients. After injection, the corticosteroid was found in the deltoid muscle just superficial to the subacromial-subdeltoid (SA-SD) bursa in 7 group 1 patients. It was found within a tendon in 6 patients, in the SA-SD bursa in 3, and in both the deltoid muscle and the SA-SD bursa in 3. No steroid was detected in 1 patient.

All of the group 2 patients had corticosteroid delivered accurately. However, 6 weeks after injection in 1 patient, it was found in the deltoid muscle and SA-SD bursa, and in 1 it was in the SA-SD bursa and a supraspinatus tendon tear.

Conclusion.—The best way to achieve accurate injection of corticosteroid in patients with painful shoulder was shown to be under sonographic guidance. This method is especially needed in patients who had a poor response to previous blind injection to ensure that medication is placed accurately.

► Studies like these are humbling. I have previously commented about the inaccuracy of our so-called "intra-articular" and soft tissue injections. But I have always thought that, as my kids used to say, they were like horseshoes and hand grenades: It was OK if you were close. This article not only reaffirms that even the best rheumatologists will frequently miss anatomical sites but further shows that there may be clinical consequences with suboptimal therapeutic responses. However, I'm skeptical that injection therapy offers lasting benefit, and at our medical center, like many in the states, musculoskeletal US is not readily available (too time-consuming and expensive). So I will probably continue to do what I've always done: do my best with local injections and repeat them if clinical benefit was incomplete.

R. S. Panush, MD

Outcome Expectancies, Functional Outcomes, and Expectancy Fulfillment for Patients With Shoulder Problems

O'Malley KJ, Roddey TS, Gartsman GM, et al (Baylor College of Medicine, Houston; Texas Woman's Univ, Houston; Univ of Texas; Houston; et al)

Med Care 42:139-146, 2004 6–22

Introduction.—Patient outcome expectancies are considered to be patients' perceptions that an outcome of medical care is likely to occur. Few trials have examined outcome expectations in persons treated for shoulder problems. The association between patient outcome expectancies, perceived shoulder function changes, and perceptions of expectancy fulfillment was investigated.

Methods.—One hundred ninety-nine patients consecutively recruited during a 4-month period (May-August) who were being treated for shoulder problems at 1 orthopedic surgeon's office completed a baseline survey. The survey addressed measures of outcome expectancies, shoulder function, health status, and demographics. At 1 month, 2 months, and 3 months, patients completed a mailed follow-up survey addressing all of the baseline measurements except demographic variables.

A measure of expectancy fulfillment was added to the 3-month follow-up survey (Table 1). A general linear modeling approach was used to evaluate the significance and effect size of (1) outcome expectancies on changes in shoulder function and (2) outcome expectancies, shoulder function changes, and their interaction on perceptions of expectancy fulfillment.

Results.—Outcome expectancies significantly predicted changes in shoulder function. They accounted for 10% of variance in functional improve-

TABLE 1.—Sample Characteristics

Variables	Mean (SD) for Continuous Variables Percentage for Categorical Variables
Demographics	
Age (yr)	51.6 (15.7)
Gender (% female)	47%
Health status	
Physical Health Status (PCS)	39.0 (8.6)
Mental Health Status (PCS)	45.6 (9.5)
Clinical features	
Diagnoses	
Arthritis	11%
Dislocation	16%
Nerve injury	5%
Rotator cuff	30%
Sprain	34%
Other	4%
Existing chronic condition	67%
Previous physical therapy	44%
Previous shoulder surgery	35%
Previous medications	73%
Surgery	16%
Physical therapy	40%
New course of medications	45%
Patient self-report variables	
Baseline shoulder function	26.2 (5.4)
Three-month shoulder function	29.6 (7.9)
Expectancy fulfillment	11.4 (4.7)
Outcome expectancies	11.7 (4.3)
Shoulder function changes	3.4 (7.5)

Note: Physical Component Summary (*PCS*) and Mental Component Summary (*MCS*) scores range from 0 to 100, with higher scores indicating better physical and mental health. Shoulder function was assessed with the Flexilevel Scale of Shoulder Function, with scores ranging from 1 to 50 and higher scores indicating better function. Expectancy fulfillment and outcome expectancies were measured by the Patient Shoulder Expectancy Fulfillment and Patient Shoulder Outcome Expectancies measures, respectively. Scores on both expectancy measures ranged from 0 to 18, with higher scores indicating greater expectancy fulfillment and more positive expectancies, respectively.

(Courtesy of O'Malley KJ, Roddey TS, Gartsman GM, et al: Outcome expectancies, functional outcomes, and expectancy fulfillment for patients with shoulder problems. *Med Care* 42(2):139-146, 2004.)

ment. The improvement difference between patients with high expectancies versus those with low expectancies was clinically important (4.57 points), since it was greater than the minimal clinically important difference (3.02 points). Outcome expectancies and shoulder function changes were significantly predictive of patients' perceptions of fulfillment expectancies. Their interaction was not statistically relevant.

Conclusion.—Patient expectations are important in medical encounters. There is a need for interventions that target patient expectancies, including discussions regarding expectancy in patient-physician negotiations of therapeutic plans. There is also a need to develop better measures of outcome expectancies and expectancy fulfillment.

► This is a complex analysis that touches on an issue of considerable clinical importance. The patient is never passive in any therapeutic contract. For many in rheumatology, the therapeutic contract is formulating with both the patient and physician aware of the variability in outcomes. For much that we do, there is a considerable placebo effect. For some, there is a placebo effect. For example, if the attitude of the physician prescribing any agent is tentative or emphasizes side effects, the patient is far more likely to find the drug intolerable. We are slowly learning how to dissect the role of attitudes and expectations in therapeutic contracts. This article is such an exercise.

Of all the variables listed in the table, only 2 were strongly associated with a higher likelihood of a palliative outcome—age and attitude (outcome expectancy) prior to therapy—whereas previous surgery was the only "clinical feature" that was associated and not as strongly. Those patients that expected to do well were more likely to perceive they had done well a posteriori. Now we need to learn how to "treat" expectancy so that many of the interventions might be circumvented.

N. M. Hadler, MD

Diagnostic Values of Tests for Acromioclavicular Joint Pain

Walton J, Mahajan S, Paxinos A, et al (Univ of New South Wales, Sydney)

J Bone Joint Surg Am 86-A:807-812, 2004 6–23

Introduction.—Several clinical diagnostic tests have been created for the physical examination of the acromioclavicular (AC) joint. The predictive value of clinical tests and imaging modalities for diagnosing AC joint pain was examined; these were compared with the Paxinos test, a clinical test in which the clavicle and acromion are compressed together.

Methods.—Of 1037 patients with shoulder pain, 113 mapped pain within an area bounded by the midpart of the clavicle and the deltoid insertion and were eligible for inclusion. Of the 42 who agreed to participate, 4 were lost to follow-up. All patients underwent 20 clinical tests, radiography, bone scanning, MRI, and an AC joint injection test. Patients were grouped according to whether they had a 50% or more reduction in pain after AC joint injection. The diagnostic effectiveness of the various tests was analyzed.

Results.—AC joint pain was verified in 28 of 38 patients. The most sensitive tests were evaluated for AC tenderness (96% sensitivity), the Paxinos test (79%), MRI (85%), and bone scanning (82%); these trials had low specificity. With the response to the injection used as the dependent variable, bone scanning and the Paxinos test were the only independent variables retained. Patients who had a positive Paxinos test and a positive bone scan had high posttest odds (55:1) and a 99% posttest probability of experiencing pain caused by pathologic changes in the AC joint. The likelihood ratio for participants with 1 negative test and 1 positive test was indeterminate (0.4:1). Patients who had both a negative Paxinos test and a negative bone scan had a likelihood ratio of 0.03:1 for having AC joint pain, which basically rules out the disorder.

Conclusion.—The tests that were highly sensitive had low specificity; those with high specificity had low sensitivity. The combination of a positive Paxinos test and a positive bone scan were predictive of damage to the AC joint as the cause of shoulder pain with a high degree of confidence.

► Far be it for me to criticize any honest attempt to test a clinical inference, particularly a clinical inference that drives one's own approach to surgical practice. The third author, Dr Paxinos, convinced himself that shoulder pain can be ascribed to disease of the AC joint if he could elicit pain by compressing that joint. In keeping with a tradition that still survives in orthopedics, he coined the eponym "Paxinos test" to lay claim to the observation. However, in modern times such claims, eponymous or not, are soon forgotten unless they withstand scientific testing. Hence, this article.

Dr Paxinos and his colleagues soon discovered that designing rigorous testing was not so straight forward. First, they had to define the population to be studied, a population in which they presumed a higher prior probability of pathogenetic AC disease. They chose to study a stratum defined by a particular location of shoulder pain illustrated in Figure 1 in the original article. We lack the data as to the reliability of this stratification, particularly because only 10% of patients with shoulder pain qualified.

The next issue is a "gold standard"; how do we know which of these patients really have pathogenetic AC disease? They chose a response to an intra-articular injection of lidocaine and steroids; "pain had been alleviated by at least 50% within 10 minutes...." However, there is no attempt to validate this response, for example, by injecting a sample of the 90% of patients who did not recognize their predicament as displayed in Figure 1 in the original article.

Table 1 in the original article displays the diagnostic test characteristics generated by comparing the patients stratified by their response with injection. Note that radiographs will lead you to many a false-negative result because of limited sensitivity and joint tenderness to many a false-positive result because of limited specificity. The latter pertains to scintiscanning and MRI.

I have no reason to learn to perform a Paxinos test. As for ascribing shoulder pain to the AC joint, caveat emptor.

N. M. Hadler, MD

Arthrographic Joint Distension With Saline and Steroid Improves Function and Reduces Pain in Patients With Painful Stiff Shoulder: Results of a Randomised, Double Blind, Placebo Controlled Trial

Buchbinder R, Green S, Forbes A, et al (Cabrini Med Centre, Malvern, Victoria, Australia)

Ann Rheum Dis 63:302-309, 2004 6–24

Introduction.—Painful stiff shoulder (also termed frozen shoulder or adhesive capsulitis) is a frequent cause of shoulder pain that affects between 2% and 5% of the general population. There is some evidence that arthrographic joint distension with saline and steroid improves shoulder function and decreases pain in patients with painful, stiff shoulder. A randomized, double-blind, controlled trial was performed to determine whether this approach improves function, decreases pain, and enhances range of motion (ROM) at 3, 6, and 12 weeks after treatment.

Methods.—Forty-six patients were randomly assigned to either active treatment or placebo. Both participants and outcome assessors were blinded to treatment allocation. Patients underwent a shoulder-specific disability measure (SPADI), a patient preference measure (Problem Elicitation Technique [PET]), and evaluations of pain and active ROM at 3, 6, and 12 weeks of treatment. Four patients in the placebo group withdrew after the 3 weeks evaluation; 3 subsequently underwent distension.

Results.—At the 3-week follow-up, significantly greater improvements in SPADI ($P = .005$), PET, overall pain, active total shoulder abduction, and hand behind back were observed in the joint distension and steroid group, compared with placebo. At 6 weeks, the results of the intention to treat analysis favored joint distension; between-group differences were significant only for PET (difference in mean change in PET, 45.9 [95% CI, 3.2-88.7]). Excluding the 4 patients who withdrew, the between-group differences of disability and pain measures significantly favored joint distension over placebo. At 12 weeks, both intention to treat analysis and an analysis excluding the 4 withdrawals revealed a significantly greater improvement in PET score for the distension group.

Conclusion.—Arthrographic distension with normal saline and corticosteroid versus placebo was efficacious for at least 3 months in measures of function, pain, and ROM in patients with painful stiff shoulder.

► They are talking about that will-o'-the-wisp, the "frozen shoulder" or "adhesive capsulitis." There is a debate as to its prevalence. Many people have restriction in shoulder mobility, and many people have intermittently associated pain. Many people do not have "frozen shoulder." This is a special entity, part of "reflex sympathetic dystrophy." It can be suspected if the range of glenohumeral motion itself is restricted, ie, internal rotation from neutral. All other arcs of motion are more complex and can be restricted by virtue of periarticular disorders. They, too, are restricted in "frozen shoulder."

If you find patients with "frozen shoulder," the duration of illness is measured in years, not months. It is a more pervasive illness in terms of pain and incapacity. Patience will be rewarded, but it requires considerable patience. This trial recruited patients with a mean age of about 50 years and a mean duration of shoulder pain of 4 months.

One of the diagnostic features of "frozen shoulder" relates to arthrography; the joint is far less capacious. Forcing fluid into the glenohumeral joint to rupture the capsule has been attempted for years as a less invasive option than surgically manipulating the joint under anesthesia. The older literature is not encouraging. This study is not either.

N. M. Hadler, MD

Predicting the Onset of Forearm Pain: A Prospective Study Across 12 Occupational Groups

Nahit ES, Taylor S, Hunt IM, et al (Univ of Manchester, England)
Arthritis Rheum 49:519-525, 2003 6–25

Introduction.—The etiology of diffuse, nonspecific forearm pain is controversial. The relative contribution of mechanical exposure and psychosocial factors has yet to be determined and was, thus, prospectively examined in 782 newly employed workers from 12 occupational groups.

Methods.—At baseline, a cohort of 782 workers free of forearm pain were identified and underwent evaluation of physical and psychosocial aspects of their job and working environment. Participants were recontacted after 1 year to ascertain whether they had a new onset of forearm pain. A sample of individuals reporting new onset forearm pain underwent a structured examination of the upper limb.

TABLE 1.—Participation Rates and Prevalence of Forearm Pain at Follow-up

Occupation	Baseline Total*	Followup Participation *N* (%)	Forearm Pain at Followup *N* (%)
All groups	782	666 (85)	55 (8.3)
Firefighters	135	120 (89)	6 (5.0)
Shipbuilders	92	79 (86)	6 (7.6)
Retail workers	87	74 (85)	10 (13.6)
Dentists	76	71 (93)	4 (5.6)
Nurses	68	59 (87)	3 (5.1)
Podiatrists	58	53 (91)	7 (13.2)
Army clerks	57	53 (93)	6 (11.3)
Army officers	56	46 (82)	2 (4.4)
Postal workers	51	35 (69)	1 (2.9)
Army infantry	43	25 (58)	7 (28.0)
Police	38	34 (89)	0 (0.0)
Forestry	21	17 (81)	3 (17.7)

*Free of forearm pain.

(Courtesy of Nahit ES, Taylor S, Hunt IM, et al: Predicting the onset of forearm pain: A prospective study across 12 occupational groups. *Arthritis Rheum* 49:519-525, 2003. Reprinted by permission of John Wiley & Sons, Inc.)

Results.—At 1 year after baseline, 666 participants (85%) were recontacted for follow-up. Fifty-five participants (8.3%) reported a new onset of forearm pain. The prevalence was higher in women than in men (10.0% vs 7.2%; $P = .22$) and highest in the youngest age group (11.9%, 20 years or younger; 7.3%, 21-23 years; 6.0%, 24-27 years; 7.9%, 28 years or older; $P = .26$). The incidence varied widely among occupational groups (Table 1). The most important mechanical risk factor was frequent repetitive movements of the arm or wrist (odds ratio [OR], 2.9; 95% CI, 1.6-5.2). The most important psychosocial risk factors were work considered monotonous at least half of the time (OR, 3.0; 95% CI, 1.6-5.7) or work with little autonomy (OR, 2.6; 95% CI, 1.1-6.1). Three independent risk factors distinguished groups of participants at markedly different risks of onset: monotonous work, repetitive wrist movements, and working with hands above the shoulder level.

Conclusion.—Along with repetitive movements of the arms and wrists, mechanical postural factors and psychosocial factors are important risk factors for development of forearm pain. The risks for the onset of forearm pain are multifactorial in nature.

► There is no doubt that all of us will experience intermittent and remittent regional musculoskeletal disorders. There is no doubt that backaches,[1] arm pain,[2] and knee pain[3] will color our lives frequently. There is no doubt that every episode will present biomechanical challenges at home and at work. Most of us most of the time cope so effectively that the episode is soon forgotten, without medical assistance. Some of us some of the time have more difficulty coping, so the episode is more memorable and seeking assistance is more appealing. This study attempts to probe the influences that impede coping and, therefore, perturb this aspect of life. It is not an easy task.

At the inception of the pain-free cohort, the workers were asked about their perceptions of the physical demands of their tasks the day before and their perceptions of the psychosocial context in which they work in general. The outcome was whether they were hurting on the day they were surveyed a year later. Look at the occupations in Table 1. Can you imagine anything constant over the course of the year in terms of the physical demands of their tasks or the psychosocial context of working in these occupations? Perhaps dentists and maybe postal workers have tasks that demand more constant upper extremity usage, but these groups were less likely to be hurting on the day of the survey.

Life is complex, and regional musculoskeletal disorders are ubiquitous. Sorting out elements, either physical or psychosocial, in occupations such as those listed in Table 1 tests the very limits of epidemiology. When the physical demands of tasks are highly stereotypical throughout the day, every day, it is possible to test the hypothesis that these tasks thwart coping. Studies of workers whose job descriptions principally entail the use of a keyboard or handheld vibrating tools, as in dentistry and the like, have discerned a hazard to the upper extremity.

N. M. Hadler, MD

References

1. Hadler NM: The semiotics of backache. *Spine*, in press.
2. Hadler NM: The semiotics of "upper limb musculoskeletal disorders in workers." *J Clin Epidemiol* 56:937-939, 2003.
3. Hadler NM: *Occupational Musculoskeletal Disorders*, ed 3. Philadelphia, Lippincott Williams & Wilkins, in press.

Ulnar and Median Nerve Palsy in Long-distance Cyclists: A Prospective Study

Patterson JMM, Jaggars MM, Boyer MI (Washington Univ, St Louis)
Am J Sports Med 31:585-589, 2003 6–26

Introduction.—Several case studies and descriptions of cyclist's palsy have been reported in the literature. There are no known prospective trials that have assessed the occurrence of cyclist's palsy. The incidence of ulnar and medial nerve palsy was prospectively evaluated in 25 long-distance cyclists.

Methods.—Twenty-five road or mountain bike riders answered a questionnaire and underwent physical examination and interview before and after a 600-kg bicycle ride.

Results.—Twenty-three of the 25 cyclists had either motor or sensory symptoms, or both after the ride. Eleven cyclists (36%) had motor symptoms alone. There were no significant differences in the incidence of motor symptoms among cyclists of various experience levels or handlebar types (mountain bike vs road bike). Sensory symptoms alone occurred in 4 cyclists (10%); most of these were along the ulnar distribution. A significantly higher proportion of mountain bikers experienced sensory deficits, compared with road bikers. No significant differences in the incidence of sensory deficits were based on the level of experience. A total of 24% of hands (8 cyclists) had a combination of motor and sensory symptoms, which were equally distributed between road bike riders and riders of various experience levels.

Conclusion.—Cyclist's palsy is observed at high rates in both experienced and inexperienced cyclists. Cyclists can reduce the incidence of this disorder by wearing cycling gloves, ensuring proper bicycle fit, and frequent changing of the hand position.

► Because long-distance cycling is my hobby, this article caught my eye. I don't race, nor have I completed 4 centuries (100 mile rides) in 4 consecutive days—though I have come close to the latter at a more leisurely pace than those who are hell bent for the finish line. And that may be the difference; I stop and pause and vary my posture. But then I have nothing to prove, certainly nothing that warrants inducing neuropathic symptoms even if they are not associated with permanent damage. This article is not a description of "cyclist's palsy"; it is a description of "hell bent for the finish line cyclist's palsy."

N. M. Hadler, MD

Lower Extremity Pain

Impact of Type of Meniscal Tear on Radiographic and Symptomatic Knee Osteoarthritis: A Sixteen-Year Followup of Meniscectomy With Matched Controls

Englund M, Roos EM, Lohmander LS (Lund Univ, Sweden)
Arthritis Rheum 48:2178-2187, 2003 6–27

Introduction.—A meniscal tear with its resulting meniscal surgery is a well-known risk factor for osteoarthritis (OA) of the knee. The long-term radiographic and patient-associated outcomes of isolated limited meniscectomy in stable knees were examined in a controlled, retrospective cohort investigation.

Results.—One hundred fifty-five patients (mean age, 54 years) with intact cruciate ligaments who had undergone meniscectomy an average of 16 years earlier were examined with the use of standardized radiography and a validated self-administered questionnaires. Knee-associated symptoms were quantified with the use of the Knee Injury and Osteoarthritis Outcome Score (KOOS). Sixty-eight control subjects matched for age, sex, and body mass index were used to determine relative risks.

Results.—Radiographic tibiofemoral OA (Kellgren/Lawrence grade, ≥ 2) was observed in 66 index knees (43%), 39 of which were deemed symptomatic according to the KOOS. Seventy-seven patients (50%) had symptomatic index knees. A multivariate model revealed that degenerative meniscal tears were correlated with both radiographic OA ($P = .030$) and combined radiographic and symptomatic OA ($P \leq .015$). The relative risks for combined radiographic and symptomatic OA after degenerative and traumatic meniscal tears were 7.0 (95% CI, 2.1-23.5) and 2.7 (95% CI, 0.9-7.7), respectively, compared with matched control subjects.

Conclusion.—An isolated meniscal tear treated by limited meniscectomy is linked with a high risk of radiographic and symptomatic tibiofemoral OA at a 16-year follow-up. Degenerative meniscal lesions and extensive resections were linked with worse outcomes. Degenerative meniscal tears may be related to incipient OA. The meniscal tear may be the first symptom of this disease.

► An alternative explanation exists for this observation. The data are as consistent with the hypothesis that open meniscectomy predisposes to symptomatic OA of the knee and that these patients would have done as well if not better without surgery. I would raise the same specter regarding arthroscopic meniscectomy. It is unconscionable that these procedures are being performed without first documenting a favorable risk–benefit ratio. That would require a randomized trial with an appropriate control group (ie, sham surgery). There is precedent in arthroscopic surgery for knee OA in elderly men; the arthroscopic debridement proved to be a sham. It is unethical that we stand by while elective surgery is promulgated on wave after wave of hubris.

N. M. Hadler, MD

Joint Laxity and the Benign Joint Hypermobility Syndrome in Student and Professional Ballet Dancers

McCormack M, Briggs J, Hakim A, et al (Whipps Cross Univ, London; Univ College London)

J Rheumatol 31:173-178, 2004 6–28

Introduction.—Injury is an important hazard that can jeopardize careers in ballet dancers. During the past 25 years, it has become apparent that hypermobility may signify the presence of a heritable connective tissue disorder known as the benign joint hypermobility syndrome (BJHS). The prevalence of hypermobility and BJHS in male and female student and professional ballet dancers was examined, along with whether BJHS has any impact on a dance career.

Methods.—Students from the Royal Ballet School and professional dancers from the Royal Ballet Company, London, were compared with teenagers and adults, respectively, from a local secondary school and the Royal Opera House who acted as control subjects. Data were documented concerning anthropometric variables, the Beighton score, and clinical characteristics of BJHS. Odds ratios (ORs) for hypermobility and BJHS in dancers were determined. The prevalence and distribution of BJHS were assessed.

Results.—Hypermobility and BJHS were common in ballet school and professional company male and female dancers, compared with teenage and adult control subjects. An OR of 11.0 (95% CI, 3.3-31.8) was observed for hypermobility in dancers from both groups. The prevalence of BJHS diminished both from student to professional and within the ballet company from corps de ballet to Principal. ORs were significant in student dancers (OR, 3.9; 95% CI, 1.3-11.3) and not in professional dancers (OR, 1.7; 95% CI, 0.6-4.7). Arthralgia was common among dancers and was reported more frequently in male versus female dancers. In female dancers, pain was reported most by dancers with other characteristics of BJHS, especially stretchy skin.

Conclusion.—Hypermobility and BJHS are frequently found in male and female student and professional ballet dancers. The drop in prevalence, and the greater reporting of arthralgia in other characteristics of BJHS in young female dancers, indicates that BJHS may have substantial negative influences, which may impact training. The same pattern was not seen in male dancers, indicating that their pain-reporting and injury are associated with factors other than BJHS.

► There is a component of Rodney Grahame's career that I envy—the opportunity to carve investigative issues out of the glory that is ballet. However, studies of performers, ballet or music or sports, is far more challenging than one might assume. These are demanding career choices in ways that render the physical demands secondary. There are demands that relate to competition that are keener and more unforgiving than almost any other pursuit. Studying any health outcome short of tissue damage is fraught with psychosocial confounders.

I still remain unconvinced that there is anything worthy of the labels hypermobility syndrome, let alone the acronym BJHS for "benign joint hypermobility syndrome." Despite the consensus that hypermobility syndrome is a form of Ehlers-Danlos syndrome (Type III), I remain skeptical. This may still be the medicalization of healthy youngsters who can move many joints through a range of motion that titillates their peers. Certainly, there are many youngsters who are more mobile than others, as were many of their parents before them. This bodes no evil in the population at large. However, it does offer options in life that take advantage of this particular phenotype, including ballet. There is no surprise that highly selective organizations such as the Royal Ballet School find their student pool enriched by people who are hypermobile. The issues raised by Rodney Grahame and his collaborators are whether these peculiarly agile youngsters are placed at risk of harm by the rigors of professional dancing.

This study does not answer that question. True professional dancers are less likely to meet criteria for the hypermobility syndrome. True, also, professional dancers are older and have less need to impress their peers with the extraordinary nature of their range of motion. They only have to impress their peers with their technical prowess. They need not represent "survivor bias," ie, those who are more hypermobile were winnowed out.

Rodney Grahame is undertaking longitudinal studies to address these issues. I will be surprised to learn that my interpretation was wrong.

N. M. Hadler, MD

Extracorporeal Shock Wave Therapy for Plantar Fasciitis: Randomised Controlled Multicentre Trial

Haake M, Buch M, Schoellner C, et al (Universität Regensburg, Bad Abbach, Germany; Orthopädische Klinik Kassel, Germany; Universität Mainz, Germany; et al)

BMJ 327:75-77, 2003 6–29

Background.—Plantar fasciitis causes heel pain in about 10% of the general population. The cause is an injury at the origin of the plantar fascia or biomechanical abnormalities of the foot. Conservative treatment is successful in 90% of cases. In the 10% that fail to respond, surgery is eventually recommended, but this fails in 2% to 35% of cases. Local corticosteroids may reduce the pain for short periods. Insertion tendinopathies have been treated with extracorporeal shock wave therapy, which is believed to provide lasting analgesia and to stimulate healing. Whether extracorporeal shock wave therapy would be efficacious in the treatment of chronic plantar fasciitis was investigated.

Methods.—The study used 272 patients from 9 hospitals and 1 outpatient clinic in Germany. All had shown no improvement with conservative therapy for a minimum of 6 months. Extracorporeal shock wave therapy was used for 135 patients and placebo was used for 137. The Roles and Maudsley score was determined for each patient after 12 weeks of the intervention. Subjective pain ratings and walking ability for up to 1 year after the last intervention were also determined.

Results.—No significant differences in success rates were achieved in the 2 groups. The therapy group had a success rate of 34%, and the placebo group's rate was 30%. After 1 year, the Roles and Maudsley scores were 1 or 2 in 81% of the therapy group and 76% of the placebo group. No additional treatment was undertaken by 36% of the therapy group or 56% of the placebo group. One patient in each group had surgery. Eighteen percent of the therapy group and 9% of the placebo group reported side effects. Included were skin reddening, pain, and local swelling. Hematoma, nausea, dizziness, hair loss, and sleep disturbance were reported less often.

Conclusion.—Patients with chronic plantar fasciitis treated with extracorporeal shock wave therapy had no better outcomes than patients treated with placebo.

▶ This confirms observations reported in last year's YEAR BOOK.[1]

R. S. Panush, MD

Reference

1. 2004 YEAR BOOK OF RHEUMATOLOGY, ARTHRITIS, AND MUSCULOSKELETAL DISEASE, pp 295-297.

Chronic Widespread Pain and Fibromyalgia

Medically Unexplained Symptoms in Patients Referred to a Specialist Rheumatology Service: Prevalence and Associations

Maiden NL, Hurst NP, Lochhead A, et al (Western General Hosp, Edinburgh, Scotland; Univ of Edinburgh, Scotland)
Rheumatology 42:108-112, 2003 6–30

Background.—When symptoms are not explained by organic disease, the term *medically unexplained symptoms* is applied. Patients with medically unexplained symptoms are common. Some emotional disorders are related, and frequent attenders of health services are particularly affected. The prevalence of medically unexplained rheumatic symptoms in patients newly referred to a rheumatology outpatient service and the relationship of such symptoms to pain, disability, socioeconomic factors, and emotional disorders were investigated.

Methods.—Patients newly referred to a hospital-based regional rheumatology service were asked to complete a questionnaire assessing emotional disorders, pain, health status, and socioeconomic factors. An organicity rating was developed whereby rheumatologists judged the degree to which symptoms were explained by organic disorders.

Results.—Of a possible 279 patients, 203 completed questionnaires. They ranged in age from 19 to 87 years (mean age, 50 years), and 68.5% were women. Forty-six percent had symptoms completely explained by organic disease, 26% had symptoms that were largely explained, 20% had symptoms that were somewhat explained, and 8% had symptoms not explained by organic disease. Nearly all the patients given diagnoses of inflammatory arthritis or a connective tissue disease and 81% of those with osteoarthritis had a high organicity rating. Thirty-one percent of patients who had arthralgia, back pain, or fibromyalgia had a high organicity rating. None of the patients whose diagnosis was depression had a high organicity rating. Potential emotional disorders were detected in 33.5% of the patients. No relationship was found between emotional disorders and organicity ratings. Characteristics of patients whose symptoms were not clearly explained by organic disease included younger age (mean age, 44 vs 52; $P < .001$), female sex (relative risk [RR], 1.8; 95% CI, 1.0-3.1), and reporting of more somatic symptoms (median, 2 vs 1; $P = .021$). No relationship was found between organicity ratings and the degree of pain, physical and mental health status, or disability. Unexplained symptoms exhibited an association with the following socioeconomic factors: financial hardship (RR, 1.7; 95% CI, 1.1-2.6), living in rented housing (RR, 1.8; 95% CI, 1.2-2.8), living with dependent relatives (RR, 1.6; 95% CI, 1.0-2.5), smoking (RR, 1.6; 95% CI, 1.0-2.4), and dissatisfaction with work (RR, 1.6; 95% CI, 1.0-2.2). The significant independent predictors of low organicity were identified as living in rented housing (odds ratio, 2.3; 95% CI, 1.1-4.7; $P = .02$) and female sex (odds ratio, 3.4; 95% CI, 1.5-7.7; $P = .004$).

Conclusions.—Twenty-nine percent of the patients who had just been referred to a rheumatology clinic had symptoms that were not well explained by organic disease. Symptom levels, pain, disability, and emotional factors were similar between those whose symptoms were not well explained and patients with symptoms attributable to rheumatologic disease. Some socioeconomic variables showed a relationship with the unexplained symptoms.

► I love this term *medically unexplained symptoms* (MUS), which I first came across elsewhere a few months ago. It's now among my favorites, like *lumbago* and *rheumatism*. I used to hate such terminology when I was younger and thought we should understand everything with clarity and precision. I've learned that rheumatology and, indeed, medicine and life are not that way. So I've become increasingly fond of descriptors of those poorly understood but common conditions that we encounter. I'm not surprised that nearly 30% of patients referred to rheumatologists have MUS (bet many of the others have lumbago or rheumatism).

R. S. Panush, MD

Neurophysiologic Evidence for a Central Sensitization in Patients With Fibromyalgia

Desmeules JA, Cedraschi C, Rapiti E, et al (Geneva Univ Hosp)

Arthritis Rheum 48:1420-1429, 2003 6–31

Background.—Fibromyalgia (FM) is not associated with any physical, radiologic, or biological findings that are directly related to dysfunction, and patients with FM usually appear well. The symptoms are believed to result from biochemical alterations in pain perception or altered pain modulation. An increased sensitivity to nonspecific stimuli (ie, mechanical pressure and cold or warm sensations) suggests that central pain mechanisms are acting aberrantly, possibly as a result of a CNS processing error. Whether abnormalities of central and peripheral nociceptive sensory input processing exist outside areas of spontaneous pain in patients with FM was assessed. Measures were obtained with quantitative sensory testing and a neurophysiologic paradigm independent of subjective documentation.

Methods.—Participants were outpatients with FM attending a self-management program. Eighty-five patients with FM and 40 control subjects without FM were matched for age and sex. Quantitative sensory testing was done with various stimuli (ie, thermal, mechanical, and electrical) at locations of nonspontaneous pain, and pain was assessed with the use of subjective scales and the spinal nociceptive flexion reflex (NFR), which is a specific physiologic correlate for the objective evaluation of central nociceptive pathways. Quality of life and the impact of FM were assessed by means of questionnaires.

Results.—Statistically, patients and control subjects were significantly different in all areas except for sex, age, and education. Most of the patients were women (mean age, 49 years) who had completed at least compulsory school. FM symptoms had been present for 0.5 to 49 years (mean, 8.0 years). The mean patient rating of pain was 5.6 on a 10-cm visual analog scale, and all measures indicated severe pain. Sixty-three percent of the patients were taking antidepressants, and ratings of quality of life were at the high end for depression, anxiety, and impaired quality of life. Patients with FM had significantly lower cold and heat pain thresholds, and their tolerance to cold pain was severely reduced. The mean latency period before hand withdrawal was 13 seconds for patients with FM, and 28 seconds for control subjects. The NFR threshold was 33% lower in patients with FM, and median values for the NFR among patients with FM were significantly decreased when compared with control subjects. The cutoff value of less than 27.6 mA for the NFR produced a sensitivity of 73.1% and a specificity of 80.4% for FM patients for detecting central allodynia. The NFR amplitude and the pain score were closely related; increases in reflex size were accompanied by increases in pain intensity ratings.

Conclusions.—The decline in the NFR and the subjective pain thresholds to electrical stimulation provided psychophysical evidence that there is abnormally processed input to the central nociceptive pathways in patients with FM. The results are consistent with an absence of peripheral large or small nerve fiber lesions. FM may result from modified stimulus processing by the CNS in the absence of any peripheral sources of nociceptive input or peripheral nerve dysfunction. Thus, a state of central hyperexcitability of the nociceptive system seems to exist in patients with FM.

▶ There is no doubt that there are neurophysiologic constructs that account for much that metaphysics considered to be the "mind." There is no doubt that our emotions, our educational accomplishments, our tightly held beliefs, and much more reflect neurophysiologic constructs. There is no doubt that the fashion in which we respond to life's joys and life's challenges reflect the idiosyncratic nature of these constructs. There is no doubt that there is a wide range of individual differences and heritable differences in this biology, all of which warrant being considered normal. Much is homeostatic. Much is the joy of humanity. Some is its sorrow.

Understanding neurophysiologic constructs is one of science's great frontiers. Important inroads have been forthcoming as to the basic mechanisms. Clinical investigation is stymied by the bluntness of the available methodology and is also stymied by the need to define a referent population, one that is either "normal" or distinctive. The literature that relates to FM is illustrative in this regard, and this article is an object lesson. Patients with persistent widespread pain have a set of neurophysiologic constructs that supports their illness. They are living life under a pall and are in such distress that they have sought care. In so doing, they have acquired illness behaviors and a distinctive sick role. There must be special fine structures to their neurophysiologic constructs. Some will be shared by others who live life under a pall but who do not experience persistent widespread pain or, if they do, do not choose to be patients. Some of these people have plenty of tender points and probably share the evidence for central sensitization that patients labeled with FM exhibit. Neither group likes to be poked or prodded. If one wants to probe the distinctiveness of the neurophysiologic construct that is labeled FM, what is the proper comparison group? Certainly, choosing random "normal" people would be no more appropriate than selecting people of the blithest of spirits.

N. M. Hadler, MD

Family Study of Fibromyalgia

Arnold LM, Hudson JI, Hess EV, et al (Univ of Cincinnati, Ohio; McLean Hosp, Belmont, Mass; Harvard Med School, Boston)

Arthritis Rheum 50:944-952, 2004 6–32

Introduction.—Some trials have found an increased prevalence of fibromyalgia (FM) in first-degree relatives of probands with FM, yet standard criteria for the diagnosis of FM were not consistently used and the number of relatives who chose not to participate were not reported. All trials were limited by small numbers and lack of comparison groups. Familial aggregation of FM and measures of tenderness and pain were evaluated, along with familial coaggregation of FM and major mood disorder (major depressive disorder or bipolar disorder).

Methods.—Probands fulfilling the American College of Rheumatology criteria for FM and control probands with arthritis (RA) and not lifetime diagnosis were recruited from consecutive referrals to 2 community-based rheumatology practices were included. Probands were aged 40 to 55 years and had at least 1 first-degree relative age 18 years or older available for interview and examination. Both probands and interviewed relatives underwent a dolorimeter tender point examination and a structured clinical interview. Interviewed relatives were queried concerning first-degree relatives who were not available for interview via a structured family interview. After adjusting for the correlation of observation within families, logistic and linear regression models were applied to analyze the aggregation and coaggregation effects.

Results.—Information was obtained for 533 relatives of 78 probands with FM and 272 relatives of 40 probands with RA. Fibromyalgia aggregated strongly in families. The odds ratio (OR) determining the odds of FM in a relative of a proband with FM, compared with the odds of FM in a relative of a proband with RA was 8.5 (95% CI, 2.8-26; $P = .0002$). The number of tender points was significantly higher, and the total myalgic score was significantly lower in the relatives of probands with FM versus relatives of probands with RA. Fibromyalgia coaggregated significantly with major mood disorder. The OR measuring the odds of major mood disorder in a relative of a proband with FM, compared with the odds of a major mood disorder in a relative of a proband with RA was 1.8 (95% CI, 1.1-2.9; $P = .013$).

Conclusion.—Fibromyalgia and decreased pressure pain thresholds aggregate in families; FM coaggregates with major mood disorders in families. Genetic factors may be involved in the cause of FM and in pain sensitivity. Mood disorders and FM may share some inherited factors.

► This is a thoughtful discussion of an observation that is not very surprising. Functional somatic syndromes and major mood disorders coaggregate in families. The thrust of this observation is in keeping with the many earlier observations of one of the authors, JI Hudson. There are 2 relevant literatures that the authors do not introduce into their formulations. First, there is an analysis of the heritability of chronic widespread pain in sibships in a Finnish twin registry; no genetic influence could be discerned.[1] That suggests that the tendency to somatize is learned, even though the tendency to suffer major mood disorders is largely inherited. The other literature relates to the "vulnerable child" who is instructed by parenting to have a more tenuous hold on a sense of well-being. This parenting style is not "abnormal" but is in the spectrum of normalcy and infuses the child with a risk for a functional somatic disorder. Such parents were usually raised themselves in this fashion.

So, families blighted with functional somatic syndromes (including "FM") are likely to be blighted with serious mood disorders and particular approaches to coping with unpleasant somatic experiences.

N. M. Hadler, MD

Reference

1. Mikkelsson M, Kaprio J, Salminen JJ, et al: Widespread pain among 11-year-old Finnish twin pairs. *Arthritis Rheum* 44:481-485, 2001.

Functional Imaging of Pain in Patients With Primary Fibromyalgia

Cook DB, Lange G, Ciccone DS, et al (Univ of Medicine and Dentistry of New Jersey, Newark; Veterans Affairs New Jersey Health Care, East Orange)

J Rheumatol 31:364-378, 2004 6–33

Introduction.—A limitation of earlier reports assessing nociceptive processes in patients with fibromyalgia (FM) has been the reliance on self-report measures of pain. Objective evidence of abnormal nociception is necessary to better understand the pathophysiologic processes involved in FM and give converging evidence of self-reported symptoms. The function of the nociceptive system was evaluated in patients with FM with the use of functional MRI (fMRI).

Methods.—Nine females with FM and 9 who were pain-free (controls) participated in 2 experiments. In experiment 1, the psychophysical responses to painful stimuli were evaluated and prepared patients for fMRI testing. In experiment 2, participants underwent fMRI scanning while receiving painful and nonpainful heat stimuli. Conventional and fMRI images were obtained with a 1.5-T MR scanner. Scanning was performed over 5 conditions: Condition 1 was a practice session with no stimuli; conditions 2 and 5 involved nonpainful warm stimuli; and conditions 3 and 4 involved an absolute thermal pain stimulus (47°C) and a perceptually equivalent pain stimuli delivered in counterbalance order.

Results.—Experiment 1 showed that FM participants were more sensitive to experimental heat pain, compared with controls ($P < .001$). In experiment 2, fMRI showed that the FM group exhibited greater activity, compared with controls, over multiple brain regions in response to both nonpainful and painful stimuli ($P < .01$). In response to nonpainful warm stimuli, participants with FM had significantly greater activity, compared with controls, in prefrontal, supplemental motor, insular, and anterior cingulate cortices ($P < .01$). In response to painful stimuli, participants with FM had greater activity in the contralateral insular cortex ($P < .01$). Data from the practice session demonstrated brain activity in pain-relevant areas for the FM group and not for controls.

Conclusion.—Brain responses to sensory stimuli in regions involved in sensory, cognitive, and emotional aspects of the pain experience are enhanced in persons with FM. These data support a physiologic explanation of FM pain and offers objective evidence of cortical and subcortical amplification of both painful and nonpainful thermal stimuli.

Evidence of Augmented Central Pain Processing in Idiopathic Chronic Low Back Pain

Giesecke T, Gracely RH, Grant MAB, et al (Univ of Michigan, Ann Arbor; Georgetown Univ, Washington, DC; Univ of Cologne, Germany)
Arthritis Rheum 50:613-623, 2004 6–34

Background.—Even with chronic low back pain (CLBP) affecting between 70% and 85% of individuals at some time during their lives, 90% recover, usually within 12 weeks. Patients who require longer for recovery generally experience a slow, uncertain process that takes a large toll on health care and disability systems. No cause is identified in many individuals, but sensory testing and functional MRI (fMRI) have noted generally increased pain sensitivity, hyperalgesia, and altered brain processing. These findings suggest a central augmentation of pain processing. Experimental pain testing and functional imaging were performed in 11 patients with idiopathic CLBP, and the results were compared with those of 11 healthy individuals and 16 individuals with fibromyalgia syndrome (FMS).

Methods.—The patients with CLBP had pain persisting for at least 12 months that could not be explained by MRI or radiographic findings. The pressure-pain threshold was assessed on a thumbnail in all research subjects. The same site was used for the fMRI studies, where stimuli of equal pressure (2 kg) and equal subjective pain intensity (lightly intense pain) were applied.

Results.—Using the Short-Form of the McGill Pain Questionnaire, patient groups reported significantly more clinical pain than control subjects, but the FMS and CLBP groups had similar pain levels. Patients with FMS had a greater extent of pain and more tender points than did patients with CLBP or healthy control subjects. The levels of psychological distress reported by patients with FMS were also higher than those reported by the healthy control subjects. Patients with CLBP showed a trend toward higher levels of anxiety and depression, but it was not statistically significant. On experimental pain tests, both FMS and CLBP patient groups had similar pain thresholds at the left thumb, and both were significantly lower than those of control subjects. Among patients, the suprathreshold pressure intensities sufficient to evoke moderate or slightly intense pain were significantly lower than those among control subjects. Pain thresholds were lower in both patient groups compared with control levels. A pressure of 2 kg led patients with CLBP and FMS to report moderate pain and to experience an increased fMRI signal in the contralateral primary and secondary somatosensory cortices, ipsilateral secondary cortex, inferior parietal lobule, and cerebellum. Control subjects reported only faint pain, and their fMRI signal increased only in the contralateral secondary cortical region. All patients tested with slightly intense pain stimuli had significant increases in the contralateral primary and secondary cortices, the inferior parietal lobule, the insula, the anterior cingulate cortex, and the ipsilateral secondary cortex and cerebellum.

Conclusions.—Increased pressure–pain sensitivity was found for individuals with idiopathic CLBP at a site distant from their clinical pain. Findings were confirmed on fMRI. Similar findings were found in patients with FMS. Treatment strategies for such pain, whether pharmacologic or non-pharmacologic, can be developed to address the chronic pain symptoms and syndromes.

► How can it be that patients with chronic low back pain who find themselves under the wing of the "tertiary care spine center" at Georgetown University are plagued as well by chronic widespread pain? The observation is not unique to Georgetown, or to patients whose chief complaint is back pain. Similar observations pertain to patients with persistent regional arm pain. However, nearly all these unfortunate individuals are not really "patients." They are likely to be claimants for disability awards, often indemnified by Workers' Compensation schemes. They acquire adverse illness behaviors in their iatrogenic passage toward the vortex of disability determination.[1] These perceptual and behavioral features are not the product of Galenic humors or any other vitalistic force. These perceptions of painfulness and the overwhelming superimposed suffering are in their mind. There, I said it . . . the unspeakable assertion that is heard by most Westerners as accusatory, condemning, and offensive. Dr Giesecke and his colleagues (Abstract 6–34) take refuge in such obfuscations as "central" or "non-nociceptive" pain because of "augmented central pain processing" akin to that in "fibromyalgia."

But in their mind is no longer a Cartesian abstraction. As discussed in the Commentary for Desmeules et al (Abstract 6–31), all thoughts, conceptualizations, and emotions are the result of neurophysiologic constructs in the brain. We have crude instruments available to sample these neurophysiologic constructs. Functional MRI probes for coarse changes in neural activation patterns, whereas single-photon emission computed tomography (SPECT) probes for variations in perfusion. There is a rapidly accumulating literature on patterns detected with tools such as these. For example, the images of Shakespearian scholars predictably change if they read a comedy or a tragedy. When a loved one is in pain, the caring observer has images that mimic those of the individual in pain. Joy and fear have neurophysiologic footprints. Some day, we will have instruments with the resolution to determine which of you readers finds my argument most compelling.

This article by Cook et al takes its place in this literature. Their conclusion that their "results provide further evidence for a physiologic explanation for FM pain" is a tautology. Of course, adverse illness behaviors are in their mind. That's a "no-brainer" (forgive me).

N. M. Hadler, MD

Reference

1. Hadler NM: *Occupational Musculoskeletal Disorders*, ed 3. Philadelphia, Lippincott Williams & Wilkins, 2004.

7 Miscellaneous

Lead Article

Chopstick Arthropathy: The Beijing Osteoarthritis Study

Hunter DJ, Zhang Y, Nevitt MC, et al (Boston Univ; Univ of California, San Francisco; Peking Union Med College Hosp, Beijing, China; et al)

Arthritis Rheum 50:1495-1500, 2004 7–1

Background.—Chopsticks have been used for approximately 5000 years in China. Most Chinese learn to use chopsticks with their dominant hand beginning at age 3 to 4 years, and few Chinese switch their hand of chopsticks use during their lifetime. Although the mode of operation of chopsticks varies from one person to the next, the predominant fingers involved are the thumb, index finger, and middle finger. The exposure to chopsticks use is potentially an important source of mechanical stress. Radiographic hand osteoarthritis (OA) has been reported to affect approximately 45% of elderly Chinese individuals and is associated with functional impairment when symptomatic. Whether the use of chopsticks is associated with prevalent hand OA was explored.

Methods.—A sample of persons aged 60 years and older was recruited in randomly selected neighborhoods in Beijing. The subjects answered questions about handedness, the hand with which they use chopsticks, and pincer grip activities. Bilateral posteroanterior radiographs of the hand were obtained, and each joint was graded according to the Kellgren/Lawrence (K/L) scale. Because most subjects used chopsticks with their dominant hands, analysis was also performed among subjects who reported no hand preference when performing other activities and subjects who denied other pincer grip activities.

Results.—A total of 1008 men and 1499 women were assessed (Table 2). The prevalence ratio for OA of the thumb interphalangeal (IP) joints in the chopsticks hand was 1.2 in men and 1.6 in women. The prevalence ratio for OA of the second and third proximal interphalangeal (PIP) joints was 1.5 in men and 1.4 in women; and the prevalence ratio for OA of the second and third metacarpophalangeal (MCP) joints was 1.4 in men and 1.4 in women. The prevalence ratios in these joints were greater than the ratios in other MCP, PIP, or distal IP joints from the same hand that were unlikely to be involved by chopsticks use, especially among women. Similar results were obtained with limitation of the analyses to ambidextrous subjects and subjects who did not engage in any other pincer grip activities. OA of the thumb IP joint affected 26% of the entire population studied, and chopsticks use ac-

TABLE 2.—Association Between Chopsticks Use and Prevalence of Radiographic Hand OA Among Beijing Elderly

Joint Group	Chopsticks-use Hand No. of Hands	Chopsticks-use Hand Prevalence, %	Non–chopsticks-use Hand No. of Hands	Non–chopsticks-use Hand Prevalence, %	Prevalence Ratio (95% CI)
Men					
Thumb IP joint	211	22.2	169	18.0	1.2 (1.1-1.4)
First MCP joint	44	4.3	44	4.7	0.9 (0.7-1.3)
Second and third MCP joints	136	14.3	99	10.5	1.4 (1.2-1.6)
Second and third DIP joints	91	9.6	94	10.1	1.0 (0.8-1.1)
Second and third PIP joints	42	4.4	27	2.9	1.5 (1.1-2.2)
Thumb base	124	13.1	156	16.6	0.8 (0.7-0.9)
Non–chopsticks-use joints	83	8.8	59	6.3	1.4 (1.1-1.7)
Women					
Thumb IP joint	335	23.3	211	14.8	1.6 (1.4-1.7)
First MCP joint	30	2.1	22	1.6	1.4 (0.9-2.0)
Second and third MCP joints	166	11.6	117	8.2	1.4 (1.2-1.6)
Second and third DIP joints	246	17.1	193	13.6	1.3 (1.1-1.4)
Second and third PIP joints	136	9.5	94	6.6	1.4 (1.2-1.7)
Thumb base	126	8.8	170	12.0	0.7 (0.6-0.8)
Non–chopsticks-use joints	177	12.3	156	11.0	1.1 (0.9-1.3)

Abbreviations: CI, Confidence interval; *DIP*, distal interphalangeal.

(Courtesy of Hunter DJ, Zhang Y, Nevitt MC, et al: Chopstick arthropathy: The Beijing Osteoarthritis Study. *Arthritis Rheum* 50:1495-1500, 2004. Reprinted by permission of John Wiley & Sons, Inc.)

counted for 19% of the risk of OA developing in this joint in men and 36% of the women.

Conclusions.—These findings suggest an association between chopsticks use and an increased prevalence of OA in the IP joint of the thumb as well as in the second and third PIP and MCP joints.

► Let me tell you about my trip to Japan last spring.

"What can be addressed, in the consideration of the orient, . . .is the possibility of a difference. . .in the symbolic systems. . .gardens, gestures, houses, flower arrangements, faces, arts, violence."

R Barthes. *Empire of Signs*[1]

"It's unlikely that even one foreigner in all our history has truly understood Japan."

J Michener, *Sayonara*[2]

"Both the sword and the chrysanthemum are part of the picture. The Japanese are, to the highest degree, both aggressive and unaggressive, both militaristic and aesthetic, both insolent and polite, rigid and adaptable, submissive and resentful of being pushed around, loyal and treacherous, brave and timid, conservative and hospitable to new ways. They are terribly concerned about what other people will think about their behavior, and they are also overcome by guilt when other people know nothing of their misstep. Their soldiers are disciplined to the hilt but also insubordinate."

R Benedict. *The Chrysanthemum and the Sword*[3]

Introduction and Background

During the summer of 2001 I received an invitation to visit a Japanese hospital as a clinician educator. After some thought, investigation, and negotiation to arrange a suitable time, I accepted with enthusiasm. As the visit (scheduled for May 2003) approached, I developed considerable trepidation about attending because of pressing issues at my medical center and concerns about the epidemic of severe acute respiratory syndrome in Asia, and I came very close to canceling the trip. That would have been a terrible mistake; the experience proved to be quite special—great fun and enormously educational. It provided an opportunity to live and learn in a foreign culture and to appreciate the strengths of our medical educational system.

The visit was fabulous. Our hosts at Maizuru Hospital were kind, polite, and gracious. We had the unusual opportunity of spending a weekend with them at their home in Kyoto, unusual because the Japanese almost never entertain anyone (Japanese or foreigner) at home. Indeed, all the Japanese we encountered were unfailingly courteous, from the rheumatologists at Kyoto University Medical School who invited me to spend a day with them and then took us out to a wonderful dinner, to the waitress who tried to tell us where the local supermarket was and ended up walking us there, to the residents who went with us to the bank and translated for us, to the couple we met having dinner at a restaurant who treated us to sake and then to a meal, to the student who got off his bike and took us to the building we sought at Kyoto University, to the farmers in the rice paddies who tried to help me find my way back to town when I got lost on a run, to the young woman who spent a weekend showing us around Tokyo. And especially the Maizuru Hospital residents who, when I finished a lecture early, said "Dr. Panush, there are still 20 minutes left; can you teach us more?"

Let me review pertinent geography, history, and culture pertaining to Japan for an appropriate background toward understanding clinical practice and medical education in Japan. Never having studied anything about Japan—indeed, never having taken geography or history and only token anthropology and sociology courses in college—I do not presume to offer any particular expertise. And it is certainly patently impossible to explain Japan in depth in this brief exposition. However, the following attempts to present salient and summative highlights.

Understanding Japan

Japan and Japanese are different. Very little in our Western upbringing prepares us for understanding the vast contrasts between our cultures. Appreciation of several elements are important in understanding Japan, the Japanese, and their culture.[4-18]

(i). All in the Family

The Japanese are a tribe. There is a unique sense of community and responsibility to the tribe. Japanese are dominated by their responsibility to their groups. The Japanese abhor personal confrontation. They operate by consensus. This is a source of strength to them and their society. Paradoxically, this accounts for their drive and efficiency. The only way to become a member of the tribe is to be born into it. Nonmembers of the tribe are different.

(ii). Isolation

Japan has been the most isolated major nation in history. Excepting for the post–World War II occupation, it has never been invaded. Indeed, for centuries Japan banned trade and commerce with any outside influence. Despite readiness to adopt foreign influences, most Japanese really do not welcome too much personal contact with foreigners, and in their hearts, feel superior.

(iii). Homogeneity

Japan is the most racially and culturally homogenous of major nations: 99%+ of Japanese are ethnically similar. No other major nation approaches this. Multiethnic diversity is understood but not part of Japanese culture. This enables Japan to "westernize" while preserving its unique identity.

(iv). Tribalism

Japanese society is exclusionary. Acceptance only comes by being born into their tribe. The primary commitment of the Japanese is to the well-being of their tribe, not to ideology or religion. The Japanese therefore have a moral relativism and find it easy to accept change.

(v). Imperial Divinity

Until their defeat in World War II, Japanese revered their emperor and considered him divine, part of an unbroken lineage descending from the sun god. Centuries to millennia of this belief, coupled with fervent and unswerving loyalty, molded "tribal" and cultural values.

(vi). Land and Resources

But a small portion of Japan is habitable and its natural resources are limited. The country's large population is dense, leading to certain cultural behaviors, including reverence for simplicity and beauty. Limited natural resources has surely influenced Japan's expansionist wars of the past two centuries.

(vii). Earthquakes and Typhoons

Natural disasters are common in the country. There is a calm acceptance of and resignation (fatalism) to such catastrophes.

(viii). Language

The Japanese language is complex and has been called the "devil's language." This is suitable for a people who distrust and shun straightforward communication.

Japan: Fast Facts

Japan is approximately the size of California. Its population is approximately 130 million people. The average commute to work is 2.5 hours (in the Tokyo metropolitan area). Tokyo, at 8+ million people, is the world's third largest city (after Seoul and Moscow). The average Japanese man is 5 feet, 7 inches and weighs 143 pounds, and the average woman is 5 feet, 2 inches and weighs 119 pounds. Life expectancy is 77 years for men and 84 for women, among the best in the world. Japan has the fourth most cell phones in the world (after Finland, Norway, and Sweden). The birth rate is 1.3 and age at marriage is 29 years for men, 27 for women. As noted, 99% of those living in Japan are ethnically Japanese. Governance is now a constitutional monarchy, with emperor Akihito and his descendents no longer considered divine. There is no national religion, although most practice both Shinto and Buddhism (together, as neither excludes other religious practices).[9-11]

Geography

Japan is an island nation approximately the same size in square miles as California, Montana, or Italy. Most of the country is mountainous. Its population of approximately 130 million people lives on approximately one tenth of the available land; only about one fifth of the land is usable or arable. Japan has the world's highest density of production per habitable land. In the Tokyo area the average home costs approximately 7 years' salary. One third of Tokyo housing is not greater than 11 × 11 square feet (in a survey not long ago). The climate is temperate. There are few natural resources. And, as been stated, natural calamities (earthquakes and typhoons) are expected. Japan was totally closed to trade and commerce for centuries until forcibly opened by Commodore Perry in 1853, which presaged Japan's emergence into the modern era. All of these features profoundly influenced the culture that developed.[4,5,9-11]

History

Japanese history can be extraordinarily simplified into premodern, feudal/medieval, classical/Edo, and modern eras. The premodern era featured the descension of the imperial line from the sun goddess, the development of Shintoism, and importation of Buddhism from the Asian mainland. Early baronies ultimately became nationally unified with capitals in various cities, Kyoto being the most enduring. Feudal/medieval times saw the development of the code of "bushido," a caste system, and is recognized by the warrior class of samurai. The classical/Edo period is the topic of the book/movie "Shogun," when Tokugawa seized power as military dictator (shogun), which was maintained in his family until the mid 1800s; it was at this time that the capital was moved from historic Kyoto to Edo, which became modern Tokyo. Japan entered the modern area when power was restored to the emperor Meiji and the country resolved to rapidly learn from the west and modernize. [4,5,9-11]

Culture

Japan developed as a nation and culture apart and still, to a large degree, remains that way. Cultural values include commitment to consensus and to the group. This fostered the work ethic that led to Japan's emergence as one of the world's strongest economies; individuals' responsibility to their group is such that the subordinate individual yields to expectations of the community; individuals work long, hard, diligently, and well. They seek harmony; confrontation is shunned. To Japanese, shame and guilt do not have religious connotations but reflect failure to meet cultural expectations; much of this is facilitated by following prescribed protocols of behavior. There is a very strong sense of obligation and reciprocity in Japanese society (giri/on); gifts, favors, and kindnesses must be reciprocated; there are stories, for example, of soldiers after World War II who helped destitute Japanese, but in doing so burdened those helped with obligations they could never repay and left the Japanese worse off than originally.[3-7,9-11]

Japanese culture has a strong sense of order and hierarchy; among professionals and businessmen, cards are always exchanged because these make it clear how and where everybody fits; the depth of bowing when meeting people reflects this. Japanese language and behavior are subtle; translators often report difficulty imparting thorough meanings to Japanese text because of this; so, too, are interpersonal relations highly nuanced. There is a sense of intuition to Japanese interpersonal relations that goes beyond verbal expression. There is no public physical contact; even within the home there may not be physical contact between parents and children (imagine an Italian in Japan!). Etiquette is highly formalized; there are protocols for most aspects of public behavior. "Gai-jin" (foreigners) are received with tolerance, curiosity, and courtesy; many Japanese will still avoid contact with foreigners.[3-7,9-11]

Education is valued extremely highly; beginning at early ages, children go to "cram" schools after regular school hours to prepare for entry to the best elementary and secondary schools and to prepare for those examinations that will place them in universities according to performance; Japan is in this respect a classless meritocracy. Until recently Japanese did not have a great deal of leisure time and therefore did not engage in many leisure activities. I saw few runners—at any time of day—while visiting. Ironically for a country without space (or perhaps because of this), the Japanese are obsessed with golf.[3-7,9-11]

Japan is not without problems. Its economy is now doing poorly. Individuals who previously had secure employment for life now find themselves jobless. There are homeless in Japan. And despite the beauty and elegance that characterize many aspects of Japanese culture, Japan discriminates against a minority of untouchables (burakumin—butchers, executioners, leatherworkers, and gravediggers) and has an unsavory history of exploiting young women from other southeast Asian countries to work in the sex industry.[9-11]

Language and Communication

Japan has four alphabets—kanji (ideographs), hiragana, katakana, and romaji—and English. Students must learn between 2000 and 3000 ideographs from the 50,000 that exist to be literate. The literacy rate in Japan exceeds 99%.[4,5,9-11]

The Japanese are subtle, indirect, and exceedingly polite in their communication. The Japanese, for example, will never say "no." "I see" means "no." "Ah" means "no." "Ah-ha" means "no." "Yes" means "no." "That is difficult" means "that is completely impossible." "That is very interesting" means "that's the dumbest thing I ever heard." "We will study your proposal" means "never."[12]

Food

Learning to use chopsticks can be difficult. The best set of instructions I came across were as follows. Take one chopstick and place it between the base of your thumb and your hand, extending outward between your middle and ring fingers. Grasp the other chopstick with the tips of your thumb and index finger. Now, holding the 2 sticks parallel, raise them over your head and signal to the waiter to bring you a fork.[12]

The Japanese diet is heavily based on fish and rice. Like other aspects of this culture that have evolved with limited space, with fatalism, and with a sense of immediacy, fine dining too developed as an experience to celebrate not only elegant taste, but also visual, gustatory, and tactile senses. The tea ceremony epitomizes this. It has evolved as the pursuit of a simple and pure state of mind with an esthetic and spiritual focus. It is a "once in a lifetime" encounter; it cannot be repeated (reminiscent of the Latin carpe diem). It seeks to achieve harmony (wa), respect (kei), purity (sei), and tranquility (jaku). These rituals have evolved over centuries, and some spend years studying this in an effort to achieve perfection.[9-11]

War

World War II

Paradoxically, this culture of grace, charm, elegance, and courtesy has been expansionist, aggressive, imperial, militaristic, arrogant, and barbaric. After fully modernizing in the late 1800s, Japan engaged in a successful military adventure against Russia, in the Russo-Japanese War of early 1900s. By 1910 Japan had invaded and annexed the Sakhalin, Kuril, and Ryukyu (Okinawa) island chains as well as Formosa, Korea, and Port Arthur. Japanese fabricated an incident that led to the invasion of China and occupied Manchuria by the 1930s. Who is not aware of Pearl Harbor and the American declaration of war of December 7, 1941? At its peak conquest, Japan occupied territory from the Aleutian islands to Australia to India to China to the Soviet Union, an extensive empire indeed.[13]

What led to the Japanese attack on Pearl Harbor? The simplistic answer is that this was probably a combination of many factors. It reflected the governance of Japan by a militarist clique who were dedicated to promoting and preserving the national essence (kokutai), who possessed a sense of arrogance and entitlement to the space and resources throughout Southeast Asia, who promulgated a "holy war" to free Asia from colonialism and communism, and who espoused a notion of developing a "greater east Asia co-prosperity sphere" for Asians (reflecting thinly disguised imperialism); there was also a sense of inevitability (karma) of impending conflict with the United States and an expectation that there would ultimately be a favorable negotiated peace with America. There may also have been a number of serious misunderstandings and miscommunications between Japanese and American negotiators and politicians, confounding the inability to avert the calamity of Pearl Harbor.[13]

Japan was guilty of war crimes almost as heinous as Germany's, probably the only difference being that Japan was not selectively genocidal but equally barbaric to all occupied populations and all prisoners. It is not widely appreciated that for Allied prisoners of war the death rate in the European theater was 4% while 27% in the Pacific theater. Japanese war crimes included civilian murders and rapes, death marches, forced prostitution, cannibalism, target practice, mutilation, vivisection, slavery, and human experimentation. Japanese experimented on prisoners of war with vivisection, cholera, epidemic hemorrhagic fever, plague, and frostbite in horrible violations of codes of conduct and morality. During the postwar period the Japanese were held less accountable than Germans for these crimes. There was an international military tribunal convened in Tokyo that documented numerous atrocities, found many guilty, and executed some. In the aftermath of WW II there was great concern that the Allies acquire any and all information the Japanese had and that it not find its way into the hands of the Russians; in exchange for this information, many atrocities were overlooked.[17,18]

How is it that these gentle, cultured Japanese could perpetrate such crimes? Bushido. Bushido (the warrior's code) evolved over a millennium. It was the equivalent to religion, being a system of ethical imperatives. This developed together with military feudalism over centuries of isolation and framed the Japanese national character. It combined zen (meditating to reach thoughts beyond verbal expression, contemplation, and achievement of excellence) and Shintoism (loyalty to sovereign, ancestral reverence, and filial piety). Bushido emphasized calm, fatalism, submission, disdain of life, friendliness with death, stoicism confronting calamity, rectitude, valor, courage, benevolence, politeness, veracity, honor, loyalty, and self control. Japanese committed ritual suicide rather than surrender; there was nothing but disdain for an enemy who would not do the same. Vanquished populations and prisoners therefore had no redeeming human value and need not to have been treated in human fashion (according to this cultural view).[16]

In yet another aspect of contradictory behavior, the Japanese developed a little- known secretive (fugu, named after the dangerous blowfish) plan to import European Jews and American Jewish capital to help build the "Greater East Asia Co-Prosperity Sphere" in Manchuria during the 1930s. While this plan never came to fruition, Japan nonetheless saved several thousand Jews; all Jews who reached Japan were sheltered during World War II.[14,15]

Medicine in Japan

Viewed in the context in all of the foregoing, it should not therefore be surprising that medicine in Japan also differs substantially from western practice.[19] Western medicine was first introduced into Japan by the Portuguese by the 16th century. With the banning of Christianity and the exiling of foreigners, all external influences were essentially limited to an area off the Port of Nagasaki until the mid-1800s. Traders, including Dutch physicians, were in residence but there was little western influence. The Meiji restoration of the late 19th century led the Japanese to look to the West for a new model of medicine. The Japanese selected the German model (note that German medicine then was arguably the world's best). Note also that the German medical system was extraordinarily hierarchical, authoritarian, rigid, and dominated by the professor. As it evolved in Japan this was also stultifying.[20-31]

Japan currently has 80 medical schools. Forty-three are national, 8 are public, and 29 are private. Tuition may be up to $6000 annually for national or public schools and can cost from $60,000 to $90,000 per year for private schools. There are approximately 100 students per year per school, 30% of whom are now women. The curriculum is usually 6 years after high school; increasing numbers of students attend medical school after a 4-year college education. Medicine remains perhaps the most prestigious occupation in Japan, and entry to medical school is extremely competitive.[32]

Medical school education in Japan is extraordinarily didactic. It is allmost entirely based on amphitheater lectures. There has been very little bedside or clinical teaching, and some schools and curricula offer no bedside or clinical training at all in medical school. All graduates must pass a national examination before further training or practice.[20-32]

Graduate Medical Education is virtually without organization and reminiscent of the pre-Flexner era in the United States. There are no boards, no accreditation council of graduate of medical education , and no residency review committee equivalents. There are no prescribed training programs. There are no specialty or subspecialty requirements. Much of postgraduate training is organ system oriented. Most training occurs in professorial "fiefdoms"; academic departments consist of a professor, an associate professor (or 2) and numerous acolytes; the professor controls beds, dollars, resources, appointments, doctoral degrees, physicians, careers, and dogma. Graduates essentially apprentice themselves to a professor, learn what they can, often obtain a medical doctorate in medicine (PhD), and only then may then move on in their career paths.[20-25,33-35]

Similarly, internal medicine training is unregulated, authoritarian, undefined, variably clinically oriented, noninteractive, and without the Socratic/disputative tradition with which we are accustomed. Remember that the Japanese are not trained to question but to accept authority; they will do the professor's bidding, follow the professor on rounds, and uncritically accept directives. After training, physicians have potential choices of academic careers, hoping that somebody further up the hierarchy will move or die so that a position becomes available; become full-time, salaried employees of public or government hospitals; or go into private practice.[20-25,36-41]

Against this background an unusual, innovative, iconoclastic, imaginative, independent individual—Dr. Tadashi Matsumura—developed a novel unique experiment at Maizuru Municipal Hospital.[20,22,24,31,39] Maizuru is a fishing village of approximately 100,000 people about an hour and a half north of Kyoto, well off the beaten path. It was probably both appropriate and necessary that the venue for this "experiment" in Japan be distant from the entrenched establishment. Dr. Matsumura's hope, having done some of his clinical training in this country, was to introduce Western (American) teaching to an internal medicine residency program. He wished to stimulate his residents to develop intellectual curiosity, to question, and to think independently. He sought to develop interactive/disputative/Socratic teaching. He wanted his program to be clinical and to focus at the bedside. He introduced evidence-based medicine to Japanese internal medicine education and practice. His is an extremely unconventional and visionary effort. Over the course of a little more than a decade, Dr. Matsumura has invited Western (largely American) medical educators to spend time in his program, so that there is almost always an American physician in residence modeling these practices. From an unusual program in an out-of-the-way place, internal medicine in Maizuru has come to be recognized as the best medicine training program in Japan. It attracts the best students and residents, many of whom desert presumably more prestigious university programs. Indeed, more and more academic programs are emulating the Maizuru experiment; while I was there, we entertained visitors from one of the medical schools in Osaka. Dr Matsumura's efforts have begun to stimulate widespread educational reflection and beginnings of reform in Japan. I was honored to be among a number of distinguished medical educators who have visited Maizuru. These included many academic division and department chiefs and chairs, program directors, and presidents of the Association of Program Directors in Internal Medicine.[20,22,24,31,39]

Medicine in Japan and at Maizuru Municipal Hospital was, in many respects, like medicine in this country in the 1960s and 1970s. The hospital has 209 beds, 60 general medicine beds, and up to 45 acute care beds. There are 15,000 emergency department visits annually and 950 admissions annually. The average length of stay is 4 to 6 weeks, not days. The autopsy rate is about 30%. Hospital costs for patient care exceed reimbursement, with deficits being made up by government allocation. The Department of Internal Medicine at Maizuru consisted of 6 full-time faculty. There were 10 residents (3 PGY 1s, 2 PGY 2s, 2 PGY 3s, 1 PGY 4, 1 PGY5, and 1 PGY 7) (remember there is no set training program). Students from all over the country would spend 1 to 2 weeks each in the department for assignments that were highly sought after. The work day and work week are similar to what we are accustomed to. Mornings begin with a conference, followed by work rounds, teaching rounds, and case presentations. Afternoons include a formal lecture, more teaching rounds and case presentations, and departmental/staff rounds in the late afternoon and early evening.[31,41]

Medical practice and care are facilitated by mandatory, universal health insurance. The Japanese have unrestricted access to health care. They spend approximately half of what we do (6% gross national product) on health care. Their infant mortality is half of ours and they have the world's highest life expectancy. Private practitioners do extremely well financially. They will see 60 to 100 patients daily, in a manner quite different from us, and generate considerable personal income from prescribing medications; they may also have "clinics" of up to 19 beds (at 20 beds one needs special "hospital" certification). There is essentially no peer review in the country (recall the cultural value views of conformity and absence of criticism).[24,40]

There are very real differences in legal and ethical aspects of medicine between this country and Japan. Anyone interested in leaving this country to practice in Japan would be pleased to know that malpractice actions and judgments are exceedingly rare. Because of all of the cultural issues discussed previously, the Japanese deal quite differently than we do with informed consent, living wills, advance directives, organ donation, disclosure, imparting bad news, and industry-related gifts.[42-45]

Biomedical research flourishes in Japan. Japanese technology is highly sophisticated. In the literature I read, Japanese contribute large numbers of studies to quality peer-review journals. These are largely laboratory-based investigations, and largely technologically derived incremental advances. Clinical research is not highly developed in Japan. Research is extremely dependant on the professor leading the research team. And there is no rigorous peer review. For all of these reasons, and perhaps because of other reasons of cultural conformity, Japanese clinical research is not considered to have the level of innovation or originality seen in the West.[46]

Summary and Conclusions

Japan is unique. Centuries of isolation in a crowded, overpopulated land ruled by a divinity and frequented by natural disasters forged a unique culture. These ethnically homogeneous people were fatalistic; revered their emperor; embraced their shared history and destiny; sacrificed individualism for the common good; developed ritualistic social mores in response to the exigencies of their lives; and learned to value simplicity, beauty, and elegance.

So, too, did medicine evolve differently in Japan than in the West. Outside influences were introduced barely a century ago. Modern Japanese medicine was modeled on German tradition, a rigidly hierarchical and authoritarian method, which fit smoothly into Japanese culture. Consequences of this now are a system of medical education that is didactic, chaotic, unregulated, intellectually stifling, devoid of disputative/disputative dialogue, without peer review, and without bedside/clinical teaching. Yet health insurance in Japan is universal, care is available to all, and certain outcomes (infant mortality and life expectancy) are the best in the world at half the percentage of gross national product the United States spends on health care.

The iconoclastic experiment at Maizuru, bringing American-style clinical teaching to the Japanese bedside in internal medicine, is an exciting one; nonconformity is not tolerated in Japan and it took special vision and courage to implement this innovation. And, judging by the excellent performance of the Maizuru residents and the growing interest of other teaching programs in Japan in emulating the Maizuru experience, it is a resounding success in at least those terms. It was an honor to participate in the endeavor, and enormous fun.

It is tempting to conclude that Japan needs more of this, that Japanese medicine (and culture) is curious but inferior to America's, that our ways (including medical education) are the standards that the rest of the world should adopt. Perhaps. Perhaps not. Beware cultural imperialism. Different is not lesser value or less worth. Somehow the different Japanese system of health care produces certain better outcomes than ours at less societal cost. Is this causal? Would they do even better adopting our methods? Would we do less well with other approaches? I don't know, but it invites caution in assuming ours is necessarily the only way to do things.

The real lesson of this experience is, I think, that fundamentally "Japanese are no different than us,"[2] even though our cultures may be. During the month we were all doctors, surely with different backgrounds, but all doctors, teaching and learning, trying to provide the best possible care to patients. I know I learned at least as much from my Japanese hosts as (I hope) they did from me.

"Japanese are no different than us."

J Michener, *Sayonara*[2]

"For the first-time gai-jin, Japan is an underachiever's fantasy of success, a place where you can have recognition without effort. If you are young, tall, or blond, you are treated as if you are a movie star. It can easily go to your head. I've seen numerous Westerners come to believe they are as glamorous, brilliant, and important as Japanese pretend they are—whether you are applauded or criticized, as a foreigner in Japan you're never invisible."

C Davidson, *36 Views of Mount Fuji*[7]

R. S. Panush, MD

References

1. Barthes R: *Empire of signs*, New York, 1982, Hill and Wang.
2. Michener JA: *Sayonara*, New York, 1953, Random House.
3. Benedict R: *The chrysanthemum and the sword: Patterns of Japanese culture*, Boston, 1989, Mariner Books.
4. Reischauer EO: *The Japanese*, Cambridge, 1977, Harvard University Press.
5. Christopher RC: *The Japanese mind: The Goliath explained*, New York, 1983, Simon and Schuster.
6. Field N: *In the realm of a dying Emperor. A portrait of Japan at century's end*, New York, 1991, Random House.
7. Davidson CN: *36 Views of Mount Fuji*, New York, 1993, Dutton/Penguin Books.

8. Oe K: *A personal matter*, Grove, NY, 1969.
9. Florence M: *Kyoto*, Oakland, California, 1999, Lonely Planet Publications.
10. Reiber B, Spencer J: *Frommer's Japan*, ed 5, New York, 2000, IDG Books.
11. Norbury P: *Culture smart! Japan*, Portland, Oregon, 2003, Graphic Arts Center Publishing.
12. Barry D: *Dave Barry does Japan*, New York, 1992, Random House.
13. Toland J: *The rising sun: The decline and fall of the Japanese empire, 1936-1945*, New York, 1970, Modern Library.
14. Tokayer M, Swartz M: *The Fugu plan: The untold story of the Japanese and the Jews during World War II*, New York, 1979, Paddington Press.
15. Ben-Dasan I: *The Japanese and the Jews*, Weatherhill, NY, 1972.
16. Niboe I: *Bushido: The warrior's code*, Santa Clarita, CA, 1979, Ohara Publications.
17. Gold H: *Unit 731 testimony: Japan's wartime human experimentation program*, Singapore, 1996, Yen Books.
18. Russell L: *The knights of bushido: A short history of Japanese war crimes*, Cassell & Co LTD, London, 2002.
19. Schor JD: "Wabi-Sabi." *JAMA* 252:3173, 1984.
20. Mori W, Homma S: *Medical science and health care in the coming century: A report from Japan*, New York, 1987, Elsevier.
21. Nakagawa Y: Adoption of western medicine in Japan. *Clio Medical* 21:113-118, 1987-1988
22. Hadler NM: An American medical educator at the Japanese bedside. *Pharos Alpha Omega Alpha Med Soc* 57:9-13, 1988.
23. Roberts WC: Japan and Japanese medicine. *Am J Cardiol* 60:427-430, 1987.
24. Tierney LM: An experience in Japanese academic medicine. *West J Med* 160:139-145, 1994.
25. Talwalkar YB: Virtues and vagaries of Japanese postgraduate medical education. *Neurol Therapeutics* 10:545-552, 1993.
26. Muraki Y: A Japanese medical student in a medical clerkship program in North Carolina. *N C Med J* 62:163-165, 2001.
27. Hefelfinger DC: International medical education. Graduate medical education at Chubu hospital, Okinawa, Japan. *Acad Med* 73:1274-1276, 1998.
28. Gillespie CA, Gillespie HE, Carr JE: Contrasts between Japanese and American medical education. *Mil Med* 149:393-396, 1984.
29. Ginoza M: A rotation in a Japanese hospital. *Hawaii Med J* 47:494, 1988.
30. Gibbons RB: Medical education in Japan. *Newsletter of the Association of Program Directors in Internal Medicine* 10:6-7, 1993.
31. Matsumura RL. Personal communication, 2002.
32. Kozu T: Undergraduate and postgraduate clinical education in Japan: The present and future situations. *Kobe J Med Sci* 43:216-235, 1997.
33. Ushiba D: Trends of medical education in Japan. *Med Educ* 19:258-265, 1985.
34. Yanto E, Yamaoka K, Sugita S, et al: Comparing postgraduate medical education at university and non-university hospitals in Japan. *Acad Med* 67:54-58, 1992.
35. Maruo T: Undergraduate and postgraduate clinical education in Kobe university school of medicine. *Kobe J Med Sci* 43:237-242, 1997.
36. Otaki J: International medical education. Considering primary care in Japan. *Acad Med* 73:662-668, 1998.
37. Ohtaki J, Fujisaki K, Terasaki H, et al: Specialty choice and understanding of primary care among Japanese medical students. *Med Educ* 30:378-384, 1996.
38. Seo M, Tamura K, Morioka E, et al: Impact of medical round on patients' and residents' perceptions at a university hospital in Japan. *Med Educ* 34:409-411, 2000.
39. Stein GH: Creative thinking-clinical problem solving resident physician training program at Kameda medical center. *Jpn Hosp* 14:35-37, 1995.
40. Rodnick JE, Werdegar D: Impressions of health care and medical education in Japan. *Fam Med* 17:166-169, 1985.

41. Yamaoka K, Kobayashi Y, Yano E: Length of in-patient stay in teaching hospitals in Japan. *Med Educ* 27:280-285, 1993.
42. Matsue T, Ozawa T, Orimo H, et al: The difference between Japan and other countries, in particular the United Kingdom, in views regarding the teaching of geriatrics to undergraduate medical students. *Med Educ* 33:140-144, 1999.
43. Asai A, Kishino M, Fukui T, et al: Postgraduate education in medical ethics in Japan. *Med Educ* 32:100-104, 1996.
44. Long SO, Long BD: Curable cancers and fatal ulcers. Attitudes toward cancer in Japan. *Soc Sci Med* 16:2101-2108, 1982.
45. Tsuruoka K, Tsuruoka Y, Kajii E: Complementary medicine education in Japanese medical schools: A survey. *Complement Ther Med* 9:28-33, 2001.
46. Imamura K: A critical look at health research in Japan. *Lancet* 342:279-282, 1993.

Spondyloarthropathies

Long-term Efficacy and Safety of Infliximab in the Treatment of Ankylosing Spondylitis: An Open, Observational, Extension Study of a Three-Month, Randomized, Placebo-Controlled Trial

Braun J, Brandt J, Listing J, et al (Free Univ, Berlin; Rheumatology Med Ctr Ruhrgebiet, Herne, Germany; German Rheumatism Research Ctr, Berlin; et al)
Arthritis Rheum 48:2224-2233, 2003 7–2

Introduction.—The treatment of ankylosing spondylitis (AS) with infliximab, an anti–tumor necrosis factor α monoclonal antibody, was efficacious in patients with active disease during a 3-month evaluation period. The efficacy and safety of infliximab treatment of AS was assessed for a 1-year evaluation period in an open, observational, extension trial of a 3-month, randomized, placebo-controlled investigation.

Methods.—All patients who tolerated infliximab (infliximab/infliximab group) or placebo (placebo/infliximab 12-week crossover group) therapy for 3 months were included in the open extension trial. Infliximab (5 mg/kg) was administered every 6 weeks after the induction phase (weeks 0, 2, and 6). The major end point was a 50% improvement in the Bath Ankylosing Spondylitis Disease Activity Index (BASDAI).

Results.—At week 54, 54 of 69 patients (78%) were still taking infliximab. The intent-to-treat primary efficacy analysis at week 54 revealed that 47% of the infliximab/infliximab group (95% CI, 31%-63%) and 51% of the placebo/infliximab group (95% CI, 36%-67%) achieved a 50% improvement in BASDAI scores (Fig 2). An analysis of those who completed the trial showed that the BASDAI scores improved between weeks 0 and 54 in both treatment groups: from 6.6 to 2.4 in the infliximab/infliximab group and from 6.3 to 2.6 in the placebo/infliximab group. The dosage of nonsteroidal anti-inflammatory drugs was decreased in nearly 70% of patients. Significant improvements were seen in measures of functioning, metrologic variables, and quality of life. Between weeks 12 and 54, 4 patients experienced serious adverse events, possibly associated with infliximab, which resulted in their elimination from the trial.

Conclusion.—Infliximab therapy in patients with AS produced a rapid and significant improvement in BASDAI scores (>50% improvement) and a

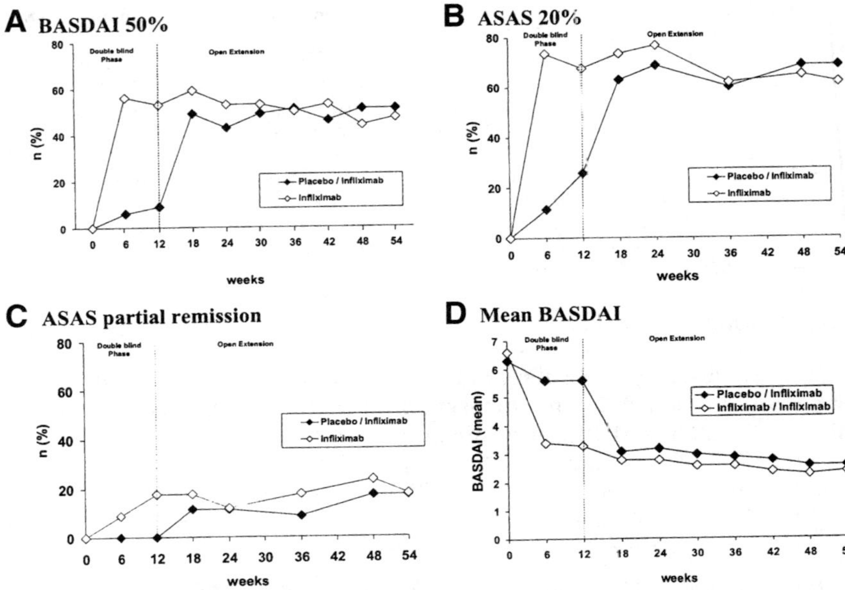

FIGURE 2.—Response to treatment, as measured by **A**, the Bath Ankylosing Spondylitis Disease Activity Index (BASDAI) scores at the 50% improvement level, **B**, the Assessment of Ankylosing Spondylitis (ASAS) criteria for 20% improvement, **C**, the ASAS criteria for partial remission, and **D**, the mean BASDAI scores. Only the 54 patients who completed week 54 of study are shown. Intent-to-treat analyses were performed on the data shown in **A-C**. (Courtesy of Braun J, Brandt J, Listing J, et al: Long-term efficacy and safety of infliximab in the treatment of ankylosing spondylitis: An open, observational, extension study of a three-month, randomized, placebo-controlled trial. *Arthritis Rheum* 48:2224-2233, 2003. Reprinted by permission from John Wiley & Sons, Inc.)

durable response for 1 year. The safety profile of infliximab in AS was comparable with that seen in the postmarketing experience for the approved indications.

▶ This was a pivotal study in the decision by the US Food and Drug Administration to add AS to the licensed indications for therapy with tumor necrosis factor (TNF)-α inhibitors. Before that decision, a conference was convened of investigators, purveyors, and "thought leaders" to discuss the indications for such therapy. I was invited, I guess in the third category (or in a fourth category of inveterate critics of therapeutic zeal).

The data, such as in this article, that infliximab offers an impressive short-term benefit to patients with inflammatory symptoms of AS is impressive (Fig 2). However, for most patients, AS is a mild disease characterized by intermittent gentle flares of backache that are no more frequent than the episodes of regional back pain suffered by all and no more likely to be associated with a loss of suppleness. Even for most patients with moderately severe spondylitis, exercises and nonsteroidal anti-inflammatory drugs prove a match. It is hard to justify long-term exposure to the long-term uncertainties of TNF-α inhibitors in either of these strata of severity of spondylitis.

The agent should be reserved for patients with recalcitrant inflammatory disease or for those with progressive syndesmophyte formation.

N. M. Hadler, MD

Recombinant Human Tumor Necrosis Factor Receptor (Etanercept) for Treating Ankylosing Spondylitis: A Randomized, Controlled Trial

Davis JC Jr, for the Enbrel Ankylosing Spondylitis Study Group (Univ of California, San Francisco; Univ Hosp, Maastricht, The Netherlands; Herne, Germany; et al)

Arthritis Rheum 48:3230-3236, 2003 7–3

Background.—Approximately 350,000 individuals in the United States are afflicted with ankylosing spondylitis, an inflammatory arthritis and enthesitis that involves the spine and peripheral joints. Traditional therapies, which include disease-modifying antirheumatic drugs, nonsteroidal anti-inflammatory drugs, and corticosteroids, do not adequately control disease activity in most patients. Thus, safe and effective therapy is needed for patients with ankylosing spondylitis. Tumor necrosis factor is important in the pathogenesis of ankylosing spondylitis. Tumor necrosis factor concentrations are elevated in the serum and synovial tissue of patients with this disease. Etanercept has been shown to substantially reduce disease activity in patients with spondyloarthropathies. Etanercept was compared with placebo in patients with moderate to severe active ankylosing spondylitis.

Methods.—A total of 277 patients were enrolled in this multicenter, randomized, placebo-controlled, double-blind trial. Patients were treated with etanercept (138 patients) or placebo (139 patients) subcutaneously twice a week for 24 weeks. The main outcome measure was the percentage of patients achieving the Assessments in Ankylosing Spondylitis 20% response (ASAS20) at weeks 12 and 24. Other outcome measures included the percentage of patients that achieved higher ASAS responses and the safety of etanercept in patients with ankylosing spondylitis. Outcome measures were assessed at 2, 4, 8, 12, and 24 weeks.

Results.—A dramatic improvement was observed in patients who were treated with etanercept. The ASAS20 was achieved by 59% of patients in the etanercept group and by 28% of patients in the placebo group at week 12 and by 57% and 22% of patients, respectively, at week 24 (Fig 2). Significant improvements were seen in all individual ASAS components, in early-phase reactant levels, and in spinal mobility measures. The safety profile of etanercept was similar to that reported in studies of patients with RA or psoriatic arthritis. Adverse events that occurred significantly more often in the treatment group than in the placebo group were injection-site reactions, accidental injuries, and upper respiratory tract infections.

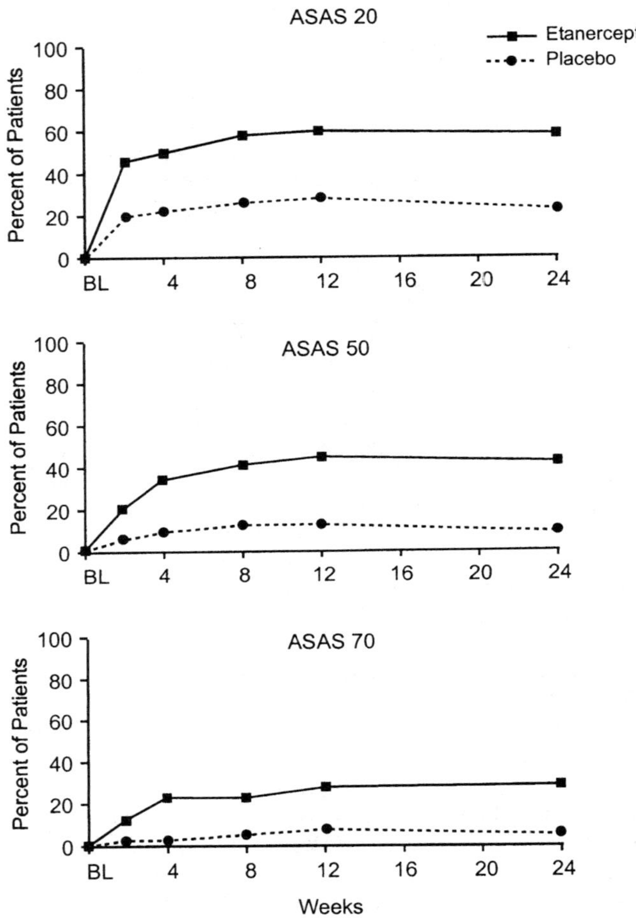

FIGURE 2.—Achievement of the Assessments in Ankylosing Spondylitis 20% response (ASAS20), the ASAS50, and the ASAS70 in patients with ankylosing spondylitis treated with etanercept or placebo, by length of treatment. $P < .01$ at all time points for all analyses. (Courtesy of Davis JC Jr, for the Enbrel Ankylosing Spondylitis Study Group: Recombinant human tumor necrosis factor receptor (etanercept) for treating ankylosing spondylitis: A randomized, controlled trial. *Arthritis Rheum* 48:3230-3236, 2003. Reprinted by permission of John Wiley & Sons, Inc.)

Conclusions.— For patients with active ankylosing spondylitis, etanercept seems to be a highly effective and well-tolerated treatment.

▶ Clearly, this is a therapeutic breakthrough. However, I was invited to participate in a meeting that was designed to inform the US Food and Drug Administration of issues that relate to licensing etanercept for this indication. There are several.

Most patients with ankylosing spondylitis have mild disease. The majority of cases go undiagnosed. Many are diagnosed based on incidental findings on radiographs. The patients all have episodes of backache, but don't we all? In fact, an article from Bath, England, suggests that many a "flare" in patients with an established diagnosis of ankylosing spondylitis represents a coincidental regional musculoskeletal disorder. How are we to determine which patient with ankylosing spondylitis is a candidate for etanercept? The agent is expensive, and its long-term toxic effects (which are relevant in this disease) have yet to be defined.

The consensus is that the agent should be reserved for patients with overt radiographic involvement faced with persistent high level symptoms. These were the patients enrolled in this trial.

N. M. Hadler, MD

Infliximab Therapy for Rheumatic Diseases in Patients With Chronic Hepatitis B or C

Oniankitan O, Duvoux C, Challine D, et al (Henri Mondor Teaching Hosp, Créteil, France)

J Rheumatol 31:107-109, 2004 7–4

Introduction.—Infliximab is a monoclonal anti-tumor necrosis factor–α (TNF-α) antibody with proven efficacy in the treatment of RA, Crohn's disease, and spondyloarthropathies. Since infliximab can reduce the macrophage TNF-α–dependent response, it should not be used for patients with overt infectious diseases. Chronic viral infections (ie, hepatitis B and C) are considered relative contraindications, given the extreme scarcity of data regarding the effect of infliximab for these conditions. Described was the first year of clinical and laboratory test data obtained on 2 patients with chronic inflammatory joint disease and chronic hepatitis B or C who were treated with infliximab.

Methods.—Disease activity, liver function tests, and hepatitis C virus and hepatitis B virus status were assessed before infliximab therapy was initiated. These parameters were reassessed before every infusion. Both patients underwent liver biopsy before infliximab therapy was initiated.

Results.—After over 1 year of treatment with infliximab, no worsening of liver function or virologic status was seen. Dramatic clinical improvements in joint disease were observed in both patients.

Conclusion.—Infliximab therapy may be safe in some patients with concomitant severe inflammatory joint disease and quiescent or controlled chronic hepatitis B or hepatitis C virus infection.

► I only choose case reports for review when I feel they offer a wake-up call. TNF-α inhibitors are powerful biologics. It is truly remarkable and fortunate that an agent like infliximab has proved to have a positive benefit/risk ratio in RA, Crohn's, and now the spondyloarthropathies (see Abstract 7–2). That is not to say that there are no worrisome aspects to the immunomodulation, such as the serologic changes noted in Abstract 3–5. At least in the relatively short term, the infliximab has done little harm.

The agent is so widely used that it is bound to transgress the criteria established for the trials that established its efficacy. Coincident chronic hepatitis C and hepatitis B virus infection both are examples, and interesting examples at that. Both the hepatitis C and hepatitis B viruses are not cytopathic. Liver damage is thought to result from the immune response to the altered hepatocytes. These 2 case reports suggest that interfering with TNF-α biology does not enhance the cytopathic immune response. Next we need trials to see if infliximab can find a place amongst the newer agents used to treat viral hepatitis.

N. M. Hadler, MD

Crystal-induced Arthropathies

Effect of Exercise and Beer on the Plasma Concentration and Urinary Excretion of Purine Bases

Ka T, Yamamoto T, Moriwaki Y, et al (Hyogo College of Medicine, Japan)
J Rheumatol 30:1036-1042, 2003 7–5

Introduction.—Alcoholic beverages, particularly beer, increase the level of uric acid in serum because ethanol ingestion increases adenosine triphosphate degradation in the liver. Exercise enhances adenosine triphosphate degradation in muscles. The effects of exercise and beer ingestion, separately and combined, on the plasma concentration of purine bases was examined in 6 healthy men.

Methods.—The participant age range was 30 to 39 years. During 3 different experiments, participants exercised for 30 minutes (at 70% of maximum oxygen uptake) and ingested beer (10 mg/kg body weight) or performed each activity separately, with each experiment performed at 2-week intervals.

Results.—The plasma concentration of uric acid was increased by 12% ($P < .05$), 8% ($P < .01$), and 29% ($P < .01$) with exercise, beer ingestion, and a combination of exercise and beer ingestion, respectively (Fig 2), which demonstrated that it increased synergistically in the combination experiment. The fractional excretion of uric acid was diminished by 44% ($P < .01$) and 52% ($P < .01$) with exercise alone and with a combination of exercise and beer ingestion, respectively; it was increased by 15% ($P < .01$) with beer ingestion alone.

Creatinine clearance was diminished by 16% ($P < .01$) with both exercise alone and a combination of exercise and beer ingestion; it was not modified with beer ingestion alone. The increase in the plasma concentration of xanthine during the beer ingestion experiment was 2.1-fold greater than during the combination ($P < .05$). The increase in urinary excretion of xanthine caused by beer ingestion was 2.5-fold greater than that caused by beer and exercise combined ($P < .05$). Exercise alone, together with a combination of beer and exercise, increased the blood concentration of lactic acid and NH_3. Beer alone reduced the concentration of pyruvic acid.

Conclusion.—The production of uric acid caused by both exercise and beer ingestion, along with the inhibition of urinary uric acid excretion from a high blood lactic acid concentration, were the primary contributors to the

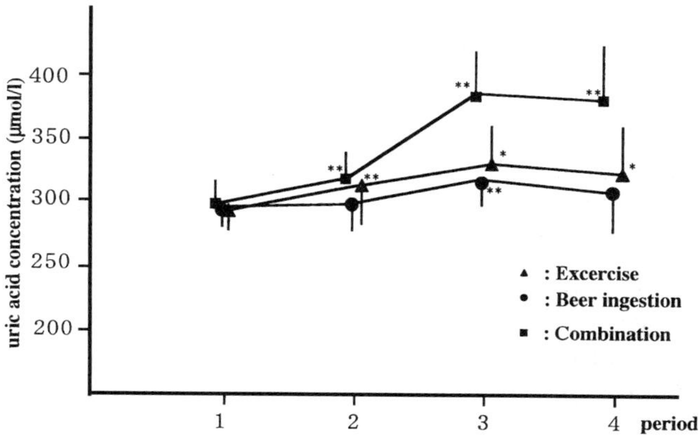

FIGURE 2.—Plasma concentration of uric acid in the 3 experiments (beer ingestion, exercise, and combination). In the exercise experiment, the plasma concentration of uric acid increased by 8%, 12%, and 11% in the second, third, and fourth periods, respectively, as compared with the reference value in the first period. In the beer ingestion experiment, it also increased by 8% in the third period. In the combination experiment as well, the plasma concentration of uric acid increased by 9%, 29%, and 27% in the second, third, and fourth periods, respectively. *Single asterisk* indicates $P < .05$; *double asterisk*, $P < .01$. (Courtesy of Ka T, Yamamoto T, Moriwaki Y, et al: Effect of exercise and beer on the plasma concentration and urinary excretion of purine bases. *J Rheumatol* 30:1036-1042, 2003.)

synergistic effect on the increase in plasma uric acid concentration. A reduction in creatinine clearance also contributed to the effect. It is likely that pyruvic acid and NH_3 produced in the muscles after exercise relieved the beer-induced increase in the plasma concentration and urinary excretion of xanthine. This may have had a minor role in the increase in plasma uric acid concentration.

▶ Interesting. I guess if you have gout, or maybe hyperuricemia, don't drink beer after exercising. Since this study is from Japan, it is worth pointing out that Japanese are smaller than Americans and their beer cans and bottles are packaged in larger containers than ours (personal observations, May 2003).

R. S. Panush, MD

The Cervical Spine in Calcium Pyrophosphate Dihydrate Deposition Disease: A Prevalent Case-Control Study

Finckh A, van Linthoudt D, Duvoisin B, et al (Univ Hosp of Vaud, Lausanne, Switzerland; Community Hosp of La Chaux-de-Fonds, Switzerland; Brigham and Women's Hosp, Boston)

J Rheumatol 31:545-549, 2004 7–6

Background.—Calcium pyrophosphate dihydrate (CPPD) deposition disease is a common rheumatologic disorder, particularly among elderly patients. CPPD is rare with people less than 50 years old, but the incidence ranges from 10% to 15% in persons 65 to 80 years, and more than 20% for persons 80 years or older. CPPD deposition disease is often considered a disorder of the peripheral joints. However, involvement of the spine is not uncommon. In the cervical spine, calcified deposits have been reported in almost every anatomical structure, including the transverse ligament of the atlas (TLA). The presence of CPPD crystals in these locations can trigger various conditions, causing neck pain. The hypothesis that CPPD deposition may also be a risk factor for neck pain was tested.

Methods.—A prevalent case-control study was conducted to assess cervical calcifications and neck pain between patients with and without known peripheral CPPD deposition disease. Cases were included if diagnosed with CPPD deposition of peripheral joints, and excluded if the chief complaint was neck pain. Cervical calcifications were assessed by lateral cervical radiographs and CT scans of the upper cervical spine. Neck pain and cervical function were appraised by a validated questionnaire.

Results.—Cervical calcifications were identified in 24 (69%) of 35 patients in the CPPD group, compared with 4 (11%) of 35 patients in the control group. Significantly more neck pain and discomfort were reported by patients with CPPD deposition disease compared with that of control subjects, and the patients with CPPD disease were 5 times more likely to report any neck pain. Among male patients, the presence of more extensive cervical calcified deposits was correlated with more severe neck pain.

Conclusions.—The cervical spine is frequently involved in CPPD deposition disease, and this involvement may be associated with the development of neck pain.

► I didn't appreciate that neck involvement, with symptoms, was this prevalent with CPPD. I will think about this when I see these patients.

R. S. Panush, MD

Infectious Arthritis and Lyme Disease

How Can We Prevent Lyme Disease?

Hayes EB, Piesman J (Ctrs for Disease Control and Prevention, Fort Collins, Colo)

N Engl J Med 348:2424-2430, 2003 7–7

Introduction.—The number of cases of Lyme disease in the United States has risen from 491 in 1982 to 17,029 in 2001. Nearly 60,000 cases are reported yearly in Europe. Most efforts at prevention have concentrated on spreading information regarding how Lyme disease is transmitted and on encouraging people to use repellents, wear protective clothing, and check themselves for ticks. The recommendations may have blunted the increase in Lyme disease in the United States, yet have not been adequate to decrease the number of cases. The prevention and treatment of Lyme disease were discussed, along with strategies for tick control.

Prevention and Treatment of Lyme Disease.—Most people with Lyme disease are seen with erythema migrans, a recognizable rash. About 20% will have mild infections that abate without treatment, and 90% treated for early-stage Lyme disease have an excellent response to antibiotic therapy,

TABLE 1.—Public Health Strategies to Prevent Lyme Disease in Communities

Promote daily tick checks and prompt removal of ticks
Provide guidance to clinicians on differentiating among local tick species
Encourage prophylactic treatment of bites from deer ticks under certain circumstances
Educate residents about efficacious methods of tick control, including area-wide use of acaricides and landscaping
Consider acaricides for specific host animals and exclusion or removal of deer
Train pest-control personnel and educate residents to use tick-control strategies properly so that adverse environmental effects are minimized
Encourage residents to practice or engage in at least one of the above prevention strategies

particularly amoxicillin and doxycycline. The remaining patients may experience symptoms that range from neurologic or joint abnormalities to encephalopathy, necessitating IV antibiotic therapy. Primary prevention strategies can help avert Lyme disease and other tick-borne illnesses. It is important that most people in a community adopt at least 1 prevention strategy (Table 1).

Tick Control.—There is scientific evidence that removal of an *Ixodes scapularis* (deer tick) within 36 hours of attachment will diminish the risk of *Borrelia burgdorferi* infection. A single 200-mg dose of doxycycline administered within 72 hours after a recognized *I scapularis* bite has an efficacy of 87% for preventing erythema migrans. For ticks attached for less than 36 hours, treatment of the bite is not necessary (Table 2).

The most effective strategy for decreasing the population of ticks on residential properties is to apply acaricides on vegetation where ticks live. These agents should be used sparingly due to the potential toxic effects on organisms not targeted. Removing underbrush in wooded areas exposes tick eggs

TABLE 2.—Strategies to Prevent Lyme Disease in the Clinical Setting

Educate patients to check for, and promptly remove, attached ticks
Provide prophylactic treatment of tick bites in certain situations
Within 72 hours after the discovery of a deer tick that is obviously engorged, or that was attached for more than 72 hours, on an adult from an area where Lyme disease is endemic, administer 200 mg doxycycline as a single dose
Within 72 hours after the discovery of a deer tick that was attached for 36 to 72 hours, consider 200 mg of doxycycline as a single dose
When the tick was attached for less than 36 hours, it is not necessary to treat the bite
In children, dosing and efficacy of prophylactic treatment have not been evaluated
Learn to recognize and treat promptly erythema migrans and other early manifestations of Lyme disease

to sunlight and reduces the tick population. Although not commercially available, acaricide fipronil for the treatment of rodents and ticks has potential for diminishing tick populations.

Conclusion.—The cooperation of public health officials, clinicians, and residents of affected areas is needed to reduce the incidence of Lyme disease.

Cognitive Function in Post-Treatment Lyme Disease: Do Additional Antibiotics Help?

Kaplan RF, Trevino RP, Johnson GM, et al (Univ of Connecticut, Farmington; Boston Univ; New York Med College, Valhalla; et al)
Neurology 60:1916-1922, 2003 7–8

Introduction.—Some patients experience persistent symptoms after recommended antibiotic treatment for Lyme disease. This condition, posttreatment chronic Lyme disease (PTCLD), may produce cognitive manifestations. It is not known whether additional antibiotic treatment will improve cognitive function in patients with PTCLD. Two randomized, double-blind, placebo-controlled trials were performed to ascertain whether antibiotic therapy improves cognitive function in patients with PTCLD.

Methods.—One hundred twenty-nine patients from 3 study sites in the northeast United States who had a physician-verified history of Lyme disease were evaluated. Of these, 78 were seropositive for immunoglobulin G antibodies against *Borrelia burgdorferi* and 51 were seronegative. Participants in each group were randomly assigned to receive IV, ceftriaxone 2 g daily for 30 days, then oral doxycycline, 200 mg daily for 60 days, or matching IV and oral placebos.

Patients were reevaluated at 90 and 180 days after treatment. Symptom severity was determined from the cognitive functioning, pain, and role functioning scales of the Medical Outcomes Study (MOS). Memory, attention, and executive functioning were evaluated by objective testing. Mood was evaluated by the Beck Depression Inventory and Minnesota Multiphasic Personality Inventory.

Results.—Seropositive and seronegative groups did not differ significantly at baseline. Both groups had a high incidence of MOS symptoms, depression, and somatic complaints; baseline neuropsychosocial test scores were normal. The combined groups demonstrated significant reductions in MOS symptoms, higher objective test scores, and improved mood between baseline and 90 days. There were no significant differences between recipients of antibiotics compared with those receiving placebo (Fig 2).

Conclusion.—There is no objective evidence of cognitive impairment in patients with PTCLD with symptoms and no evidence of persistent *B burgdorferi* infection.

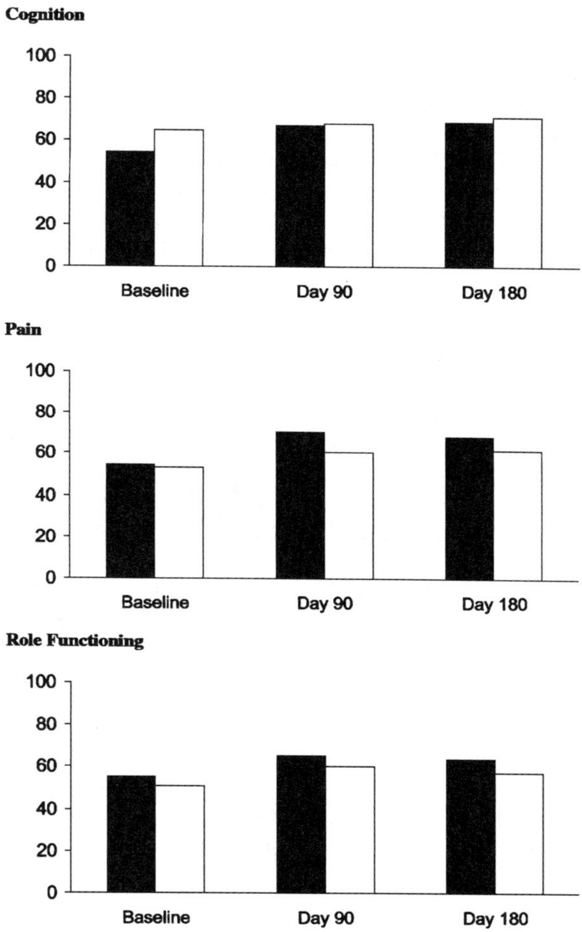

FIGURE 2.—Medical Outcomes Study scales for patients receiving antibiotics (*black bars*) and those receiving placebo (*white bars*). For each scale, the range of scores was 0 to 100, with higher scores indicating better cognitive functioning, less pain, and fewer limitations in daily functioning. (Courtesy of Kaplan RF, Trevino RP, Johnson GM, et al: Cognitive function in post-treatment Lyme disease: Do antibiotics help? *Neurology* 60(2):1916-1922, 2003.)

Study and Treatment of Post Lyme Disease (STOP-LD): A Randomized Double Masked Clinical Trial

Krupp LB, Hyman LG, Grimson R, et al (Stony Brook Univ, NY)
Neurology 60:1923-1930, 2003 7–9

Background.—Most patients with Lyme disease are cured by a simple antibiotic regimen. Some patients' complaints remain after 1 or more courses of treatment, and these are classified as having post–Lyme syndrome. Whether the ongoing symptoms of post–Lyme syndrome can be successfully managed with antibiotics was assessed by determining the clinical improvement in severe fatigue and cognitive speed and clearance of a potential biological marker of infection.

Methods.—The 55 patients with Lyme disease had persistent severe fatigue lasting at least 6 months after antibiotic therapy. Twenty-eight patients were randomly assigned to receive ceftriaxone and 27 to receive placebo. Measures included improvement in fatigue, which was defined by a change of at least 0.7 points on an 11-item fatigue questionnaire, and improvement in cognitive function, which was defined as a change of 25% or greater on a test of reaction time. An experimental measure of CSF infection, outer surface protein A, was the primary laboratory outcome and was determined at the 6-month evaluation.

Results.—Sixty-four percent of patients taking ceftriaxone and 18.5% of those taking placebo had improved fatigue levels. Improvement was present at 1 month in both groups but was maintained only in the ceftriaxone group. The most significant improvements were noted in patients who had a positive Western blot, no previous IV therapy, and less pain (visual analogue scale score of less than 5.7). The effect on fatigue remained significant, even when adjustments were made for psychiatric disorder, depressive symptoms, pain, and age.

Neither ceftriaxone nor placebo had any effect on cognitive speed or overall performance on a neuropsychological battery. Verbal memory, attention, and cognitive processing speed showed no group differences. Only 16% of the patients had outer surface protein A antigen at baseline, and its clearance did not differ between the 2 groups after 6 months. No significant differences in the frequency of serious or minor adverse events were noted between the groups, although 43% of those taking ceftriaxone and only 25% of those taking placebo had diarrhea.

Conclusion.—Ceftriaxone treatment for 28 days produced improvement in fatigue but not in cognitive function among patients with persistent Lyme disease. The improvement was noted in the first month, as was improvement with placebo, but only the treatment group continued to have improvement at 6 months. Patients who had had oral therapy only in the past had better results than those who had previous IV therapy. Thus, the repeated courses of antibiotics sometimes used for persistent Lyme disease appear not to be justified by the outcomes and run the risk of serious adverse effects related to the antibiotics administered.

Long-term Follow-up of Patients With Culture-Confirmed Lyme Disease

Nowakowski J, Nadelman RB, Sell R, et al (New York Med College, Valhalla; Westchester Med Ctr, Valhalla, NY)

Am J Med 115:91-96, 2003 7–10

Background.—Erythema migrans was found in over 90% of patients who met the criteria of the Centers for Disease Control and Prevention (CDC) for Lyme disease. Not all patients who seem to have erythema migrans are infected with *Borrelia burgdorferi*. In some cases, patients have a tick-bite hypersensitivity reaction or infection caused by another tick-borne organism. Thus, culture is required to verify *B burgdorferi* infection. A prospective evaluation of patients with culture-confirmed erythema migrans from an area highly endemic for Lyme disease was undertaken.

Methods.—Data from a highly endemic area in New York State covered 94 patients (96 episodes) diagnosed with early Lyme disease between 1991 and 1994. Assessments were carried out at baseline and after 7 to 10 days, 21 to 28 days, 3 months, 6 months, 1 year, and annually after that point. Follow-up extended for a mean of 4.9 years. The patients received antibiotics when their disease was diagnosed.

Results.—Eighty-seven cases were treated with a first-line oral antimicrobial regimen or IV ceftriaxone for 10 to 21 days. In nine cases, the treatment was a 7-day course of azithromycin. All but 2 patients who did not return after the baseline visit had documented improvement in their condition. Two patients required additional treatment for continuing symptoms, 1 after 3 months and 6 months and 1 after 6 years. No demonstrable clinical response was achieved in these cases. All 94 patients who were evaluated showed resolution of the erythema migrans rash within 3 weeks of treatment. Ten percent of the patients were symptomatic at their final visit, which was a mean of 5.6 years after their treatment. Three patients had consistent symptoms; the other 5 patients had intermittent symptoms.

In 71% of the 7 cases evaluated, symptoms were mild. Forty-seven percent of the patients reported intercurrent tick bites. In 14 patients, erythema migrans developed a second time, and 3 patients were reinfected a third time. Four patients seroconverted after 2 to 5 years, even though they had no change in symptoms or erythema migrans recurrence. Development of symptoms during follow-up was statistically linked to more numerous and more severe symptoms at baseline and multiple erythema migrans skin lesions at presentation. No correlation with outcome was found for baseline or current seropositivity or for the duration of erythema migrans before antibiotics were received.

Conclusion.—The 96 cases reported had excellent outcomes. The lesions of erythema migrans resolved within 3 weeks, and by 3 months, 85% of the patients were asymptomatic or had returned to their previous health status. After 6 months, 92% of the patients had returned to their previous health status. Eight patients were symptomatic after 1 year, but only 3 were consistently symptomatic from baseline on. Thus, the long-term outcome of patients whose early Lyme disease is treated with antibiotics is excellent, although these patients remain at high risk of repeated tick bites and reinfection related to their geographic area.

► Fortunately, I have only seen 1 "pseudo-Lyme" disease patient recently. Interestingly, she had had classic clinical features of polychondritis for many years. But since she had an intercurrent illness which could have been (treated) Lyme infection, she and her family chose to believe that she had "chronic" Lyme disease and sought (and received) long-term antibiotics. I encountered her in the hospital, where she landed because of complications of her antibiotic treatment. Unfortunately, like so many of these patients who adopt a belief system incompatible with current science and biology, she was lost to follow-up, presumably returning to someone who would inappropriately care for her inappropriate diagnosis. I like these articles (Abstracts 7–7 through 7–10), which emphasize the need to address Lyme disease by prevention and underscore the increasingly clear data indicating that prolonged antibiotics for Lyme disease are worthless.

R. S. Panush, MD

Septic Arthritis of the Pubic Symphysis: Review of 100 Cases

Ross JJ, Hu LT (Caritas Saint Elizabeth's Med Ctr, Boston; New England Med Ctr, Boston)

Medicine 82:340-345, 2003 7–11

Introduction.—Septic arthritis of the pubic symphysis is uncommon. The first known case of *Streptococcus pneumoniae* infection of the pubic symphysis was reported. Ninety-nine cases of septic arthritis of the pubic symphysis reported since 1973 were reviewed.

Case Report.—Woman, 37, was seen in the emergency department for acute onset of fever, nausea, vomiting, and diarrhea. She was treated for viral gastroenteritis and discharged. The patient returned 2 days later with persistent symptoms and reported new lower abdominal pain. She had a 3-month history of right hip and suprapubic pain after a trial of labor resulted in an emergency cesarean section. Her temperature was 29.2°C, blood pressure was 80/60 mm Hg, and heart rate was 100 beats/min. Her abdomen was diffusely tender with no rebound or guarding. The patient had full range of motion of both hips and no tenderness. Her chest radiograph results were normal, her serum white blood cell count was 17,100 cells/mm^3, and the erythrocyte sedimentation rate was 70 mm/h.

She was admitted to the ICU. Blood cultures grew *S pneumoniae* and were sensitive to penicillin. Abdominal CT showed mucosal thickening and edema of the ileum; there was fluid within the symphysis pubis. Pelvic MRI showed gadolinium enhancement of the pubic symphysis, pubic bones, and adjacent muscle and soft tissue.

The patient's hypotension responded to IV fluid. She remained febrile with temperatures up to 39.5°C for 1 week, despite appropriate treatment with vancomycin and piperacillin/tazobactam, then ceftriaxone. The patient experienced severe suprapubic tenderness on weight-bearing. All subsequent blood cultures were negative. After 1 week, she defervesced and the abdominal pain with weight-bearing abated. She fully recovered after 8 weeks of IV ceftriaxone.

TABLE 1.—Clinical Characteristics of 100 Patients With Septic Arthritis of the Symphysis Pubis

Characteristic	No. of Patients (%)
Female	51/97 (53)
Male	46/97 (47)
Pubic pain	53/78 (68)
Groin pain	32/78 (41)
Thigh pain	12/78 (15)
Hip pain	9/78 (12)
Fever >38 °C	53/72 (74)
Pubic tenderness	69/78 (88)
Painful (antalgic) gait	46/78 (59)
Pain with hip motion	35/78 (45)
WBC >11 $\times 10^9$	22/62 (35)
Bacteremia	32/44 (73)
Pubic osteomyelitis	97/100 (97)
Surgery performed	55/100 (55)
Mortality	2/100 (2)

Note: Denominators reflect the number of patients reported with adequate data.

(Courtesy of Ross JJ, Hu LT: Septic arthritis of the pubic symphysis: Review of 100 cases. *Medicine* 82(5):340-345, 2003.)

Methods.—All reports of septic arthritis of the pubis symphysis during the past 30 years were identified from the PubMed search engine.

Results.—The mean age of 100 patients with septic arthritis of the symphysis pubis was 48 years (range, 7-86 years). The most frequent patient complaint was pubic pain (68%). Seventy-eight percent had a fever of 38.0°C or higher, 88% had pubic tenderness, 59% had painful gait, and 45% had pain with hip movement (Table 1). The mean period of symptoms before diagnosis was 29 days (range, 1-180 days). There were 4 major risk groups: women having recently undergone incontinence surgery; athletes, usually in sports requiring forceful hip adduction; patients with pelvic malignancy; and IV drug users (Table 2).

TABLE 2.—Predisposing Conditions Among 100 Adults With Septic Arthritis of the Symphysis Pubis

Predisposing Condition	No. of Patients
Female incontinence surgery	24
Athlete	19
Pelvic malignancy	17
Intravenous drug use	15
None (previously healthy)	10
Male incontinence surgery	3
Postpartum	2
Cardiac catheterization	2
Herniorrhaphy	2
Miscellaneous*	6

*Miscellaneous conditions included renal transplantation, decubitus ulcer, infected penile prosthesis, transvesical urethrolithotomy, pubic erosion from a Foley catheter, and Sjögren syndrome (1 patient each).

(Courtesy of Ross JJ, Hu LT: Septic arthritis of the pubic symphysis: Review of 100 cases. *Medicine* 82(5):340-345, 2003.)

TABLE 3.—Organisms Isolated in 100 Cases of Septic Arthritis of the Symphysis Pubis

Organism	No. of Isolates
Staphylococcus aureus	34
Pseudomonas aeruginosa	24
Polymicrobial	19
Escherichia coli	5
Enterococcus sp.	5
Mycobacterium tuberculosis	3
Streptococcus agalactiae	1
Streptococcus pneumoniae	1
Miscellaneous*	8

*Miscellaneous organisms included *Serratia marcensens*, *Brucella melitensis*, *Bacteroides fragilis*, *Fusobacterium necrophorum*, *Citrobacter* sp, *Peptostreptococcus* sp, *Staphylococcus saprophyticus*, and lactobacilli (1 patient each).

(Courtesy of Ross JJ, Hu LT: Septic arthritis of the pubic symphysis: Review of 100 cases. *Medicine* 82(5):340-345, 2003.)

The most common pathogens isolated in these patients were *Staphylococcus aureus* and *Pseudomonas aeruginosa* (Table 3). Fifty-five percent of patients needed surgery. Pubic osteomyelitis was observed in 97 patients. Adverse outcomes were common in women who underwent incontinence surgery; In 21% (5/24) of women, chronic urinary incontinence developed, and in another 8% (2/24), chronic pelvic pain developed.

Conclusion.—Patients with septic arthritis of the pubic symphysis experience characteristic clinical, laboratory, and imaging findings. Patients can be divided into 4 major risk groups, each with different causative organisms.

► I've not made this diagnosis and hope I haven't missed it. I am familiar with this as it happened to a friend, one of our rheumatology colleagues (who must remain nameless [HIPAA, you know]), presumably associated with running. The association with sports is peculiar, perhaps facilitated by sports-related osteitis pubis.

R. S. Panush, MD

Ethics, Education, Science, and Society

No More Free Lunches: Patients Will Benefit From Doctors and Drug Companies Disentangling

Abbasi K, Smith R

BMJ 326:1155-1156, 2003 7–12

Background.—From small "freebies" such as pens and pizza lunches to significant gifts such as courtesy golf and unaffordable vacation trips, pharmaceutical companies have entwined themselves with the medical profession in what has been described as "an embrace of avarice and excess, an embrace that distorts medical information and patient care." The extent of the relationship between physicians and the pharmaceutical industry, the effects of this relationship on research and on prescribing, and the consequences of this relationship for patients were examined.

Overview.—It is vital that physicians and pharmaceutical companies work together, but the practice by these companies of providing transportation, luxury accommodations, and banquets at conferences and educational seminars can result in bias in decisions made regarding patient care. Some countries and professional organizations have recognized the dangers of this relationship and have developed codes of practice. However, these codes of practice are meaningless unless they are explicit and vigorously observed. British and North American researchers have reported evidence that the prescribing habits of physicians are influenced by drug companies. In addition, the pharmaceutical industry has exerted an increasing influence on research and publication. A systematic review by researchers in North America has reported that studies sponsored by pharmaceutical companies are 4 times as likely to have outcomes favoring the sponsor than are studies funded by nonindustry sources.

Conclusions.—Greater distance between physicians and pharmaceutical companies would benefit all parties, including (and most importantly), the patient.

Why I No Longer Accept Pens [or Other Gifts] From Industry [And Why You Shouldn't Either]

► "If market research by large industrial companies had suggested that the returns were not adequate, these activities would not take place . . . doctors were either unwilling to admit to the powerful influence of commercial pressure or unconscious of it . . . some . . . declared that they would retain virgin intellectual purity . . . such a belief may preserve self-respect, but it is a delusion."[1]

"The degree to which the profession, mainly composed of honorable and decent men, can practice such self-deceit is quite extraordinary. No big company gives away its shareholders' money in an act of disinterested generosity."[2]

"We have already established what you are. We are only quibbling about your price."

Anonymous

"What choice should a man make? That which leads to honor . . . Where there are no men, strive to be an honorable man."

Talmud, Avot 2:1 and 2:5

There's really not much I'd change if I could do my career over again. But there are a couple of things. Like most of us, perhaps, there are some things I would do differently and some memories that still haunt me that I wish I could exorcise. One is the horrible, unconscionable operations we performed as second-year medical students on dogs in the labs: I still have nightmares about this. I wish I then had the courage to protest that aspect of our curriculum, but I now do what I can in my way to make amends. Another regret is the naiveté with which I interacted with drug companies as a younger academician.

There was a time when I eagerly accepted gifts from drug companies. It began early in my professional life. I was running a division, training fellows, getting government and industry grants to find the causes and cures for rheumatic diseases, presenting my data at national and international meetings, and generally doing the things that advance an academic career. I was flattered by the attention of the drug reps. I felt entitled to whatever they handed out; after all, I had worked hard to be in a position to take those perks (also they were neat and my kids often had stuff that nonphysicians' kids didn't). At one point a colleague photographed some of the Pfizer memorabilia we had proudly accumulated (after the introduction of Piroxicam), which included calendars, notepads, pens, watches, gym bags, hats, umbrellas, T-shirts, backpacks, calculators, calendars, paper clips, magnets, and of course slides. The company even featured this in some of its promotional material. I collected these as if they really reflected meaningful achievement, as if stature could be measured by the number and value of gifts awarded by drug companies. I don't think my attitude was unique (I hope it wasn't!). In those days one of the desirable "prizes" was an invitation to speak at a drug company–sponsored extravaganza ("meeting"), accompanied by first-class travel for one's spouse, at a luxurious resort abroad (eg, Monaco) with a continuing open invitation to serve on the company's "advisory board" (with additional financial rewards). The accompanying speaking invitations and number of frequent flier miles were considered (by some) as equivalent to being identified as someone important in rheumatology, and everyone important, it seemed, was "on the circuit," not only in rheumatology but in other specialties as well. Of course I knew that more fundamental achievements really defined academic/professional accomplishment, but industry gifts and perks seemed almost like a surrogate for these. I am now profoundly embarrassed by the prominence of industry-related influences in my activities and by what I now consider the misguided, immature, unprofessional sense of values they reflected.

I evolved to a very different perspective, albeit slowly. My epiphany occurred at the October 2003 American College of Rheumatology (ACR) meeting. It may have been when, walking to an early evening activity at one of the headquarter hotels, I passed a limousine at the entrance-way whose driver was holding a sign with the names of two prominent leaders in rheumatology (and I am confident these rheumatologists do not normally travel by limo). Or it may have come later that same night when, returning to my hotel and walking through the lobby, I passed a group of other distinguished rheumatologists being extravagantly entertained by a pharmaceutical company in one of the off-the-lobby restaurants. Perhaps it was when virtually none of my rheumatology colleagues was ever free for dinner during the meeting because of invitations to lavish industry-sponsored affairs. Or maybe it was when, at the Journal of Rheumatology reception (which many internationally-recognized rheumatologists visited), the Editor lamented that none of the post-doctoral fellows would come and avail themselves of an opportunity to meet leaders in their field because fellows' time was preempted by the company sponsoring their attendance at the meeting. Not only did I find these events intellectually and emotionally repugnant but also viscerally disturbing.

A character in Brecht's *Galileo* asks, "why should we go out of our way to look for things that can only strike a discord in this ineffable harmony?" Why rail at industry gifts? Are not most trivial? Are they not necessary for our research and education? Do they not subsidize our meetings? Are they not essential for many academic programs? Do we not have codes of conduct to sanction and satisfactorily regulate these activities? Are we not impervious to their (implied) blandishments? Colleagues say, "C'mon, Rich, you're overreacting; don't we deserve to enjoy an occasional nice meal or accept a trifle at industry largesse? Are we not capable of making unbiased decisions? I think the correct answer is a resounding "No" to all.

Let me explain. Accepting industry gifts is unethical, unprofessional, and pernicious. And unnecessary. Gifts differ from contracts or grants. Gift exchange exemplifies the potentially problematic individual and professional relationships with industry. "Gifts," in this context, is used to reflect relationships from which personal or organizational benefit may accrue. Medicine is humane science inextricably bound to an ethical lattice. It is a moral enterprise[3]. Individual physicians and their professional association(s) must be committed to promote the welfare of those we serve. They should affirm the moral imperatives from which authenticity and integrity derive by conforming to the highest possible standards of ethical and professional conduct. Opportunities for professional associations and their individual members to accept monetary support and/or gifts, to generate income, and to partner with industry in order to promote their interests, perceived privileges, and sense of entitlement challenge our ability to recognize moral dilemmas and to subordinate self-interest to that of our patients. Medicine, however, is not about physicians, our practices, institutions, organizations or individual organization, needs, research, careers, prerequisites, prerogatives, agendas, or perceived entitlements. It is about dedication and devotion to our patients and to their welfare even at personal and professional risk to profit, pride, and position[4-16].

Gifts are powerful symbols throughout cultures used to initiate and sustain relationships. Gifts are used ubiquitously to seduce and influence physicians. Companies are motivated by profit, not altruism. Contemporary society has lost sight of—or ignored—the importance of gifts as regulators of human relationships. Offering a gift proffers friendship. Accepting a gift initiates or reinforces a relationship. Accepting a gift assumes social obligations of grateful conduct, grateful use, reciprocation, and response. While gift-giving is an act of apparent generosity it serves the self-interest of the giver. Formal contracts can be dissolved but gift relationships are subtle and less well defined. Remember, companies' ultimate goals are to increase profit to shareholders. "If market research by large industrial companies had suggested that the returns were not adequate, these activities would not take place . . . doctors were either unwilling to admit to the powerful influence of commercial pressure or unconscious of it . . . some . . . declared that they would retain virgin intellectual purity . . . such a belief may preserve self-respect, but it is a delusion."[1] "The degree to which the profession, mainly composed of honorable and decent men, can practice such self-deceit is quite extraordinary. No big company gives away its shareholders' money in an act of disinterested generosity."[2] A recent editorial, by a former editor of the New England Journal of Medicine, called for more stringent, not softer, conflict-of-interest guidelines, emphasizing grave concern that "close and remunerative collaboration . . . naturally breeds goodwill . . . and the hope that the [beneficial relationship] will continue. This attitude can subtly influence . . . judgment . . . Can we really believe that clinical researchers (or individual physicians or organizational leadership or organizations/institutions) are more immune to self-interest than other people?"[13]

Gift exchange absolutely reflects relationships with reciprocal obligations, even though many do not consciously recognize this. The act of accepting gifts of any value violates fundamental bioethical and professional precepts. What are these? They are simple, really; profound, too, but simple. Several ethical problems arise for individual physicians with regard to gifts (Table 1). Gifts obligate. Gifts influence behavior. And gifts violate the ethical precepts of distributive justice (unfairly allocating resources without patients' knowledge or consent), beneficence (eroding physician's fiduciary relations as trustees of patients' welfare above all else), non-maleficence (transferring costs to patients and increasing costs of care), fidelity (obligating physicians to companies), and of self-improvement/professionalism (presuming an entitlement for subsidies or gifts as incentives for continuing education)[4-16]. Also, we learn much about drug (product) prescribing, our most common activity, from sources that stand to profit from our choices. We abdicate our responsibility to educate ourselves impartially. We sell access to our young (students, residents, and fellows) when they are most impressionable in exchange for institutional and personal prerequisites. We risk losing the trust of society and our patients through ethically inappropriate relationships that other fiduciaries (i.e., bankers, judges, journalists, or purchasing agents) would not accept. And we invite outside regulation to curb perceived excesses and costs if we don't do this ourselves. A recent editorial noted that quantity or quality of gifts was

TABLE 1.—Problems With Gifts

- Ethical
  - Gifts obligate
  - Gifts influence behavior
  - Gifts conflict with fundamental ethical precepts:
  - Distributive justice: unfair allocation of resources without patients' knowledge or consent
  - Beneficence: erodes physicians' fiduciary relationship as trustee of patients' welfare above all else
  - Nonmaleficence: costs transferred to patients and increases costs of care
  - Fidelity: obligates physicians to companies
  - Self-improvement/professionalism: perception of "entitlement" for subsidies or need for gifts or incentives for continuing education is pernicious
- Professional
  - Altruism: patients' best interests must be foremost, not self-interest
  - Honor and integrity: avoiding conflict of interest and relationships that might allow personal gain to supersede patients' best interests, or even perceptions of this
  - Respect for others: absolutely no advantage is to be taken from relationships
- Other
  - Public image
  - Societal trust
  - High cost of medical care and drugs
  - Unbiased/impartial continuing medical education
  - Access to our "young" (students, residents, fellows)
  - Pride
  - Honor
  - Dignity
  - Self-respect
- Threat of outside (eg, government/regulatory) intervention

irrelevant. Individuals adopt those "notions that favor their own interests . . . [and] drastically underestimate how strong their bias would be." "Disclosure may have perverse effects"; "the implication for industry gifts is straightforward: they should be prohibited."[17]

But surely we are not susceptible to outside influences. Others, perhaps, but not us. Nonsense. Compelling and considerable scientific data document that this notion is delusional. So do the pervasive industry marketing practices. Once again, all together now, "No big company gives away its shareholders' money in an act of disinterested generosity."[2] These data are briefly summarized in Table 2 and have been reviewed extensively elsewhere by myself and others, and they don't change[4,5,8,9]. Selected examples from a growing and robust literature include the following. Physicians' prescribing habits reflect a preponderance of commercial over scientific influence. Physicians' requests to add drugs to formularies were strongly associated with physicians' interactions with companies manufacturing the drug. Of articles published in literature, more articles with drug company support than without were likely to favor the drug of interest. Authors supporting calcium channel blockers during a recent controversy were more likely to have financial relationships with manufacturers than other authors. Significant increase in physician prescribing followed all-expense-paid educational meetings at luxury resorts, etc.[4,5,8,9]

Many professional societies have adopted positions about this. The interested reader is referred elsewhere for details. In general, these variably discourage or recommend limitations to acceptance of industry gifts that others might perceive as inappropriate, recommend disclosure of any relationships, caution about clinical trials methodology and objectivity, and urge that control of continuing medical education activities not be compromised[4,5,8,9]. Virtually all tolerate some degree of gift acceptance and are therefore ethically unacceptable. There is an extensive array of additional opinions well worth reading[4,5].

TABLE 2.—Can Physicians Be Bought, Rented, or Influenced?[5]

Physicians' prescribing habits reflected a preponderance of commercial over scientific influence
Physicians' requests to add drugs to formularies were strongly and specifically associated with physicians' interactions with companies manufacturing the drugs
Of articles published in the literature, more with drug company support than without were likely to favor drug of interest
Authors supporting calcium channel blockers, during a recent controversy, were much more likely to have financial relationships to the manufacturers than other authors
Significant increases in physicians' prescribing followed all-expenses-paid "educational" meetings at luxurious resorts
Faculty and residents who were surveyed changed their prescribing habits and recommended formulary additions based on contacts with drug representatives
Funding sources introduced bias into CME programs favoring sponsors
Some chief residents considered reliability of drug representatives superior to the medical literature
Not all drug representatives' statements were accurate or complied with FDA requirements

While there is a growing literature about ethical behavior for individual physicians, there is substantially less pertaining to the ethics of professional societies. Guidelines for medical organizations have been suggested[3]. These are quite stringent and would not be met by most societies. They include admonition about dangers of focusing unduly on the economic concerns of members to the detriment of transcendent obligations to patients and the public, warning against being self-serving and subordinating patients' interests to those of members, expecting financial support solely from members' dues (as support from or deals with the healthcare industry inevitably risk and create unacceptable conflicts of interest), and having scientific meetings free of industry sponsorship, even if that sponsorship is offered as unrestricted and for general education purposes.

How did we get here, so seemingly inextricably involved with industry? The seduction began subtly in medical school, continued during residency and fellowship, and was complete thereafter. We learned from our elders and peers and, for the most part, came to expect that it was our due to get free pens, notepads, calendars, samples, meals, educational events, trips, and then grants, stipends and honoraria. From whence came this sense of entitlement, the arrogance to presume that we physicians should expect these things—particularly so-called educational events and subsidizations of meetings—that no other self-respecting professionals would claim? Where and when did we learn that we needn't pay for meals or our own continuing education? From naivete, ignorance, lack of education and sensitization, a sense of entitlement, and probably some degree of greed. Do we want our behavior to recall the story of the Hollywood producer attempting to buy the favors of a beautiful movie star for a trivial sum, which offer she refused indignantly; however, when the producer was prepared to pay her as much as a million dollars, she was ready to accept. He then opined, "We have already established what you are. The only thing we are quibbling about is your price"?

Have things changed? I think so. Editorialists, opinion leaders, the public, the government, some organizations, and increasing numbers of physicians are beginning to recognize the improprieties of our relationships with industry. Continuing medical education requirements are becoming more stringent. Mine is not the only department, or medical center, to have a strict code of conduct eschewing all gift relationships with industry. Organizations like No Free Lunch have sprung up with a growing voice[18]. The May 2003 issue of the British Medical Journal was devoted entirely to this topic, and extremely critical of the cozy relationships that had evolved and been accepted between physicians and industry[19]. Recent editorials in The Lancet addressed continuing medical education ("what is of most concern here is the fact that so much continuing medical education comes through the filter of industry"[20]) and the "corrosive example of . . . commercial influence," and concluded by asking how tainted by commercial conflicts has medicine become? Heavily, and damagingly so, is the answer and they challenged "do those doctors who support this culture for the best of intentions . . . have the courage to oppose practices that bring the whole of medicine into disrepute?"[21] Former editors of the New England Journal of Medicine have argued compellingly against industry relationships. I quote them at some length because, for good reason, they are articulate thought leaders in medicine. Kassirer wrote, ". . . nearly all . . . went into medicine with high-minded motives and that financial gain was only a secondary consideration. . . . nearly all had been exposed in medical school to lectures and small group discussions about appropriate professional behavior. Yet the culture in academic medical centers becomes a major determinant of professional behavior once students enter the clinical years and later when they become house officers. Some of this acculturation is promoted by faculty members who themselves are exploiting their academic status for financial gain. But much of it, I suspect, is a consequence simply of inattention to the issue. Most students and house officers have not been challenged to consider that their relations with pharmaceutical companies might compromise their judgment . . . Some resist, but others develop a sense of entitlement . . . A colleague who graduated from medical school almost 30 years ago once told me he never forgot that a certain company had given him his very first medical bag. Deans of medical schools and training program directors must do a better job of addressing conflict of interest. Where professionalism is concerned, they must teach that there is no free lunch. No free dinner. Or textbooks. Or even a ballpoint pen."[14] Relman wrote, "To its shame, the medical establishment tolerates . . . continuing education programs [which] accept grants from the pharmaceutical industry and frequently allow the industry to suggest topics and speakers and help with preparation of the programs. They are reluctant to do anything that would jeopardize the industry's support . . . As for the doctors attending these industry-sponsored education programs, they like the slick presentations, which often use industry-supplied teaching materials. They also like the low or nonexistent fees, the free food, and the numerous small gifts given out at the commercial exhibits that often accompany big education events. And naturally they are confident that their own independence is wholly unaffected by all of this—although surveys reveal that they are less sanguine about other doctor's ability to resist industry's blandishments. But the companies providing the support wouldn't pour money into education unless they were confident of a return on their investment . . . Until the Medical Schools (and hospitals) insist that the pharmaceutical industry stick to its own business (which can include advertising but not education) we are unlikely to get the help we need from our doctors in controlling runaway drug expenditures."[22]

The issues have been framed eloquently. It is not unreasonable to consider gifts broadly and together with industry-sponsored continuing medical education, as the issues are certainly overlapping if not identical. Accepting gifts coarsens our sensibilities and declares our values. Some have suggested that the way to consider these issues is to ask how we would feel if our patients or the public were aware of what we did. I reject that approach: real character is reflected by what we do when no one is watching. Some in leadership at my medical center used to remonstrate with me from time to time about the potential cost savings, in the era of budget deficits, of not having to buy pens, note paper, lunches, bagels, coffee, prescription pads, and the like if I would but relent and accept these ubiquitous industry gifts. I remained steadfast in my refusal (and also remained employed, as of this writing). I suggest that the challenge is to uphold our ethics, our professionalism[23], our pride, our integrity, our image, our identity, our fiduciary responsibilities, our commitment to patients' and public welfare, indeed our very soul, especially in difficult circumstances. Character is also reflected in how we respond to adversity. Every gift we accept, every item, every paper clip, every meal, every speaker, every event erodes these and diminishes us. Every act of refusal, every pen not taken, every notepad not used, every dinner forgone is an emphatic statement affirming of our collective ideals. It is past time to reclaim our honor, our dignity, and our self-respect, and to remember why it is we chose our profession.

"May neither avarice nor miserliness, nor thirst for glory or for a great reputation engage my mind; for the enemies of truth and philanthropy may easily deceive me and make me forgetful of my lofty aim and doing good for thy children."

Prayer of Maimonides

Acknowledgment

Some drafts of and notes for the manuscript were written with generic pens and pencils on generic paper, perhaps to the disappointment of some industry companies or representatives. I have delivered presentations on this topic at Grand Rounds settings, but received no honoraria or even travel reimbursements (the talks were local, though). My medical center still accepts occasional unrestricted grants for certain educational activities, but we're working on that. My wife would like to see our mortgage paid off and my parents would like to see me driving a car that isn't 11 years old, but I think they understand, as it was they who instilled in me the belief that one should aspire to high standards.

R. S. Panush, MD

Reprinted from *J Rheumatol* 31:1478-1482, 2004, with permission.

References

1. Opren scandal [editorial]. *Lancet* 1:219-220, 1983.
2. Rawlins MD: Doctors and the drug makers. *Lancet* 2:276-278, 1984.
3. Pellegrino ED, Relman AS: Professional medical associations: Ethical and practical guidelines. *JAMA* 282:984-986, 1999.
4. Panush RS: Introduction to miscellaneous topics. In: Panush RS, editor. *YEAR BOOK OF RHEUMATOLOGY, ARTHRITIS, AND MUSCULOSKELETAL DISEASES*. St Louis, 2001, Mosby, pp 349-359.
5. Panush RS: Not for sale, not even for rent: Just say no. Thoughts about The American College of Rheumatology adopting a code of ethics. *J Rheumatol* 29:1049-1057, 2002.
6. Panush RS: Reply. *J Rheumatol* 30:202-203, 2003.
7. Panush RS: Professionalism—it's all about the patient. And respect. *Rounds,* Livingston, NJ, 2003, Saint Barnabas Health Care System, pp 1-2.
8. Panush RS, Kavanaugh A, Romain P: Ethical issues in rheumatologic practice and investigation. In: Smolen JS, Lipsky PE, editors. *Biological therapy in rheumatology.* London, 2003, Martin Dunitz, pp 639-651.
9. Dendi P, Desai S, Jacobs FM, et al: Why ethics are important to the busy practitioner caring for patients with rheumatologic and musculoskeletal disorders. *Bull Rheum Dis* 52:1-7, 2003.
10. Panush RS, Sergent JS: A rude awakening. *JAMA* 277:515-516, 1997.
11. Relman AS: Separating continuing medical education from pharmaceutical marketing. *JAMA* 285:2009-2012, 2001.

12. Hadler NM: Hubris for sale or rent. Rheuma21st Archived Reports, 1999. Available from: http://www.rheuma21st.com/archives/ACR99.html. Accessed April 5, 2004.
13. Angell M: Is academic medicine for sale? *N Engl J Med* 342:1516-1518, 2000.
14. Kassirer JP: Financial indigestion. *JAMA* 284:2156-2157, 2000.
15. Korn D: Conflicts of interest in biomedical research. *JAMA* 284:2234-2236, 2000.
16. DeAngelis CD: Conflict of interest and the public trust. *JAMA* 284:2237-2238, 2000.
17. Dana J, Loewenstein G: A social science perspective on gifts to physicians from industry. *JAMA* 290:252-255, 2003.
18. Carrasquillo O, Goodman RL: Pharma's bad karma. Resistance is not futile. *J Gen Intern Med* 18:315-316, 2003.
19. Time to untangle doctors from drug companies [theme issue]. *BMJ* 346:1155-1210, 2003.
20. Just how tainted has medicine become [editorial]? *Lancet* 59:1167, 2002.
21. Drug-company influence on medical education in USA [editorial]. *Lancet* 356:781, 2000.
21. Relman A: Your doctor's drug problem. *New York Times* Nov 18, 2003.
22. Stobo JD, Cohen JJ, Kimball HR, et al: *Project professionalism.* Philadelphia, 1995, American Board of Internal Medicine, pp 1-29.

Thoughts for New Medical Students at a New Medical School

Smith R (London)
BMJ 327:1430-1433, 2003

7–13

Introduction.—When asked to speak to new medical students at a new medical school, the Hull York Medical School, Richard Smith prepared a presentation he hoped would spark a rich debate concerning the importance of what physicians do. A mix of the ideas of Smith, members of *BMJ*'s editorial board (Box 1), and David Sackett ("the father of evidence-based medicine") (Box 2), as well as advice from the literature for young persons in general was presented (Box 3) (Box 4) (Box 5) (Box 7).

Advice for Medical Students.—Wanting to be the very best of something guarantees it will not happen. The aim is to be a good enough medical student and physician. Being good enough is to be good. Having stereotypes of physicians can prompt a lifetime of trying to be something not possible. There is much physicians do not know. It is not possible to know it all. Besides, large volumes of new information are generated every day.

It is important to use information tools to augment personal knowledge. "I don't know" are the 3 most important words in medical education. Know what you don't know and don't feel bad about it. There is no question too stupid to ask; someone else in the room will be glad you asked it. Medical students must be willing to adapt since they may not be practicing medicine in the same world in which they were educated. A clear set of values and an enthusiasm for learning, however, should be maintained if medicine is to mean anything (Box 6).

Although physicians and health systems claim to put patients first, there is ample evidence that patients do not feel that is true. Putting patients first, actively listening to them, and working with them as partners will help patients feel like people rather than cases. Integrity must come first; it is a daily

- Learn to cope with uncertainty
- Challenge what you are taught, especially if it seems inconsistent or incoherent
- Regard your knowledge with humility
- Be yourself at all times
- Enjoy yourself
- Try to practise medicine with the same ethics and principles you believed in when you started medical school
- Never be afraid to admit your ignorance
- Medicine is not only clinical work but is also concerned with relationships, team work, systems, communication skills, research, publishing, and critical appraisal
- Treat your patients with the same care and respect as if they were your loved friends or family
- Cure is not what everyone is expecting from you: your patients and their families may be just seeking support, a friendly hand, a caring soul
- Outside the family there are no closer ties than between doctors and patients
- Don't believe what you read in medical journals and newspapers
- Aim at knowing how to learn, how to get useful medical information, and how to critically assess information
- The first 10 times you do anything—present a patient, put in an intravenous catheter, sew up a laceration—will be difficult, so get through the first 10 times as quickly as possible
- Although you should not be afraid to say "I don't know" when appropriate, also do not be afraid to be wrong
- Cherish every rotation during your training, even if you do not intend to pursue that specialty, because you are getting to do things and share experiences that are special
- When you have a bad day because you are tired stressed, overworked, and underappreciated, never forget that things are much worse for the person on the cold end of the stethoscope. Your day may be lousy, but you don't have pancreatic cancer

BOX 1.—Advice to young doctors from members of the *BJM*'s editorial board. More advice can be found on bmj.com. (Courtesy of Smith R: Thoughts for new medical students at a new medical school. *BMJ* 327:1430-1433, 2003. With permission from the BMJ Publishing Group.)

- The most powerful therapeutic tool you'll ever have is your own personality
- Half of what you'll learn in medical school will be shown to be either dead wrong or out of date within five years of your graduation; the trouble is that nobody can tell you which half–so the most important thing to learn is how to learn on your own
- Remember that your teachers are as full of bullshit as your parents
- You are in for more fun than you can possibly imagine

BOX 2.—Advice from Dave Sackett, the father of evidence-based medicine. (Courtesy of Smith R: Thoughts for new medical students at a new medical school. *BMJ* 327:1430-1433, 2003. With permission from the BMJ Publishing Group.)

Give every man thy ear, but few thy voice;
Take each man's censure, but reserve the judgement.
Costly thy habit as thy purse can buy,
But not express'd in fancy; rich, not gaudy;
For the apparel oft proclaims the man,
And they in France of the best rank and station
Are of a most select and generous chief in that.
Neither a borrower nor a lender be;
For loan oft loses both itself and friend,
And borrowing dulls the edge of husbandry.
This above all: to thine own self be true,
And it must follow, as the night the day,
Thou canst not then be false to any man.

BOX 3.—Advice from Polonius to his son Laertes. (Courtesy of Smith R: Thoughts for new medical students at a new medical school. *BMJ* 327:1430-1433, 2003. With permission from the BMJ Publishing Group.)

If you can dream—and not make dreams your master,
If you can think—and not make thoughts your aim;
If you can meet with Triumph and Disaster
And treat those two impostors just the same

BOX 4.—Advice from Rudyard Kipling's *If*. (Courtesy of Smith R: Thoughts for new medical students at a new medical school. *BMJ* 327:1430-1433, 2003. With permission from the BMJ Publishing Group.)

Take things more easily. Don't ask yourself so much whether this or that is good for you. Don't question your conscience so much—it will get out of tune, like a strummed piano. Keep it for great occasions. Don't try so much to form your character—it's like trying to pull open a rosebud. Live as you like best, and your character will form itself. Most things are good for you; the exceptions are very rare. Spread your wings; rise above the ground. It's never wrong to do that.

BOX 5.—Ralph Touchett, who is close to death, advises Isabel Archer in Henry James' *Portrait of a Lady*. (Courtesy of Smith R: Thoughts for new medical students at a new medical school. *BMJ* 327:1430-1433, 2003. With permission from the BMJ Publishing Group.)

The best thing for being sad is to learn something. That is the only thing that never fails. You may grow old and trembling in your anatomies, you may lie awake at night listening to the disorder of your veins, you may miss your only love, you may see the world about you devastated by evil lunatics, or know your honour trampled in the sewers of baser minds. There is only one thing for it then—to learn. Learn why the world wags and what wags it. This is the only thing which the mind can never exhaust, never alienate, never be tortured by, never fear or distrust, and never dream of regretting.

BOX 7.—Advice on the importance of learning from T H White in *The Once and Future King*. (Courtesy of Smith R: Thoughts for new medical students at a new medical school. *BMJ* 327:1430-1433, 2003. With permission from the BMJ Publishing Group.)

- Clear ethical values
- Being clear about the purpose of your organisation
- Putting patients first
- Constantly trying to improve
- Basing what we do on evidence
- Leadership
- Education and learning

BOX 6.—As the world changes, what should persist? (Courtesy of Smith R: Thoughts for new medical students at a new medical school. *BMJ* 327:1430-1433, 2003. With permission from the BMJ Publishing Group.)

and constant challenge to be honest. Integrity has been defined as a destination, not a state.

Final Thoughts.—What may be a Texan prayer has worthy wisdom: In one pocket keep a message that says: "You are just dust and ashes;" in the other pocket, keep one that says: "The world was created just for you." Both of these messages may be equally true. Final advice: Never forget the value of learning, not only for chasing after wisdom but also because it may be the ultimate balm.

HARLOT plc: An Amalgamation of the World's Two Oldest Professions

Sackett DL, for HARLOT plc (Trout Research and Education Ctr, Markdale, Ont, Canada; et al)
BMJ 327:1442-1445, 2003 7–14

Introduction.—Although written "tongue in cheek," this description of services of HARLOT plc, a combination of the world's oldest and second oldest professions, may contain some uncomfortable truth concerning how to "maximize the profits of manufacturers of dodgy drugs and devices." The promoters of HARLOT plc decided it was time to find out whether being bad pays better than being good. They specialize in "How to Achieve Positive Results Without Actually Lying to Overcome the Truth."

It's the Money, Dummy.—HARLOT plc provides a comprehensive package of services to the discriminating trial sponsors who wish not to risk the acceptance and application of their products and policies "amid the uncertainties of dispassionate science." These services are for manufacturers who are seeking to increase the market shares of their dodgy drugs and devices, for health professional guilds wanting to increase the demand for their unnecessary diagnostic and therapeutic services, and for national health departments seeking to implement irrational and self- serving health policies.

Data can be cooked in an individual randomized trial (Table 1) to achieve desired results. There is an array of aftercare services available to keep the truth from interfering with sales and implementation (Table 2). For customers who cannot afford these services, there are some nonelite offerings (Table 3). Although limited space permits the individual description of only a few services of HARLOT plc, references for all of them are available by subpoena from the legal department.

TABLE 1.—Stepped Care for "Me Too" Drugs or Devices and Useless Screening Tests

Step	Bias to be Exploited	Strategies for Applying this Bias (While Hiding Your Intentions and Actions)	Payment
E—Zee-me-Too Protocols			
1	Selective, non-systematic reviews	Cite just those reports that support your product, proposal, or policy (and slag all your competitors)	£
2	Substituting placebos for established effective treatment	Invoke fallacious "placebo effects" and "assay-sensitivity" arguments in order to avoid head to head comparisons	$
3	Unconcealed allocation to ensure better prognoses in "experimental" patients	Provide updatable wall posters for displaying the group to which the next patient will be allocated, see-through allocation envelope systems, etc	€
4	"Mini-max" manipulation of your competitor's product	Give insufficient ("mini") doses of your competitor's product, accompanied by scary ("max") warnings about its (but not yours) side effects and toxicity	Ocean-front property in New Jersey
5	Incorporating irrelevant surrogate and composite end points	Concoct an invalid inflation of event rates (especially among control patients)	Lapis lazuli
6	"Shifting the goal posts" for "superiority" and "non-inferiority"	Require trivially better outcomes for "superiority" but massively worse outcomes for "inferiority"	Diamonds
Ethics-R-Us			
7	Uninformed consent	Create consent forms in which study patients sign a "waiver of right to receive information" about the nature of, risks of, or alternatives to your product	¥
RATs (Research Administration Teams)			
8	Adding efficacious co-interventions to (just) your product	Give (just) the experimental patients additional treatments of known efficacy, find and treat their comorbidity, etc	Ocean-front property in California
9	Unblinded outcome assessment	Provide encouragement of (only) experimental patients' functional capacity performance or symptom scores, and ignore their minor strokes, heart failure, and side effects	Insider trading before publication
10	Repeated interim analyses	Scan repeated early analyses for spurious but favourable trends that justify terminating the trial in your favour	Rubies
FPSU (Find the Pony Statistical Unit)			
11	Munchausen's statistical grid (looking for the pony)	Execute sub^{n}-group analysis where n=keep going until you find a statistically significant effect in your favour	n×10^{3} shares of stock
12	Overinterpretation of a positive trial	Report just the (impressive) relative risk reduction while suppressing the (unimpressive) absolute risk reduction and number needed to treat	0.5% of net sales
13	Overinterpretation of an indeterminate trial	Report a too small trial with a huge 95% confidence interval (that includes 0) as "negative," thereby "proving" that there is a "no difference" between your product and the (better) one produced by your competitor	0.5% of gross sales

(Courtesy of Sackett DL for HARLOT plc: HARLOT plc: An amalgamation of the world's two oldest professions. *BMJ* 327:1442-1445, 2003. With permission from the BMJ Publishing Group.)

TABLE 2.—Aftercare Program

Designation	Strategy	Tactic
SAFE (Say Anything For a Euro) Panel of "experts"	Provide generous research grants, first class travel, luxurious accommodations, exorbitant honorariums, and gargantuan ongoing "consultant" fees to "experts" who (surprise) favour your product, screening test, or programme	Get SAFE experts to generate the guidelines, write the editorials, pick the keynote speakers, referee for the key journals, etc
SCUM (Sick Celebrities to Use in the Media)	Hire stars of stage and screen, famous athletes, and washed up politicians who will "disease monger" and tout your product or screening test	Get them on to talk shows, into gossip magazines, and into the front lines of parades on any issue
PPCT (Pay the Piper and Call the Tune)	Give generous "journalism" awards for articles that monger your disease or praise your product in the lay media	Continue to feed media new diseases and products to push
RCAF (Rabid Citizens Against Facts)	Secretly fund "patients' action" groups to attack any counter-evidence that shows your product, programme, or screening test is useless or harmful	Denounce detractors with testimonials and threats
DISARM (DIScourage Arguments with Research Money)	Disarm your critics by funding an evaluation of your new screening test or health programme	Then stop the funding, ignore the results as out of date, or abandon the test or programme for a new, equally untested one
FYP (Foundation in Your Pocket)	Build beautiful headquarters and conference centres for health foundations	Smooth the way for infiltrating SAFE experts into their leadership and programme development
MTM (Move the Ministry)	Lobby to shift responsibility for the approval of new drugs and devices from the Ministry of Health to the Ministry of Industry	Shift the objective from healthy patients to healthy national economies
GFGC (Get the Fox to Guard the Chicken house)	Purchase a pharmaceutical benefits management organisation	Control the selection and purchasing of drugs while preserving the illusion of a market
BOSS (Bureau Of Secret Surveillance)	Buy confidential information from pharmacists as to exactly who is prescribing exactly what	Tailor drug reps' visits to focus on just the prescribing habits that need to be changed to your benefit
SOW Save/Sacrifice Our Workers)	Threaten to move your product development and manufacture to another country	Launch media and lobbying blitzes that exaggerate how many jobs will be lost if you leave (see cigarette manufacturers' ploys)
SHARKS (Striking Horror And Retreat through Killer Solicitors)	Hire all the really good lawyers	Use them to threaten nay-sayers, members of drug review boards, etc with frivolous but expensive libel lawsuits. Suppress negative health technology assessment reports until you've met your sales targets

(Courtesy of Sackett DL for HARLOT plc: HARLOT plc: An amalgamation of the world's two oldest professions. *BMJ* 327:1442-1445, 2003. With permission from the BMJ Publishing Group.)

TABLE 3.—Non-Elite Services

Customers	Services	What We Can Do for You
Governments, health insurance companies, and health maintenance organisations	OUR (Opportunistic Use of Research) support	We can find whatever research there is that supports your views and trash any research that is in conflict with your views. (Note: if you change your views, there will be an additional charge for this service.) We can also help you to design evaluations that will take as long as you want. In the rare event that one of our studies does not give you the answers you want, we will give you ample warning so that you can cut the study's funding and suppress its findings
Professional organisations	POMP (Professional Opportunities to Maximise Profit)	We can find whatever research there is to support aggressive use of your guild's services and trash any research that suggests that your services are not highly effective
Clinicians and hospitals who might get sued	TIT (Trials in the Interest of Treating) for clinicians and hospitals	Our package of preventive services includes our generic informed consent forms, modelled after the forms we use to get study patients to waive their right to receive information. When you are sued, we can provide you with the evidence you need to defend yourself and your staff, regardless of whether you were right or wrong, and we can trash the plaintiff's evidence
Patients and patient organisations who might want to sue	TAT (Trials for Advocating Treatments) for patients and patient organisations	If you want to sue your care giver, we can provide you with the evidence you need and trash the defendants' evidence. If your organisation wants to demand a treatment, no matter how useless it might be, we can provide you with the evidence you need to support your claims
Lawyers	EWOCs (Expert Witnesses On Call)	We can provide you with expert witnesses and the research to back their testimony, and we can attack the credibility of the other side's experts. (Note: if we are asked to provide witnesses for both sides, we guarantee results only for the side that offers us the largest fee)
Academics	SALAMI (our how to Succeed in Academic Life Advice and Mentoring Institute)	We can teach you how to pad your curriculum vitae, raise your profile, exploit your trainees, and slice your research results into a minimum of one article per enrolled patient

(Courtesy of Sackett DL for HARLOT plc: HARLOT plc: An amalgamation of the world's two oldest professions. *BMJ* 327:1442-1445, 2003. With permission from the BMJ Publishing Group.)

Conclusion.—In summary, HARLOT plc cashes in on its years of clinical research experience and as yet untarnished reputation to "protect your worthless product as we shepherd it through the mindfields sewn by objective scientists, fussy ethics committees, conscientious journal editors, writers of evidence based guidelines, and licensing bodies." If the advice of HARLOT is faithfully followed, drugs and products should "sell like hotcakes," at which point HARLOT plc reserves the right to refund all fees in return for 0.5% of gross sales in perpetuity.

Parachute Use to Prevent Death and Major Trauma Related to Gravitational Challenge: Systematic Review of Randomised Controlled Trials

Smith GCS, Pell JP (Cambridge Univ, England; Greater Glasgow NHS Board, Glasgow, Scotland)

BMJ 327:1459-1461, 2003 7–15

Background.—Parachutes are used to reduce major trauma related to the effects of gravity. However, not all cases in which parachutes are used are free of major trauma, and not all cases in which parachutes are not used have an adverse outcome. A systematic review was undertaken to determine the results of randomized, controlled trials on this topic.

Methods.—Data were sought from Medline, the Web of Science, Embase, and the Cochrane Library databases as well as suitable Internet sites and citation lists. The goal was to identify randomized, controlled trials showing the effects of using a parachute during a free fall. Major trauma, defined as an injury severity score over 15, or death were the outcome measure.

Results.—No randomized, controlled trials covered the performance of parachutes.

Conclusion.—Advocates of evidence-based medicine frown on the practice of adopting interventions that are only supported by observational information. However, parachutes are indeed used without any supporting data from randomized, controlled trials. The logical conclusion is that common sense must be applied in a consideration of risks and benefits of parachute use or that parachutes should not be used outside of the context of a properly conducted trial until evidence-based support can be obtained. The suggested protocol was a double blind, randomized, placebo controlled, crossover trial.

► The *BMJ* is one the journals I peruse periodically in my library. I find reading it quite enjoyable. Good brief articles on an interesting variety of topics, provocative essays and social commentary, and refreshing editorials. Too much of my journal reading is timid, confirmatory, unimaginative science in dull, turgid prose. A special treat was the Christmas issue replete with some great contributions and wonderfully clever satire. I've selected examples of both. They deserve to be read in their originals, as the summaries do not do them justice.

Richard Smith's piece (Abstract 7–13) is one I wish I had written. It is full of pithy, sage advice to new medical students. (See boxes 1 to 7.) In the second selection (Abstract 7–14), David Sackett, a needy academician whose name is synonymous with evidence-based medicine, proposes a new enterprise (HARLOT) designed to reap huge profits for the authors by providing clinical trial sponsors whatever results they wish, as summarized in Tables 1 to 3. The last article (Abstract 7–15) challenges the premise that parachutes prevent major trauma related to gravitational challenge by utilizing principles of evidence-based medicine, and finding no randomized, controlled trials of parachute intervention.

R. S. Panush, MD

Occam's Razor Versus Saint's Triad

Hilliard AA, Weinberger SE, Tierney LM Jr, et al (Mayo Clinic and Mayo Found, Rochester, Minn; Harvard Med School, Boston; Univ of California, San Francisco; et al)

N Engl J Med 350:599-603, 2004 7–16

Purpose.—Occam's razor—referring to the advice, "Among competing hypotheses, favor the simplest one"—is a truism of modern medical practice. The less well-known Saint's triad—referring to the association of a hiatal hernia, gallbladder disease, and diverticulosis—reminds physicians to consider the possibility that more than one diagnosis may be present at once. These 2 medical adages are discussed in the context of a patient with 2 distinct causes of a single symptom.

Or Hickam's Dictum?—A woman had a 10-day history of worsening dyspnea. She had RA and was taking immunosuppressive medications. As the dyspnea progressed, the patient also had a fever, tachypnea, and hypoxemia. Possible diagnoses included pulmonary or other infections, a secondary process involving the lungs, or a noninfectious inflammatory process. The patient was given empirical antibiotic therapy while sputum cultures were performed. She underwent a chest spiral CT scan, which revealed large emboli in the pulmonary arteries along with extensive ground-glass infiltrates. She was then given heparin therapy, and her condition stabilized. Bronchoscopy demonstrated the presence of *Pneumocystis carinii* pneumonia. Her condition improved rapidly with antibiotics, corticosteroids, and heparin.

Discussion.—In this case, immunosuppression placed the patient at risk of opportunistic *P carinii* infection. Her symptoms may have made her reduce her physical activity, thus predisposing her to venous thromboembolism. Thus, a single symptom of dyspnea may have had 2 distinct causes. The authors urge that both Occam's razor and Saint's triad be borne in mind when considering complex diagnostic situations, along with Hickam's dictum: "A patient can have as many diagnoses as he darn well pleases."

► I knew about Occam's razor and have tried to use this on rounds to display my erudition. But it is becoming a cliché, and students and residents increasingly nod their heads in recognition when I ask, "Do you know Occam's razor?" However, I never knew the original Latin from the 14th century attributed to William of Occam: "Pluralitas non est ponenda sine necessitate" ("Plurality must not be posited without necessity"). I never heard of Saint's triad (ie, hiatal hernia, gallbladder disease, and diverticulosis), named for the South African surgeon who emphasized the importance of considering multiple diagnoses. Then there is the apocryphal Hickam's dictum: "A patient can have as many diagnoses as he darn well pleases." Now, unless my students and residents have read this article (which is doubtful), I may be able to impress them again.

R. S. Panush, MD

PowerPoint: Shot With Its Own Bullets

Norvig P (Mountain View, Calif)

Lancet 362:343-344, 2003 7–17

Introduction.—Recent articles have critiqued the popular PowerPoint presentation software for inhibiting open exchange between presenters and audience and for making it difficult to present more complex ideas. This commentary makes the suggestion that PowerPoint may even contribute to poor decision making.

PowerPoint and Decision-Making.—Cited is the example of George Low, a NASA program manager, who suggested, presented, and gained approval for a plan to make the first Moon orbit with Apollo 8. The ambitious decision, with its engineering challenges and national security implications, was made in a single day. A recent article suggested that efforts to make complex information fit into PowerPoint templates may have even contributed to poor decision making, leading to the explosion of the space shuttle Columbia. Good decisions should be reached by cooperative discussion among "knowledgeable and passionate" experts rather than by preformatting all information.

Discussion.—Generic presentations may not only bore an audience but also contribute to poor decisions. A call is made for collaborative discussions with the goal of reaching the best decision rather than persuading one's audience.

▶ May I have the first slide please—whoops, wrong presentation; this is a written comment about PowerPoint (ppt) presentations. I'm very proud of myself. Because my institution has had to invoke austerity budgets, I've been forced to learn ppt, either that or speak and lecture without visual aids, which seems unthinkable (and hard!). I've actually enjoyed preparing ppt presentations: there's a certain Zen satisfaction and creativity and immediacy to it, although it does take time. I got a kick out of this piece and will use ppt selectively, recognizing that ppt may oversimplify (read the example of a ppt version of the Gettysburg Address in the original article) and inhibit meaningful dialogue.

R. S. Panush, MD

Is There a July Phenomenon? The Effect of July Admission on Intensive Care Mortality and Length of Stay in Teaching Hospitals

Barry WA, Rosenthal GE (Iowa City VA Med Ctr, Iowa; Univ of Iowa, Iowa City)

J Gen Intern Med 18:639-645, 2003 7–18

Introduction.—Every July, teaching hospitals have an influx of new physicians recently graduated from medical schools who are supervised by senior residents and fellows. The delivery of care by less experienced physicians brings into question the quality of care delivered early in the academic year, well known as the "July phenomenon." Few trials have examined the July phenomenon and none have investigated its effect in intensive care patients, a group that may be especially susceptible to deficiencies in management stemming from housestaff inexperience. Hospital mortality and length of stay in ICU admissions from July to September were compared with admissions during other months. That relationship was then compared in teaching and nonteaching hospitals and in surgical versus nonsurgical patients.

Methods.—A retrospective cohort analysis of 156,136 consecutive eligible patients admitted to 38 ICUs in 28 hospitals in Northeast Ohio between March 1, 1991, and March 31, 1997, was performed.

Results.—After adjusting for admission illness severity via Acute Physiology and Chronic Health Evaluation III methodology, the odds of death was similar for admissions from July through September, relative to the mean for all months in major (odds ratio [OR], 0.96; 95% confidence interval [CI], 0.91-1.02; $P = .18$) (Fig 2), minor (OR, 1.02; 95% CI, 0.93-1.10; $P = .66$), and nonteaching hospitals (OR, 0.96; 95% CI, 0.91-1.01; $P = .09$). These findings were similar when individual month and academic year were evalu-

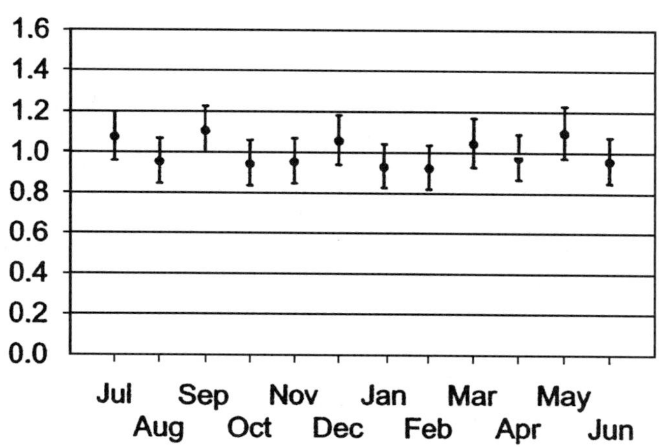

FIGURE 2.—Odds of death and associated 95% confidence intervals in major teaching hospitals during individual months of the academic year. (Courtesy of Barry WA, Rosenthal GE: Is there a July phenomenon? The effect of July admission on intensive care mortality and length of stay in teaching hospitals. *J Gen Intern Med* 18:639-645, 2003. Reprinted by permission of Blackwell Publishing.)

ated separately and in stratified analyses of surgical and nonsurgical patients.

Conclusion.—There was no evidence to support the existence of a July phenomenon in a large series of ICU patients. Future trials should evaluate the organizational factors that permit hospitals and residency programs to compensate for the inexperience of new house staff early in the academic year.

Strategies for Improving Attendance at Medical Grand Rounds at an Academic Medical Center

Mueller PS, Litin SC, Sowden ML, et al (Mayo Clinic, Rochester, Minn)
Mayo Clin Proc 78:549-553, 2003 7–19

Background.—Medical grand rounds (MGRs) served a central teaching function beginning in the late 19th century, but this has changed significantly over the past few decades. What used to be a survey of diagnostic and therapeutic approaches to patients at bedside is now lacking patients and including histories only as a prelude to lectures. Most academic medical centers continue to regard MGRs as an important educational activity, although little is known about whether participation changes practice or improves the quality of medical care.

The Department of Medicine at the Mayo Clinic in Rochester, Minnesota conducts MGRs as a weekly 1-hour conference at lunchtime in which faculty, fellows, residents, medical students, and others receive updates on advances in internal medicine practice, research, and education. It can also be viewed at 2 on-campus locations via live teleconference. Faculty participants earn continuing medical education credit; fellows and residents are required to attend in some cases. Strategies implemented before, during, and after 1998 to encourage attendance at MGRs were reviewed, along with the results achieved.

Methods.—The 5 strategies employed for improving MGR attendance were use of electronic card readers to help understand attendance patterns; use of yearly needs assessment surveys; development of sessions having topical interest; increasing formal participation by residents and faculty researchers; and increasing publicity. Card readers were used to document the attendance at MGRs of faculty, fellows, residents, and others from 1998 to 2001.

Results.—MGR attendance increased each year with the implementation of the strategies. The mean increase in attendance was 39% overall; that of faculty, fellows, and resident full-time–equivalent staff increased 12%. The special topics sessions had no statistically significant increase in attendance over other sessions. Higher attendance was noted at sessions in which the topic was of special importance or timeliness, such as a bioterrorism session. Moving the MGRs to another location negatively influenced attendance. Fifty percent of attendees were department of medicine faculty, and most of the others were fellows or residents.

Almost half of the MGR attendees participated by live teleconference. It was not the speakers who drew most attendees, but rather the specific topics addressed. Barriers to attendance included departmental meetings scheduled at the same time and lack of food. Almost half of the faculty attendees used participation for continuing medical education credit, and 90% of the attendees reported favorable impressions of the clinical images and research vignettes. E-mail announcements of the sessions were also highly appreciated.

Conclusion.—When an organized effort was made to improve the interest in and attendance at MGRs, attendance improved. Strategies that were successful included identifying attendance patterns, using needs assessment surveys, developing and implementing special topics sessions, guiding speakers on topic selection, including internal medicine residents and researchers, and using various means of advertising the sessions.

► As a department chair at a large medical center with responsibility for a residency program I found these 2 selections (Abstracts 7–18 and 7–19) of particular interest. We've always thought (or at least I've certainly heard) that it's not safe to get sick and be hospitalized and cared for by new residents in July. That seems not to be the case, at least in terms of ICU mortality and length of stay. I'm not convinced, though, about elsewhere in the hospital; ICU's are usually managed by upper level, experienced residents.

I worry about our MGRs and appreciated the approach taken at the Mayo Clinic to sustain theirs. We surveyed our resident and faculty/staff physicians and found that our attendance and interest really hadn't changed a lot over the years. In our community, we find the quality and content of MGRs are less an issue than are the problems of medicine generally today: ennui; lack of time; global frustration; lack of time; subspecialization; "eurekopenia;" lack of time; and conflicting loyalties, affiliatiations, activities, and imperatives. There are no easy fixes for this. Maybe a new generation will simply face medicine with a different perspective than ours.

R. S. Panush, MD

Eurekapenia: A Disease of Medical Residency Training Programs?
Hellmann DB (Johns Hopkins Univ, Baltimore, Md)
The Pharos Spring:24-26, 2003 7–20

Background.—Many types of experiences go into molding a doctor, but among the most important are "eureka moments" when one experiences the power and pleasure of making a discovery while on a difficult search or journey. These eureka moments can occur at any point in evaluating a patient and add drama, fun, excitement, and meaning to the practice of medicine. Such moments confirm that no matter how limited ones knowledge and skills, one can still make a difference in the life of a patient. They make one *want* to be a physician. However, medical practice has changed to the degree that these experiences may be lacking now, leading to "eurekapenia."

Method.—Four assistant chief residents reviewed 50 charts comprising 25 from 1982 and 25 from 1997. Each admission was evaluated for length of the intern's initial history and physical examination. Interns were assigned a "eureka score" of 1 point when an assessment and plan were longer than 1 page, 1 point for quoting or referencing the medical literature or textbooks, and 1 point for performing a diagnostic test, for a maximum of 3.0 points.

Results.—The average intern's admission note was 8 pages long in 1992; it was 4 pages long in 1997. The average eureka score in 1982 was 1.4; it was 0.7 in 1997. Factors identified as contributing to this eurekapenia included the increased number of patients admitted each year, with little time to evaluate each one thoroughly; the adoption of universal standards that preclude having a house staff laboratory on each floor because of the danger to patients; the rise of resistant organisms; and adoption of policies that ensure tests are performed correctly and interpreted accurately. The latter 2 are responsible for the fact that residents rarely personally perform these tests.

Conclusion.—Eurekapenia appears to be widespread. However, it may be treatable. Proposals include encouraging faculty to model the search for eureka moments by doing clinical rounds at the bedside and reviewing primary data whenever possible. Residents need more time to talk with and examine patients. Creative solutions are also needed: using technological advances to search medical literature, analyze or establish patient databases, and consult experts. Technology can also help to revise the doctor's black bag to include portable US devices, oximeters, and personal digital assistants to facilitate ordering tests and reporting results. Residents and faculty need to work together to create and explore opportunities for eureka moments.

► What a great article! And by one of our editors! Kudos, David. I think the problem is more us than the system. It is incumbent upon those of us who are medical educators to rise above the exigencies of daily medicine and communicate the fun and excitement of doing clinical medicine well.[1,2] There followed, in the next issue of *The Pharos*, a number of letters from individuals describing their moments of "eureka."

I can quickly recount several, many recent: the first time as a junior resident responsible for the presentation to our chair (Dr Stead), preparing the student all night long, having him present, and then watching Dr Stead reflect, pause, and say "Let's go on to the next patient since it's obvious you understand what's going on here"; the positive Watson Schwartz test on our patient who owned North Carolina's largest still and was suspected of being lead intoxicated; diagnosing a ruptured Baker's cyst with pseudothrombophlebitis on ward rounds, which had not been appreciated; recently picking up unrecognized myxedema with prolonged deep tendon reflex relaxation phase on rounds a couple of months ago; instantly identifying relapsing seronegative symmetrical synovitis with pitting edema unappreciated by multiple other examiners in the office last week; and watching the pattern evolve during double-blind, placebo-controlled challenges that documented milk-induced synovitis in the patient we reported some years ago.[3]

These moments are there; they are but to be recognized and savored. They validate what we do and transmit our legacy to a new generation.

R. S. Panush, MD

References

1. Panush RS: The new academic year. *Am J Med* 99:98, 1995.
2. Panush RS: A higher standard. *Am J Med* 98:211-212, 1995.
3. Panush RS, Stroud RM, Webster EM: Food-induced (allergic) arthritis: Inflammatory arthritis exacerbated by milk. *Arthritis Rheum* 29:220-226, 1986.

On the Value of an Old Dress Code in the New Millennium

Brandt LJ (Albert Einstein College of Medicine, Bronx, NY)

Arch Intern Med 163:1277-1281, 2003 7–21

Background.—Medical students no longer follow the traditional dress code of a white laboratory coat over dress clothing. To determine whether dress makes a difference in perceived care, 31 articles were reviewed.

Methods.—The available literature was searched via electronic databases to find articles dealing with dress codes, professional attire, physician attitudes, the traditional white coat, and other references to clothing.

Results.—The 3 top reasons for wearing a white coat were to be easily recognized by colleagues and patients, to carry needed medical items, and to keep the underlying clothes clean. Physicians choosing not to wear traditional white coats were generally in psychiatry or pediatrics and half were seeking to avoid any perceived negative effect of the coat on establishing rapport with their patients. A danger of wearing the white coat was microbiological contamination. A "plateau effect" was identified in which a steady state of maximal microbiological contamination was reached in the first week of use of the coat and did not change significantly after that point. Coats worn during the physical examination of patients should not be worn in nonclinical areas, such as the cafeteria or library, to limit the spread of microorganisms.

Studies have found that the phenomenon of white coat hypertension actually occurs in far fewer patients than previously suspected and occurs when blood pressure is measured by a physician rather than a technician, regardless of attire. Various questionnaires and studies revealed most respondents had positive responses to traditional attire and negative responses to casual attire. Younger physicians were less supportive of traditional attire than older physicians. Patients tended to be more relaxed about their physicians' attire but positively viewed name tags, visible stethoscopes, and groomed moustaches. A multiple-choice questionnaire given to 200 patients in Boston and San Francisco revealed that 65% of the respondents believed white coats should be worn, 7% believed they should not, and about one third had no preferences.

With respect to female physicians, 34% of patients preferred they wear a skirt or dress and 27% had no preference. A female physician in green scrubs was seen as inspiring trust and confidence because she was not confused for a secretary or other worker. Disapproval was expressed toward blue jeans (53%) and tennis shoes (27%). Of 74 physician respondents in 1 study, 91% never wore blue jeans and 57% never wore tennis shoes while seeing patients; 44% always wore a tie, 77% always wore a white coat, and 49% sometimes wore a white coat.

Patients feel physician attire has an impact on their level of trust and satisfaction and believe physicians should have a professional appearance. A significant number of patients, especially older ones, dress specifically to see their doctor. In pediatric settings, physicians dressed formally were more positively perceived and those dressed informally were more negatively perceived. Patient satisfaction is not purely influenced by attire, with studies emphasizing the desirability of professionalism and approachability.

Conclusion.—Patients care about their health care provider's appearance regardless of age, geographic location, or culture. A neat, clean appearance is valued more than specific attire, but a white coat and name tag are important. Physicians themselves are more conservative about attire than are patients. Personal traits, such as gentleness, concern, friendliness, and empathy, are ranked as most important for any physician.

► I always like finding articles that confirm my biases and prejudices. One of these is that attire is important to physicians. Indeed, I do not let my residents wear scrubs during the workday (I relent at night). I expect them to look professional because I think it facilitates them to act professionally. I ask them to consider how they would feel about consulting another professional (clergyman, banker, financial planner, attorney) who was wearing the equivalent of pajamas.

I've never understood why health care professionals feel compelled to undress and change into scrubs for work; I don't accept that it is to protect garments; it was unthinkable for us as medical residents to have access to scrubs. White coats provided adequate protection to our clothes and we did all sorts of things residents no longer do (now done by others). But those were the days when boats were iron and men were too. I love Abba Eban's comment ". . .do we not carry informality of dress and speech to a point in which untidiness of form yields untidiness of thought. . .?"

R. S. Panush, MD

A Levels and Intelligence as Predictors of Medical Careers in UK Doctors: 20 Year Prospective Study

McManus IC, Smithers E, Partridge P, et al (Univ College London)
BMJ 327:139-142, 2003 7–22

Introduction.—The selection of medical students in the United Kingdom primarily depends on grades achieved in school-leaving examinations, including A levels. Intelligence shows stability through life. Achievement tests depend primarily on recent educational experiences. Whether A level grades (achievement) and intelligence (ability) predict physicians' careers was determined in a prospective cohort examination with a 20-year follow-up.

Methods.—Five hundred and eleven physicians who entered Westminster Medical School as clinical students between 1975 and 1982 were followed-up with the use of a postal questionnaire in January 2002. The main outcome measures were time taken to achieve various career grades in hospital or general practice, postgraduate qualifications obtained (ie, membership/fellowships, diplomas, and higher academic degrees), number of research publications, and measures of stress and burnout associated with A level grades and intelligence (result of AH5 intelligence test) at entry to clinical school. The general health questionnaire, the Maslach burnout inventory, and a questionnaire concerning satisfaction with one's career at follow-up were used.

Results.—Forty-seven physicians (9%) were no longer listed on the Medical Register. They had lower A level grades than those who remained on the register ($P < .001$). A levels were predictive of performance in undergraduate education, performance in postregistration house officer posts, and time to achieve membership qualifications ($P < .001$). Intelligence was not independently predictive of no longer being listed on the register, career outcomes, or other measures. A level grades were not predictive of a diploma or higher academic qualifications, research publications, or stress or burnout. Diplomas, higher academic degrees, and research publications were significantly associated with personality measures.

Conclusion.—A level grades (achievement), which are particularly used for selecting students in the UK, have long-term predictive validity for undergraduate and postgraduate medical careers. The AH5 (test of ability or aptitude) was of little predictive value for subsequent medical careers.

► One of the responsibilities I struggle with is selecting residents. I don't know how to find those who will "succeed." There is literature about this (see 2004 YEAR BOOK, pp 329-330). Available data suggest good test taking ability predicts good test taking ability, that there is a requirement for a threshold of intelligence beyond that it is probably overrated, and the "EQ" (emotional quotient) are important. This study tends to confirm my impressions that achievement predicts achievement better than ability or aptitude. ". . .What's past is prologue. . ." (Shakespeare, Tempest II.1.253-254).

R. S. Panush, MD

Length of Patient's Monologue, Rate of Completion, and Relation to Other Components of the Clinical Encounter: Observational Intervention Study in Primary Care

Rabinowitz I, Luzzatti R, Tamir A, et al (Technion-Israel Inst of Technology, Haifa, Israel)

BMJ 328:501-502, 2004 7–23

Background.—In a consultation, the patient's opening statement, or monologue, is an important part of history taking, and doctors are encouraged not to interrupt the patient. However, they often do, most likely because they think that the patient's monologue is time consuming. When interrupted, patients usually conclude their monologue in less than 30 seconds in primary care and in about 90 seconds in consultant settings. Discussions with patients in primary care that included a new clinical problem before and after doctors were instructed not to interrupt were assessed, and the length and rate of completion of patients' monologues were recorded.

Methods.—Consecutive encounters between 8 family physicians and their patients were recorded on 2 days in 6 family clinics in northern Israel. All of the doctors were videotaped on both days. The doctors were told that the study focused on the interaction between the doctor and the patient. The patients were given this explanation through a written notice on the door of the consulting room and also orally by the doctor when required. At the start of the second day, the doctors were handed a written note that advised them that when the patients start to speak, the doctor should not interrupt them until the physician is satisfied that the patients have finished. The 8 doctors were a convenience sample, and all had completed their residency program.

TABLE.—Characteristics of Consultations Before and After Doctors Were Instructed Not to Interrupt the Patient's Opening Statement

Variable	Day 1 (Before Instruction)	Day 2 (After Instruction)
No (%) of encounters with new clinical problem	58	54
Length of patient's monologue (seconds)		
Mean (SD)	26 (28.5)	28 (26.9)
Median (range)	15 (1-120)	21 (2-123)
No (%) of monologues completed	18/56 (32)	32/49 (65)*
Physical examinations:		
No (%) of encounters	53 (91)	45 (83)
Mean (range; SD) length (seconds)	89 (5-215; 62)	88 (5-296; 84)
No (%) of encounters with tests or referrals	18 (31)	21 (39)
No (%) of encounters resulting in diagnosis	56 (97)	52 (96)
No (%) of encounters resulting in prescription	30 (52)	24 (44)
Mean length (range; SD) of encounter (minutes)	10.5 (1-33.5; 5.9)	9 (2-25; 2.7)
Geometric mean (minutes)	8.9	7.8

*$P < .001$. Completion of monologue could be determined in only 105 encounters. (In a subgroup of 75 encounters in which patients were aged 10 years or over [mean age 43.8; median 40.0; SD 22.4], in 12/38 [32%] encounters on day 1 and 25/37 [68%] encounters on day 2 the monologues were completed; $P < .01$ [χ^2 and regressions, controlling for doctor].)

(Courtesy of Rabinowitz I, Lusatti R, Tamir A, et al: Length of patient's monologue, rate of completion, and relation to other components of the clinical encounter: Observational intervention study in primary care. *BMJ* 328:501-502, 2004. With permission from the BMJ Publishing Group.)

Of 235 consultations recorded, 214 were viewed. Of these 214 consultations, 112 (52%) involved a new clinical problem. These consultations were reviewed for the length of the patients' monologues, whether the monologue was completed, the duration and performance of the physical examination, and the ordering of tests.

Results.—The monologues averaged 26 seconds on day 1 and 28 seconds on day 2 (Table). After the intervention, twice as many monologues were completed, and 6 doctors accounted for this increase (80%). A physical examination was performed in 88% of the encounters, and the average duration of this examination was a minute and a half. Tests were ordered for one third of these patients, a diagnosis was provided in almost all cases, and prescriptions were issued in half the encounters. No significant difference in these figures was noted before and after the encounter.

Conclusions.—Allowing patients to complete their monologues requires little time and does not interfere with other components of the clinical encounter. In consultations that involved a new clinical problem, the number of completed monologues doubled when doctors were told not to interrupt.

► I will use this information when seeing patients and educating students, residents, and fellows. Apocryphal data have suggested that the average physician interrupts patients in about 15 seconds. These observations suggest that patients' opening monologues won't exceed 30 seconds, on average, in primary care or 90 seconds in consultative settings, and that allowing patients to complete these will lead to greater patient satisfaction with the encounter and rapport with the physician. Busy as we are, we should be able to allocate those few extra seconds.

R. S. Panush, MD

Complementary and Alternative Medicine

Effectiveness of Leech Therapy in Osteoarthritis of the Knee: A Randomized, Controlled Trial

Michalsen A, Klotz S, Lüdtke R, et al (Kliniken Essen-Mitte, Germany; Univ of Duisburg-Essen, Germany)
Ann Intern Med 139:724-730, 2003 7–24

Background.—Currently, natural leeches are used to treat postoperative local congestions after reconstructive and plastic surgery. Other traditional uses of the leech, such as the treatment of localized inflammation and pain, remain part of many ethnomedical systems. Preliminary studies have demonstrated that clinically significant pain relief can be obtained after leech therapy for osteoarthritis (OA) of the knee. The effectiveness of leech therapy for symptomatic relief of OA of the knee was evaluated.

Methods.—This randomized, controlled trial was conducted in the outpatient department for integrative medicine of an academic teaching hospital. The study group included 51 patients with OA of the knee (mean age, 62.5 ± 10.2 years) who were treated with a single treatment of 4 to 6 locally applied leeches and 27 patients with a mean age of 65.5 ± 6.7 years who

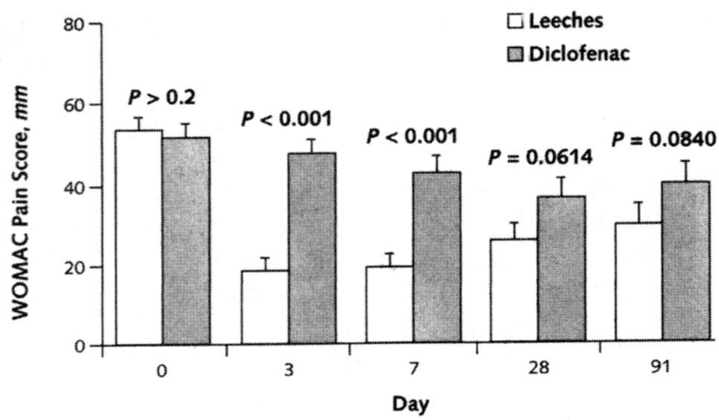

FIGURE.—Western Ontario and McMaster Universities Osteoarthritis Index (WOMAC) pain score. Mean course of WOMAC pain score in both groups in study course (mean ± SD) are based on raw [not imputed] data; *P* values were calculated from repeated-measurement analysis of variance). Complete WOMAC patient data in leech therapy and topical diclofenac treatment groups were available for 24 and 26 patients, respectively (day 7); 24 and 24 patients, respectively (day 28); and 23 and 23 patients, respectively (day 91). (Courtesy of Michalsen A, Klotz S, Lüdtke R, et al: Effectiveness of leech therapy in osteoarthritis of the knee: A randomized controlled trial. *Ann Intern Med* 139:724-730, 2003.)

were treated with a 28-day course of topical diclofenac (control group). The main outcome measures were the mean of the pain, function, and stiffness subscores of the Western Ontario and McMaster Universities Osteoarthritis Index and physical sum score of the Medical Outcomes Study 36-Item Short-Form Health Survey with group comparisons at days 3, 7, 28, and 91. The primary end point was pain at day 7.

Results.—The primary end point was reduced from a mean ± SD of 53.5 ± 13.7 to 19.3 ± 12.2 after leech therapy compared with 51.5 ± 16.8 to 4.44 ± 19.7 with topical diclofenac. The difference between the group pain scores was not significant after day 7, but differences for function, stiffness, and total symptoms remained significant in favor of leech therapy until the end of the study and for quality of life until day 28 (Figure). Expectations regarding outcome had no effect on the results.

Conclusions.—These findings support the effectiveness of leech therapy in relieving symptoms in patients with OA of the knee. However, the potential of leech therapy for the treatment of OA and the pharmacologic properties of leech saliva have yet to be clarified.

▶ What is this doing in the *Annals of Internal Medicine*? The message here is not about leeches or OA, but that complementary and alternative medicine (CAM) is now very much mainstream. Indeed, major journals actively seek out good-quality, provocative CAM-related studies to feature. I have commented extensively about this in the past, and reprise some of my thoughts here. (Panush RS: Shift happens. Complementary and alternative medicine for rheumatologists. *J Rheumatol* 29:656-658, 2002.

"If I tell you something three times, it's true."

Lewis Carroll

". . .A rip-off of the public of $2 million. . . They are screening garbage looking for diamonds...The real story is not that alternative medicine has turned the corner but that there was political meddling by insiders in Washington that created this because of their own naiveté."

V. Herbert, MD, JD

CAM: What to make of it and what to do with it? There has been a societal paradigm shift in attitude toward health and healing. Complementary and alternative medicine—called quackery only a few years ago—is now in vogue, acceptable, and trendy. Embraced by millions, supported by insurers, thriving among the hallowed hallways of the National Institutes of Health, and appearing in prestigious, scholarly publications.[1,2]

When I began my academic career, a wise mentor counseled that an important element of success was to learn something well and develop facility to say it over and over again in different ways in print. I took his advice to heart. This is my eightieth piece on some aspect of complementary and alternative medicine.

To explain how this came to pass, let me say that as a young academician CAM was the farthest topic from my mind; it was not something a serious scholar would even remotely consider. One afternoon in the late 1970s I received a call from my dean. A wealthy individual in his office was willing to donate to the university if we would study diet therapy for arthritis. Would I do it? But I was too busy in my laboratory finding the cause and cure for rheumatoid arthritis to waste time studying diet; besides, no respectable rheumatologist would want to be identified with such a study. A few years later my dean renewed the invitation. The person requesting the study was again in his office with a blank check and it would be very important for my career to do this. By now the project piqued my intellectual curiosity. And so I came to study diet and learn about CAM. However, my thoughts about CAM have evolved from ridicule[3,4] to tolerance,[5] to genuine interest and optimism,[6,7] to skepticism.[8] Let me explain.

Why the popularity? CAM appeals in part to patients' frustrations. It is seductive to many with chronic disease whose suffering is incompletely relieved, for whom therapies are inadequate, whose drugs are toxic and expensive, whose disease outcomes are unpredictable, and who consult harried physicians.[5] Others seek natural, healthy, holistic, empowering lifestyles.[9] And still other patients have psychosocial problems that lead them away from mainstream therapies.[10]

What is CAM? My simple definition: nonmainstream therapies.[11] More formally, CAM is considered a heterogeneous population of disparate practices and beliefs that vary substantially among traditions, that form no consistent body of knowledge, and that are alienated from a culture's dominant medical profession. The interested reader is referred elsewhere to an excellent exposition with a detailed taxonomy.[12] A related presentation offers a perspective of CAM today—the "paradigm shift" from antagonism to acknowledgment—as a consumer-driven reconfiguration of medical pluralism that has always existed in North America.[13]

What can rheumatology expect from CAM? I think there is less here than meets the eye. Indeed, it is of interest to note those presentations on CAM at the 2001 American College of Rheumatology Scientific Session: 14 on CAM, 8 on familial Mediterranean fever, 10 on amyloid, 16 on stem cells, 20 on Kawasaki disease, 28 on Behçet's syndrome, and 28 on gastrointestinal safety. They are of the order of magnitude of relatively rare, obscure disorders and do not begin to approach those on topical issues. I am unaware of clinically significant or "breakthrough" advances in rheumatology derived from CAM. (No, I do not consider glucosamine [or minocycline] in this category.) Nor do I see any on the horizon. I would speculate that herbal (botanical) products might offer some promise.[1,2] Indeed, The *Journal of Rheumatology* has featured encouraging studies of *Trypterygium wilfordii* Hook F,[14] a stinging nettle leaf extract,[15] and an extract from the plant *Uncaria tomentosa* (cat's claw)[16] for experimental and human rheumatic diseases. It will be of interest to see how these evolve and what utility, if any, they will provide to our patients. Lest I be misunderstood, let me state the great respect I have for friends and colleagues, like Drs David Eisenberg, Brian Berman, and Adam Perlman (at my institution) and others who are dedicated to the rigorous, scientific study of CAM. Theirs is a worthy and needed effort. I may not share their optimism about the long-term clinical importance of those efforts, at least in rheumatology, but I wouldn't be disappointed to be proven wrong.

How should rheumatologists think about CAM? By balancing a mind open to new ideas with healthy skepticism. It was probably more serendipity than science that led us to gold, antimalarials, sulfasalazine, and other important antirheumatic therapies. Aspirin and colchicine came from botanicals (willow bark and meadow saffron, respectively). Who, years ago, would have imagined using antibiotics for ulcers? And today's conventions may be tomorrow's follies—remember tonsillectomies and adenoidectomies, or irradiation for ankylosing spondylitis?[6] Consider novel hypotheses but hold them to the crucible of scientific inquiry, to the same standards demanded for any experimental question. Some mainstream therapies have not been scientifically validated (some, perhaps much, of what we do for low back pain, the iced saline lavages I administered as a resident for gastrointestinal bleeds, for example) and some nonmainstream therapies may be safe and effective (balneotherapy in our culture, for example). Ideally we should use what has been proven safe and effective, integrating this into our repertoire; this is now considered "integrative medicine." There is only one kind of good medicine, and it is derived from evidence-based science, whatever the source.

In summary, my own views of CAM:

- If it sounds too good to be true, it is.
- If you haven't read about it in the scientific literature, it's not established.
- If you first heard about it from the media, lay press, or your patients, it's not validated. There are no secrets in good science or good medicine.
- There have been no "breakthrough," important advances in rheumatology from "complementary" and "alternative" medicine.
- The question regarding trying "complementary" and "alternative" therapies shouldn't be "why not?" but "why?"
- This is reality. Deal with it. Discuss "complementary" and "alternative" therapies with patients.

- I don't believe or not believe in "complementary" and "alternative" medicine. I believe in science, scientific methods, and a single high standard of good evidence-based medicine for all patients.

"A foreboding I have—maybe ill-placed—of an America in my children's generation, and my grandchildren's generation. . .when, clutching our crystals and religiously consulting our horoscopes, our critical faculties in steep decline, unable to distinguish what's true and what feels good, we slide, almost without noticing, into superstition and darkness. . . science requires an almost complete openness to all ideas. On the other hand, it requires the most rigorous and uncompromising skepticism."

Carl Sagan

"When I speak of science, I refer not to the work of a group of people with special training but to a habit of thought that refuses to accept any propositions about the natural world without objective and verifiable evidence."

Marcia Angell, MD

R. S. Panush, MD

References

1. Panush RS, editor: Complementary and alternative therapies for rheumatic disease. *Rheum Dis Clin North Am* 25:789-968, 1999.
2. Panush RS, editor: Complementary and alternative therapies for rheumatic disease. *Rheum Dis Clin North Am* 26:1-195, 2000.
3. Dlesk A, Ettinger MP, Longley S, et al: Unconventional arthritis therapies. *Arthritis Rheum* 25:1145-1147, 1992.
4. Panush RS: Food for thought, but not for arthritis. *Primary Care Rheumatology* 2:1-5, 1992.
5. Panush RS: Reflections on unproven remedies. *Rheum Dis Clin North Am* 19:201-206, 1993.
6. Panush RS: Alternative medicine: Science or superstition [editorial]? *J Rheumatol* 21:8-9, 1994.
7. Panush RS: Complementary and alternative therapies for rheumatic diseases. *Rheum Dis Clin* 26:1-197, 2000.
8. Panush RS: Introduction to miscellaneous topics. *Year Book of Rheumatology, Arthritis, and Musculoskeletal Disease.* St Louis, 1999, Mosby, pp 293-297.
9. Astin JA: Why patients use alternative medicine: Results of a national study. *JAMA* 279:1548-1553, 1998.
10. Burstein HJ, Gelber S, Guadagnoli E, et al: Use of alternative medicine by women with early-stage breast cancer. *N Engl J Med* 340:1733-1739, 1999.
11. Panush RS: Diets, other "complementary" and "alternative" therapies, and the rheumatic diseases. In Koopman WJ, ed: *Arthritis and allied conditions. A textbook of rheumatology*, ed 14, Baltimore, 2001, Lippincott, Williams & Wilkins, pp 965-987.
12. Kaptchuk TJ, Eisenberg DM: Varieties of healing. 2. A taxonomy of unconventional healing practices. *Ann Intern Med* 135:196-204, 2001.
13. Kaptchuk TJ, Eisenberg DM. Varieties of healing. 1. Medical pluralism in the United States. *Ann Intern Med* 135:189-195, 2001.
14. Tao X, Cush JJ, Garrett, M, et al: A phase I study of ethyl acetate extract of the Chinese antirheumatic herb *Tripterygium wilfordii* Hook F in rheumatoid arthritis. *J Rheumatol* 28:2160-2167, 2001.
15. Broer J, Behnke B: Immunosuppressant effect of IDS 30, a stinging nettle leaf extract, on myeloid dendritic cells in vitro. *J Rheumatol* 29:659-666, 2002.
16. Mur E, Hartig F, Eibl G, et al: Randomized double blind trial of an extract from the pentacyclic alkaloid-chemotype of *Uncaria tomentosa* for the treatment of rheumatoid arthritis. *J Rheumatol* 29:678-681, 2002.

The Effect of Glucosamine-Chondroitin Supplementation on Glycosylated Hemoglobulin Levels in Patients With Type 2 Diabetes Mellitus: A Placebo-Controlled, Double-Blind, Randomized Clinical Trial

Scroggie DA, Albright A, Harris MD (Lackland Air Force Base, Tex; Uniformed Services Univ of the Health Sciences, Bethesda, Md)

Arch Intern Med 163:1587-1590, 2003 7–25

Background.—Type 2 diabetes mellitus and osteoarthritis not uncommonly coexist in patients over age 60 years. The therapies used for osteoarthritis, generally nonsteroidal antiinflammatory drugs, have significant potential toxic effects, and the conditions often accompanying diabetes can increase the risk of toxic effects from these agents. A combination of dietary supplements, glucosamine and chondroitin sulfate, is often used by patients with osteoarthritis who believe these therapies are safe alternative medicines. High levels of glucosamine have raised glucose levels in animal models, presenting the possibility that humans may respond similarly. A placebo-controlled, double-blind, randomized trial was undertaken to assess the clinical effect of glucosamine supplements on the serum glucose levels of patients with type 2 diabetes.

Methods.—The 38 elderly patients studied were receiving 1 or 2 drugs for glycemic control. Patients were given either 1500 mg of glucosamine hydrochloride and 1200 mg of chondroitin sulfate in daily doses for 90 days (26 patients) or placebo (12 patients). Hemoglobin A_{1c} (HBA_{1c}) levels were determined before and after the 90 days of therapy.

Results.—Four patients in the treatment group withdrew, 3 for reasons unrelated to treatment and 1 for excessive flatus, which is a possible side effect of glucosamine. Very little change was recorded in the HBA_{1c} levels in either group. On post hoc analysis, the sample sizes of 22 patients in the treatment group and 12 patients in the placebo group had a power of 80% for revealing a large difference between the groups and a power of 80% for detecting change in HBA_{1c} levels of 0.15 in the group receiving glucosamine and chondroitin.

Conclusion.—The use of oral glucosamine supplements had no adverse effect on the glycemic control of patients with type 2 diabetes.

Structural and Symptomatic Efficacy of Glucosamine and Chondroitin in Knee Osteoarthritis: A Comprehensive Meta-analysis

Richy F, Bruyere O, Ethgen O, et al (Univ of Liège, Belgium; World Health Organization, Liège, Belgium; Cochrane French Ctr, Lyon, France)

Arch Intern Med 163:1514-1522, 2003 7–26

Background.—The recent recommendations offered by the American College of Rheumatology and the European League Against Rheumatism propose classifying drugs to treat osteoarthritis as either symptom-modifying or structure-modifying agents. Symptom-modifying drugs principally improve pain and function; structure-modifying drugs mainly focus on radiographic changes and the analysis of joint space narrowing (JSN). A meta-analysis was undertaken to document the evidence of structural efficacy for glucosamine and the symptomatic effects of glucosamine plus chondroitin sulfate for patients with knee and hip osteoarthritis.

Methods.—Fifteen studies were identified as most closely addressing the main points of the study. Outcome measures included radiologic evolution assessed by JSN, evaluation of pain assessed by visual analogue scale (VAS pain), joint mobility (VAS mobility), Lequesne Index (LI), Western Ontario MacMaster University Osteoarthritis Index (WOMAC), tolerance determined by the number of adverse effects developed, and response to treatment as assessed by physicians.

Results.—The evidence derived from the studies found highly significant data to back up the structural efficacy of glucosamine on minimum JSN. By converting the effect size to natural units, the potential minimal JSN difference between the effects of placebo and those of glucosamine was found to be 0.27 mm after 3 years of daily doses of 1500 mg of glucosamine sulfate. WOMAC results were also positively influenced.

Significant changes in patients taking chondroitin and glucosamine were noted with respect to symptoms; these changes were not noted in patients taking placebo. The onset of action was 2 weeks for either of the active agents. Chondroitin proved effective on LI, VAS pain, VAS mobility, and responding status. An excellent safety profile emerged for glucosamine and chondroitin, with studies documenting low rates of serious adverse events comparable to those seen with placebo.

Conclusion.—Glucosamine was shown to have a structure-modifying effect that requires further investigation. Glucosamine produced positive effects on the JSN and WOMAC, and chondroitin produced similar effects on LI, VAS pain, VAS mobility, and responding status. Relationships among time, dose, patient baseline data, and structural efficacy remain to be explored.

► The first article (Abstract 7–25) convincingly refutes the notion that diabetics might have problems taking glucosamine. The second (Abstract 7–26) presents summary data supporting symptomatic benefit of glucosamine and maybe chondroitin. Whether glucosamine affords disease- or "structure"-modifying effect is not clear; some of the purported radiographic change may have reflected changes in joint positioning due to symptom palliation from medication.

R. S. Panush, MD

The Impact of Stretching on Sports Injury Risk: A Systematic Review of the Literature

Thacker SB, Gilchrist J, Stroup DF, et al (Ctrs for Disease Control and Prevention, Atlanta, Ga)

Med Sci Sports Exerc 36:371-378, 2004 7–27

Background.—It has long been a standard practice for athletes at all levels to stretch before participation. Athletes, coaches, trainers, physiotherapists, and physicians have recommended stretching to prevent injury and to enhance performance. A substantial body of literature has been devoted to the topic, and a variety of approaches have been developed for specific sports. However, in recent years, some investigators have questioned the routine practice of stretching, contending that little evidence is available to support the popularly held notion that pre- or postparticipation stretching prevents injury. It has been suggested that such stretching may even affect performance negatively. The evidence for the effectiveness of stretching as a tool for the prevention of injuries in sports was retrospectively investigated, and recommendations for research and prevention were made.

Methods.—Electronic databases, including MEDLINE, Current Contents, Biomedical Collection, the Cochrane Library, and SPORTDiscus were searched without language limitations, and citations from articles retrieved were identified. In addition, experts in the field were contacted. This meta-analysis was limited to randomized trials or cohort studies for interventions that included stretching. Articles were excluded if they lacked control subjects or if stretching could not be assessed independently. In 6 of the 361 articles, stretching was compared with other methods to prevent injury.

Results.—No significant association was noted between stretching and a reduction in total injuries. Similar findings were observed in the subgroup analyses.

Conclusions.—Evidence in this meta-analysis was insufficient for a recommendation for discontinuation of routine stretching before or after exercise for the prevention of injury among either professional or recreational athletes. Additional research is urgently needed, particularly in the form of well-conducted randomized controlled trials, to determine the proper role of stretching in sports.

▶ It always fun to see science dispel myth. The lack of efficacy of stretching to prevent injuries or postexercise soreness was touched upon in previous YEAR BOOKS. My take on this is that some regular stretching is valuable for athletes and recreational exercisers to maintain flexibility, elasticity of muscles, and maybe to reduce injury but should best be done when "warmed up." Similarly, vigorous exercise should follow a suitable "warm-up," which is not accomplished by merely stretching.

R. S. Panush, MD

Subject Index

A

B

C

D

E

F

G

H

I

N

O

S

T

U

V

W

Y

Author Index

G

H

I

J

K

L

T

U

V

W

X

Y

Z

Order your subscription today. Simply complete and detach this card and drop it in the mail to receive the best clinical information in your field.

YES! Please start my subscription to the **CLINICS** checked below with the ❑ first issue of the calendar year or ❑ current issues. If not completely satisfied with my first issue, I may write "cancel" on the invoice and return it within 30 days at no further obligation.

Please Print:

Name ______________________________

Address ______________________________

City ______________ State ______________ ZIP ______________

Method of Payment

❑ Check (payable to **Elsevier**; add the applicable sales tax for your area)

❑ VISA ❑ MasterCard ❑ AmEx ❑ Bill me

Card number ______________ Exp. date ______________

Signature ______________________________

Staple this to your purchase order to expedite delivery

❑ **Adolescent Medicine Clinics**
- ❑ Individual $95
- ❑ Institutions $133
- ❑ *In-training $48

❑ **Anesthesiology**
- ❑ Individual $175
- ❑ Institutions $270
- ❑ *In-training $88

❑ **Cardiology**
- ❑ Individual $170
- ❑ Institutions $266
- ❑ *In-training $85

❑ **Chest Medicine**
- ❑ Individual $185
- ❑ Institutions $285

❑ **Child and Adolescent Psychiatry**
- ❑ Individual $175
- ❑ Institutions $265
- ❑ *In-training $88

❑ **Critical Care**
- ❑ Individual $165
- ❑ Institutions $266
- ❑ *In-training $83

❑ **Dental**
- ❑ Individual $150
- ❑ Institutions $242

❑ **Emergency Medicine**
- ❑ Individual $170
- ❑ Institutions $263
- ❑ *In-training $85
- ❑ Send CME info

❑ **Facial Plastic Surgery**
- ❑ Individual $199
- ❑ Institutions $300

❑ **Foot and Ankle**
- Individual $160
- Institutions $232

❑ **Gastroenterology**
- ❑ Individual $190
- ❑ Institutions $276

❑ **Gastrointestinal Endoscopy**
- ❑ Individual $190
- ❑ Institutions $276

❑ **Hand**
- ❑ Individual $205
- ❑ Institutions $319

❑ **Heart Failure (NEW in 2005!)**
- ❑ Individual $99
- ❑ Institutions $149
- ❑ *In-training $49

❑ **Hematology/ Oncology**
- ❑ Individual $210
- ❑ Institutions $315

❑ **Immunology & Allergy**
- ❑ Individual $165
- ❑ Institutions $266

❑ **Infectious Disease**
- ❑ Individual $165
- ❑ Institutions $272

❑ **Clinics in Liver Disease**
- ❑ Individual $165
- ❑ Institutions $234

❑ **Medical**
- ❑ Individual $140
- ❑ Institutions $244
- ❑ *In-training $70
- ❑ Send CME info

❑ **MRI**
- ❑ Individual $190
- ❑ Institutions $290
- ❑ *In-training $95
- ❑ Send CME info

❑ **Neuroimaging**
- ❑ Individual $190
- ❑ Institutions $290
- ❑ *In-training $95
- ❑ Send CME inf0

❑ **Neurologic**
- ❑ Individual $175
- ❑ Institutions $275

❑ **Obstetrics & Gynecology**
- ❑ Individual $175
- ❑ Institutions $288

❑ **Occupational and Environmental Medicine**
- ❑ Individual $120
- ❑ Institutions $166
- ❑ *In-training $60

❑ **Ophthalmology**
- ❑ Individual $190
- ❑ Institutions $325

❑ **Oral & Maxillofacial Surgery**
- ❑ Individual $180
- ❑ Institutions $280
- ❑ *In-training $90

❑ **Orthopedic**
- ❑ Individual $180
- ❑ Institutions $295
- ❑ *In-training $90

❑ **Otolaryngologic**
- ❑ Individual $199
- ❑ Institutions $350

❑ **Pediatric**
- ❑ Individual $135
- ❑ Institutions $246
- ❑ *In-training $68
- ❑ Send CME info

❑ **Perinatology**
- ❑ Individual $155
- ❑ Institutions $237
- ❑ *In-training $78
- ❑ Send CME inf0

❑ **Plastic Surgery**
- ❑ Individual $245
- ❑ Institutions $370

❑ **Podiatric Medicine & Surgery**
- ❑ Individual $170
- ❑ Institutions $266

❑ **Primary Care**
- ❑ Individual $135
- ❑ Institutions $223

❑ **Psychiatric**
- ❑ Individual $170
- ❑ Institutions $288

❑ **Radiologic**
- ❑ Individual $220
- ❑ Institutions $331
- ❑ *In-training $110
- ❑ Send CME info

❑ **Sports Medicine**
- ❑ Individual $180
- ❑ Institutions $277

❑ **Surgical**
- ❑ Individual $190
- ❑ Institutions $299
- ❑ *In-training $95

❑ **Thoracic Surgery (formerly Chest Surgery)**
- ❑ Individual $175
- ❑ Institutions $255
- ❑ *In-training $88

❑ **Urologic**
- ❑ Individual $195
- ❑ Institutions $307
- ❑ *In-training $98
- ❑ Send CME info

*To receive in-training rate, orders must be accompanied by the name of affiliated institution, dates of residency and signature of coordinator on institution letterhead. Orders will be billed at the individual rate until proof of resident status is received.